Historic Landscapes and Mental Well-being

Historic Landscapes and Mental Well-being

edited by

Timothy Darvill, Kerry Barrass,
Laura Drysdale, Vanessa Heaslip
and Yvette Staelens

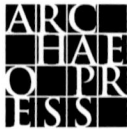

Archaeopress Publishing Ltd
Summertown Pavilion
18-24 Middle Way
Summertown
Oxford OX2 7LG
www.archaeopress.com

ISBN 978-1-78969-268-6
ISBN 978-1-78969-269-3 (e-Pdf)

© the individual authors and Archaeopress 2019

Front cover: Human Henge participants exploring a round barrow on Windmill Hill, Wiltshire. (Drawing by Donna Songhurst. Copyright reserved)

Back cover: Stonehenge, Wiltshire, a prehistoric healing centre? (Photograph by Timothy Darvill. Copyright reserved)

This publication, and the accompanied open access version, was funded by the Heritage Lottery Fund (now the National Lottery Heritage Fund) as part of its support for the Human Henge project.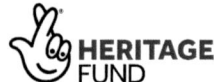

Human Henge is a trademark registered with the UK Intellectual Property Office.

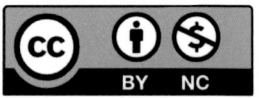

This work is licensed under a Creative Commons Attribution-NonCommercial 3.0 Unported License.

Printed in England by Oxuniprint, Oxford
This book is available direct from Archaeopress or from our website www.archaeopress.com

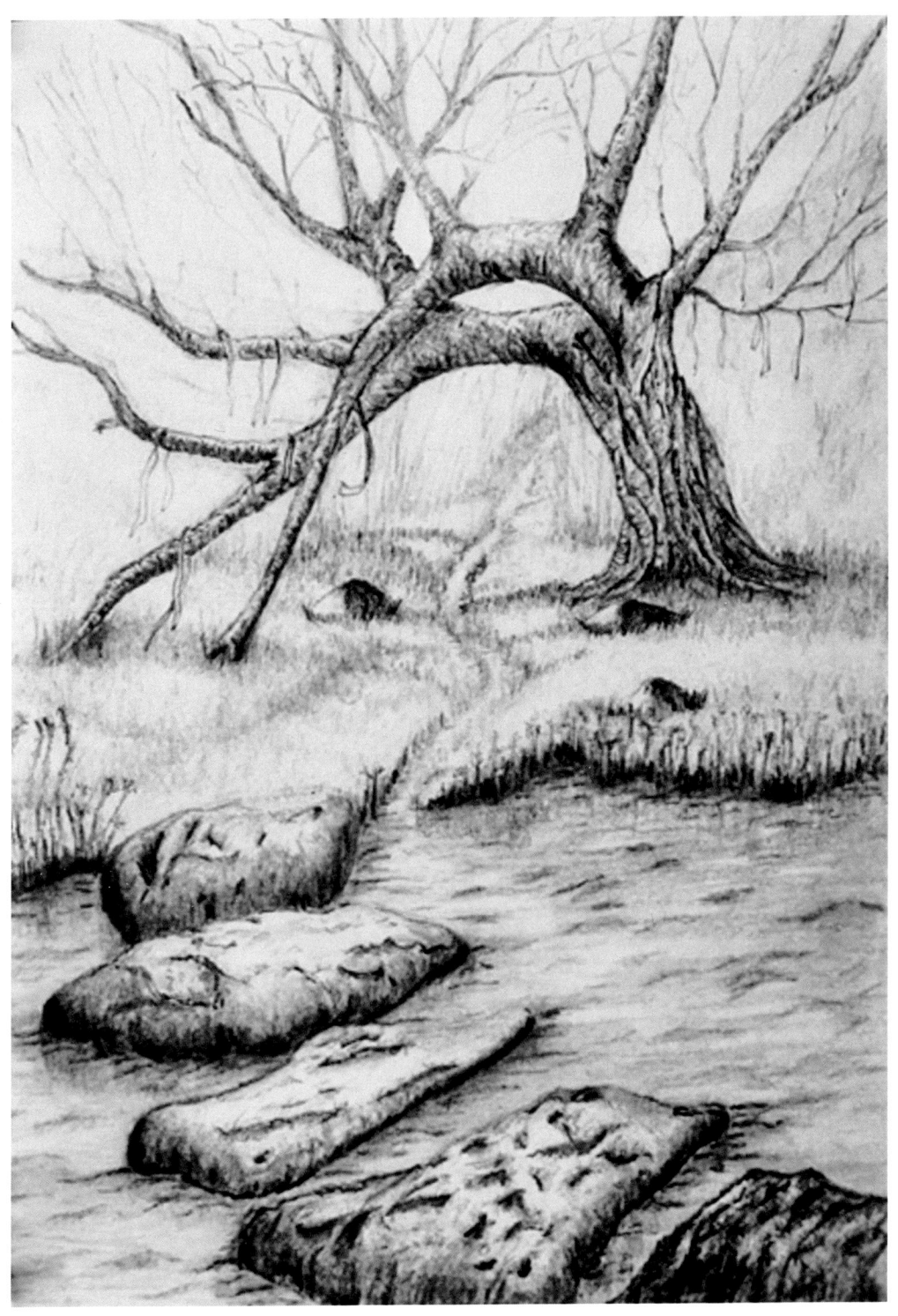

Stepping stones to other times, other places, other worlds (Drawing by Donna Songhurst)

 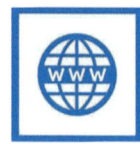

A free open-access pdf version of this book is available to download at: https://tinyurl.com/DarvillEtAl

Supporting sound files relating to Chapter 7 are available to listen to at:

https://tinyurl.com/Dutiro

https://tinyurl.com/desOiseaux

Contents

List of Figures, Tables, and Sound Files iii

Abbreviations ix

Contributor biographies xiii

Foreword xix
Sara Lunt

Chapter 1 Introduction: Heritage and well-being 1
Timothy Darvill, Kerry Barrass, Laura Drysdale, Vanessa Heaslip, and Yvette Staelens

Chapter 2 Mental well-being and historic landscapes: The heritage context 29
Liz Ellis and Alice Kershaw

Chapter 3 Therapeutic landscapes past and present: The mental health context 37
Toby Sutcliffe

Chapter 4 Inclusion and recovery: Archaeology and heritage for people with mental health problems and/or autism 44
William Rathouse

Chapter 5 Walking with intent: Culture therapy in ancient landscapes 54
Laura Drysdale

Chapter 6 Monuments for life: Building Human Henge at Stonehenge and Avebury 65
Timothy Darvill

Chapter 7 'What did you do today mummy?': Human Henge and mental well-being 85
Yvette Staelens

Chapter 8 High value, short intervention historic landscape projects: Practical considerations for voluntary mental-health providers 97
Daniel O'Donoghue

Chapter 9 Human Henge: The impact of Neolithic healing landscapes on mental health and well-being 123
Vanessa Heaslip

Chapter 10 A place to heal: Past perceptions and new opportunities for using historic sites to change lives 135
Martin Allfrey

Chapter 11 People making places making people ...144
Briony Clifton

Chapter 12 'The archaeological imagination': New ways of seeing for mental health recovery ...153
Rebecca L Hearne

Chapter 13 Prehistoric landscapes as transitional space ...163
Claire Nolan

Chapter 14 Messing about on the river: Volunteering and well-being on the Thames foreshore ...179
Helen Johnston

Chapter 15 Between the Barrows: Seeking a spirit of place ...189
Christopher Howard Elmer

Chapter 16 The Roman Baths: A place of recovery ...204
Paul Murtagh

Chapter 17 'The People Before Us' Project: Exploring heritage and well-being in a rapidly changing seaside town ...215
Lesley Hardy and Eleanor Williams

Chapter 18 Landscapes of mental health: The archaeology of St Wulstan's Local Nature Reserve, Malvern, England ...228
Andrew Hoaen, Bob Ruffle, and Helen Loney

Chapter 19 Archaeology and mental health: War memorials survey in Ceredigion ...242
William Rathouse

Chapter 20 Waterloo Uncovered: From discoveries in conflict archaeology to military veteran collaboration and recovery on one of the world's most famous battlefields ...253
Mark Evans, Stuart Eve, Vicki Haverkate-Emmerson, Tony Pollard, Eleonora Steinberg, and David Ulke

Chapter 21 Crafting, heritage and well-being: Lessons from two public engagement projects ...266
Zena Kamash

Afterword ...280
Alex Coulter

List of Figures, Tables, and Sound Files

Stepping stones to other times, other places, other worlds (Drawing by Donna Songhurst. Copyright reserved)

Chapter 1 Introduction: Heritage and well-being

Figure 1.1. Line chart showing diachronic trends for four measures of well-being between 2012 and 2018 in the UK as recorded by the Office for National Statistics using sample populations. The left-hand scale shows mean average values based on approval ratings along a gradient ranging from low (0) to high (10). (Data from ONS 2019) 9

Figure 1.2. Five ways to well-being. (Based on GOS 2008: 21) 10

Figure 1.3. A powerful landscape: West Kennet Long Barrow, near Avebury, Wiltshire. (Drawing by Donna Songhurst. Copyright reserved) 13

Figure 1.4. Being in the landscape: Participants and facilitators of the Human Henge project on King Barrow Ridge overlooking Stonehenge Wiltshire. (Photograph by Timothy Darvill, Human Henge project. Copyright reserved) 16

Chapter 5 Walking with intent: Culture therapy in ancient landscapes

Figure 5.1 The Human Henge travelling exhibition at Amesbury Town Library, May 2017. (Photograph by Timothy Darvill, Human Henge project. Copyright reserved) 56

Table 5.A A Summary of the outreach activities and media coverage relating to the Human Henge project 2017–2019 57

Figure 5.2 'Brickhenge' at the Festival of Archaeology in Salisbury, July 2017. (Photograph by Timothy Darvill, Human Henge project. Copyright reserved) 60

Chapter 6 Monuments for life: Building Human Henge at Stonehenge and Avebury

Figure 6.1. The Men-an-Tol, Ladron, Cornwall. The stones were possibly once part of a stone circle. Tradition holds that the central perforated stone has healing powers. (Photograph by Timothy Darvill. Copyright reserved) 69

Figure 6.2. The remains of St Osmond's Shrine in the south aisle of Salisbury Cathedral, Wiltshire, showing three round kneeling-holes (*foramina*) allowing pilgrims to place parts of their body close to the central sarcophagus. (Photograph by Timothy Darvill. Copyright reserved) 70

Figure 6.3 Chartwell Dutiro playing his mbira on the Cuckoo Stone, near Stonehenge, Wiltshire. (Photograph by Timothy Darvill, Human Henge project. Copyright reserved) . 76

Figure 6.4 Human Henge in motion: Dancing at the Cuckoo Stone, near Stonehenge, Wiltshire. (Photograph by Yvette Staelens, Human Henge project. Copyright reserved) .. 77

Table 6.A Summary of the venues used for Human Henge events in the first iteration of the Programme in the Stonehenge landscape, October to December 2016. 78

Table 6.B Summary of the venues used for Human Henge events in the third iteration of the Programme in the Avebury landscape, January to March 2018. 79

Figure 6.5. Maxence des Oiseaux playing a bone flute beside Stone 9 in the southwest sector at Avebury, Wiltshire. (Photograph by Timothy Darvill, Human Henge project. Copyright reserved) 80

Chapter 7 'What did you do today mummy?': Human Henge and mental well-being

Figure 7.1. Human Henge fruit and biscuits served with love. (Photograph by Yvette Staelens. Copyright reserved) 86

Sound File 1. Chartwell Dutiro playing his mbira and singing 89

Figure 7.2 Chartwell Dutiro playing mbira on the Cuckoo Stone. (Photograph by Yvette Staelens. Copyright reserved) 89

Figure 7.3. Balafons made by Alphonse Tourna and played by Human Hengers. (Photograph by Yvette Staelens. Copyright reserved) 90

Sound File 2. Maxence des Oiseaux playing his bone flute for the Human Henge project 90

Figure 7.4. Bone flute played by Maxence des Oiseaux for the Human Henge project. (Photograph by Yvette Staelens. Copyright reserved) 90

Figure 7.5. Rag-tree at Swallowhead Springs, near Avebury, Wiltshire. (Photograph by Yvette Staelens. Copyright reserved) 91

Figure 7.6. 'Skyscape inner problems recede as sense of self feels part of the endless universe'. (Photograph by Yvette Staelens. Copyright reserved) 92

Figure 7.7. Handling prehistoric collections at the Alexander Keiller Museum, Avebury. (Photograph by Yvette Staelens. Copyright reserved) 92

Figure 7.8. Clay masks made by Human Hengers at Avebury. (Photograph by Yvette Staelens. Copyright reserved) 93

Figure 7.9. Firemaking in a Neolithic home. (Photograph by Yvette Staelens. Copyright reserved) 94

Figure 7.10. The hare on the barrow. (Photograph by Yvette Staelens. Copyright reserved) ...94

Figure 7.11. 'Getting soaked and chilled — loving it.' (Photograph by Yvette Staelens. Copyright reserved) 95

Figure 7.12 'Rain in the woods. Sweet chaos. Stripping hazel.' (Photograph by Jessica Swinburne. Copyright reserved) 96

Chapter 8 High value, short intervention historic landscape projects: Practical considerations for voluntary mental-health providers

Figure 8.1. Sarsen strewn landscape at Lockeridge, Wiltshire. (Drawing by Donna Songhurst. Copyright reserved) 99

Figure 8.2. Avebury Henge, Wiltshire. (Drawing by Donna Songhurst. Copyright reserved) .110

Chapter 9 Human Henge: The impact of Neolithic healing landscapes on mental health and well-being

Table 9.A Participants' age and gender composition. 124

Figure 9.1 Data collection methods. (Illustration by Vanessa Heaslip. Copyright reserved) ...125

Table 9.B Short Warwick-Edinburgh Mental Well-being Scale. (Based on Tennant *et al.* 2007) 125

Figure 9.2 Group activity condensed into a word-cloud: Groups 1–3. (Illustration by Vanessa Heaslip. Copyright reserved) 126

Table 9.C Quantitative results 128

Figure 9.3 Creative activity outputs Groups 1–3. (Compiled by Vanessa Heaslip. Copyright reserved)...129

Chapter 11 People making places making people

Figure 11.1 Avebury mist on the West Kennet Avenue. (©National Trust/Abby George).........145

Figure 11.2 Sarsen boulders at Lockeridge Dene, Avebury. (©National Trust/Mike Robinson)..147

Figure 11.3 The Stables Gallery in front of Avebury Manor, Wiltshire. (©National Trust Images/James Dobson) 148

Figure 11.4 Clay sculpting workshop. (©National Trust/Abby George)...150

Figure 11.5 West Kennet Avenue and the road to Avebury in the snow. (©National Trust/ Mike Robinson)...151

Chapter 13 Prehistoric landscapes as transitional space

Figure 13.1 Location map of the study area. (Illustration by Elaine Jamieson. Contains Ordnance Survey data, Crown copyright, and database right 2015) 165

Figure 13.2 Research participants at the Sanctuary, near Avebury, Wiltshire. (University of Reading, used with permission) 165

Figure 13.3 Martinsell Iron Age enclosure, Wiltshire. (University of Reading, used with permission) 168

Figure 13.4 West Kennet Avenue, Avebury, Wiltshire. (University of Reading, used with permission) 171

Figure 13.5 Avebury stone circle, Wiltshire. (Photograph by Claire Nolan. Copyright reserved)..173

Chapter 14 Messing about on the river: Volunteering and well-being on the Thames foreshore

Figure 14.1 TDP volunteers recording post-medieval ship timbers reused in barge beds on the Thames foreshore in Rotherhithe, London. (Photograph by Helen Johnston. Copyright reserved)..180

Figure 14.2 Participants at the Open Foreshore event at the Tower of London foreshore (Photograph by N. Cohen. Copyright reserved)...181

Figure 14.3 Recording WWII bomb damage to the river wall upstream from the Palace of Westminster, London. (Photograph by N. Cohen. Copyright reserved)..................184

Figure 14.4 Volunteers recording a WWI Submarine Chaser in the mud at Isleworth, London. (Photograph by N. Cohen. Copyright reserved) 184

Figure 14.5 Working on the foreshore on a misty day at Charlton, London. (Photograph by N. Cohen. Copyright reserved) 185

Chapter 15 Between the Barrows: Seeking a spirit of place

Figure 15.1 The Harmony Woods site reimagined during the Bronze Age. (Artwork by David Hopkins. Reproduced by kind permission)..190

Figure 15.2 The Harmony Woods planting site with the sports pavilion in the distance. (Photograph by C. Elmer 2016. Copyright reserved) 191

Figure 15.3 School children excavating the 2016 trench. (Photograph by C. Elmer. Copyright reserved) 193

Figure 15.4 Example of a completed memory cloud. (Illustration by C. Elmer. Copyright reserved) 194

Chapter 16 The Roman Baths: A place of recovery

Figure 16.1 Participants from Phoenix Futures replacing fallen stones at the Strathclyde Park Roman Bathhouse. (Photograph by Paul Murtagh. Copyright reserved) 207

Figure 16.2 The trail emerging as we clear vegetation from the path. (Photograph by Paul Murtagh. Copyright reserved) 210

Figure 16.3 A public engagement event at the Strathclyde Park Roman bathhouse with members of the Antonine Guard. (Photograph by Paul Murtagh. Copyright reserved) 211

Chapter 17 'The People Before Us' Project: Exploring heritage and well-being in a rapidly changing seaside town

Figure 17.1 Folkestone, 1826, after Joseph Mallord William Turner (1775-1851), purchased 1988. (Photograph courtesy of Tate London, 2019. Copyright reserved) 216

Figure 17.2 A graffitied poster from Folkestone's Triennial Arts Festival (Photograph by Lesley Hardy. Copyright reserved) 218

Figure 17.3 Participant Simon recording gravestones (Photograph by Eleanor Williams. Copyright reserved) 220

Figure 17.4 Artwork created during the project by Folkestone resident Steve McCarthy. (Photograph by Eleanor Williams. Copyright reserved) 221

Figure 17.5 A drawing in response to the churchyard visit by a pupil at St Eanswythe's Primary School, Folkestone. (Drawing by a participant in school open day on July 3rd 2017. Copyright reserved) 224

Chapter 18 Landscapes of mental health: The archaeology of St Wulstan's Local Nature Reserve, Malvern, England

Figure 18.1 St Wulstan's Local Nature Reserve in 2009 showing boundaries of the former hospital and new buildings. (Based on Digimap 2018a, used under license) 229

Figure 18.2 St Wulstan's hospital site at 1955, with pre-hospital landscape trees and hedgerows shown. (Based on Digimap 2018a, used under license) 232

Figure 18.3 St Wulstan's hospital site in 1971 showing main areas of 1960s planting including orchards and hedges. (Based on Digimap 2018c, used under license) 233

Figure 18.4 Aerial photograph showing site after closure in 1992. (Courtesy of the Historic England Archive NMR SU 7481/7. Crown copyright reserved) 234

Figure 18.5 Plan of the 2018 tree survey on the 2009 Digimap aerial photo. (Based on Digimap 2018d, used under license) 236

Table 18.A Tree species identified by survey undertaken in 2018. 237

Chapter 19 Archaeology and mental health: War memorials survey in Ceredigion

Figure 19.1 Team members pose next to the memorial in the village of Goginan, west of Aberystwyth. (Photograph by William Rathouse. Copyright reserved) 244

Figure 19.2 War memorial plaques re-erected in Aberystwyth library are surveyed. (Photograph by William Rathouse. Copyright reserved) 245

Figure 19.3 Staff volunteer and service user measure and prepare scale photographs of Ysbyty Ystwyth War Memorial. (Photograph by William Rathouse. Copyright reserved)245

Figure 19.4 Preparing scale photographs and recording inscriptions. (Photograph by William Rathouse. Copyright reserved) 246

Figure 19.5 A scale drawing of a memorial we surveyed featuring an allegory of peace or victory. (Drawing by Rhys Davies. Copyright reserved) 247

Chapter 21 Crafting, heritage and well-being: Lessons from two public engagement projects

Figure 21.1 RetRo workshop in progress at the Petrie Museum, London: creative writing and drawing. (Photograph by Zena Kamash. Copyright reserved)...269

Figure 21.2 RetRo workshop in progress at the Great North Museum, Newcastle: photography. (Photograph by Zena Kamash. Copyright reserved) 269

Figure 21.3 Felting workshop in progress at Cheney School, Oxford. Karin Celestine (standing) explains the wet felting technique to the participants. (Photograph by Zena Kamash. Copyright reserved)..270

Figure 21.4 Participants of the first felting workshop with their final felted panels. (Photograph by Karin Celestine. Copyright reserved)..271

Figure 21.5 Participants of the second felting workshop with their final felted panels. (Photograph by Zena Kamash. Copyright reserved) 272

Abbreviations

AD	*Anno Domini* (in the Year of our Lord on the Christian Calender)
AHRC	Arts and Humanities Research Council
AHSW	Arts and Health South West
APPAG	All-Party Parliamentary Archaeology Group
APPGAHW	All-Party Parliamentary Group on Arts, Health and Wellbeing
ASC	Autistic spectrum condition
ATU	Andover Trees United
AWP	Avon and Wiltshire Mental Health Partnership NHS Trust
BAJR	British Archaeological Jobs Resource
BBC	British Broadcasting Corporation
BC	Before Christ (back-projected chronology based on the Christian Calender)
BGH	Breaking Ground Heritage
BU	Bournemouth University
CAVLP	Clyde and Avon Valley Landscape Partnership
CBA	Council for British Archaeology
CBT	Cognitive behavioural therapy
CEO	Chief executive officer
CHWA	Culture, Health and Wellbeing Alliance
CMHT	Community mental health team
COE	Council of Europe
DAG	Defence Archaeology Group
DCLG	Department of Communities and Local Government
DCMS	Department for Culture, Media and Sport (DDCMS from 3 July 2017)
DDCMS	Department for Digital, Culture, Media and Sport (DCMS before 3 July 2017)
DIO	Defence Infrastructure Organization
DOH	Department of Health
EC	European Commission (of the EU)
ECT	Electroconvulsive therapy
EH	English Heritage
EIP	Early intervention in psychosis

ESOL	English for speakers of other languages
EU	European Union
FMRI	Functional magnetic resonance imaging
FROG	Foreshore Recording and Observation Group
GAD	Generalized anxiety disorder
GLA	Greater London Authority
GLO	Generic learning outcome
GOS	Government Office for Science
GP	General practitioner
HACT	Housing Associations' Charitable Trust
HBMCE	Historic Buildings and Monuments Commission for England
HE	Historic England
HES	Historic Environment Scotland
HLF	Heritage Lottery Fund (National Lottery Heritage Fund from January 2019)
HMG	Her Majesty's Government
IAPT	Improving access to psychological therapies
IWM	Imperial War Museum
KCC	Kent County Council
LGBTQ	Lesbian, gay, bisexual, transgender, and queer
MA	Museums Association
MENA	Middle East and North Africa
MLA	Museums, Libraries and Archives Council
MHCLG	Ministry of Housing, Communities, and Local Government
MHP	Mental health problem
MOD	Ministry of Defence
MOLA	Museum of London Archaeology
NEF	New Economic Foundation
NHS	National Health Service
NICE	The National Institute for Health and Care Excellence
NIE	Northern Ireland Executive
NIEA	Northern Ireland Environmental Agency
NIEDOH	Northern Ireland Executive Department of Health

NLHF	National Lottery Heritage Fund (formerly Heritage Lottery Fund before January 2019)
NT	National Trust
OECD	Organization for Economic Co-operation and Development
ONS	Office for National Statistics
OT	Occupational therapy
PHE	Public Health England
PTSD	Post-traumatic stress disorder
RCAHMS	Royal Commission on the Ancient and Historical Monuments of Scotland
RCHME	Royal Commission on the Historical Monuments of England
RF	Richmond Fellowship
RNIB	Royal National Institute of Blind People
RSA	Royal Society for the Encouragement of Arts, Manufactures and Commerce
RSPB	Royal Society for the Protection of Birds
RT	Restoration Trust
RTH	Recovery Through Heritage
RVS	Royal Voluntary Service
SCMH	Sainsbury Centre for Mental Health
SPW	Service Public de Wallonie
St	Saint
SVP	Serving personnel and veterans
TB	Tuberculosis
TDP	Thames Discovery Programme
UCL	University College London
UK	United Kingdom (England, Northern Ireland, Scotland and Wales)
UN	United Nations
UNESCO	United Nations Educational, Scientific, and Cultural Organization
US	United States (of America)
WEA	Workers' Education Association
WEMWBS	Warwick-Edinburgh Mental Well-being Scale
WHO	World Health Organization

WHS	World Heritage Site
WRVS	Women's Royal Voluntary Service
WWI	World War I (First World War, 1914–1918, also known as the Great War)
WWII	World War II (Second World War, 1939–1945)
WWCW	What Works Centre for Wellbeing
WWWMP	West Wales War Memorial Project

Contributor biographies

Martin Allfrey is Senior Curator of Collections for English Heritage and responsible for leading the research, documentation, and presentation of the fine art collections, historic interiors, and archaeological artefacts in English Heritage's West territory. With over 30 years of experience as a curator, Martin has an in-depth knowledge of the management of historic properties and the wider museums and heritage sector. Martin is passionate about broadening access to historic sites and collections and is always willing to explore new ways to bring them to life.
Email: Martin.Allfrey@english-heritage.org.uk

Kerry Barrass is a Postgraduate Research Assistant in the Department of Archaeology and Anthropology at Bournemouth University. She came to work in archaeology as the fulfilment of a lifetime's interest in the subject, after more than 20 years in the IT industry. Since graduating from Bournemouth University and gaining a Masters degree from the University of Southampton, she has spent several years working in a range of archaeology-based roles. These have included research, archaeological finds management, fieldwork, teaching, editing, and post-excavation analysis. She considers her involvement with the Human Henge project as a researcher to be one of the most fulfilling roles in either of her careers.
Email: kbarrass@bournemouth.ac.uk

Briony Clifton is Assistant Archaeologist for the National Trust in the Stonehenge and Avebury World Heritage Site, providing archaeological support and advice throughout these globally significant landscapes. From time to time she works with Breaking Ground Heritage and Operation Nightingale, who use archaeology in rehabilitation programmes for serving and ex-service personnel. She was involved with the development of the Human Henge Avebury programme, supporting its delivery and leading two sessions. Briony is also a member of the Human Henge Project Board.
Email: Briony.Clifton@nationaltrust.org.uk

Alex Coulter is Secretary and Project Manager for the All-Party Parliamentary Group on Arts, Health and Wellbeing and has been the Director of Arts & Health South West (AHSW)since 2010. AHSW is the lead organization for the national Culture, Health and Wellbeing Alliance, launched in April 2018. Before joining AHSW, she managed the Arts in Hospital project at Dorset County Hospital for 15 years and worked as a freelance arts and health consultant in the acute and primary care sectors. Previous to this, she was an artist. She studied Art History at the Courtauld Institute, Fine Art at Chelsea School of Art, and for an MSc in Management Development at Bristol University.
Email: alex@ahsw.org.uk

Timothy Darvill is Professor of Archaeology in the Department of Archaeology and Anthropology at Bournemouth University. His research interests focus on the Neolithic of Northwest Europe, and archaeological resource management. He has excavated in England, Wales, Isle of Man, Germany, Malta, and Russia. In 2008 he directed excavations within the central stone settings at Stonehenge. He is leading the research team on the Human Henge project.
Email: tdarvill@bournemouth.ac.uk

Laura Drysdale is Director of the Restoration Trust and Project Manager of Human Henge. Laura managed an English Heritage collections conservation team, and was a Senior Manager at the Museums Libraries and Archive Council before supporting marginalized people at Stonham, Julian Support, and Together for Mental Health. The Restoration Trust was founded in 2014, and now runs culture therapy partnership projects involving participants with archaeology, archives, museum collections, contemporary art, and music.
Email: laura@restorationtrust.org.uk

Liz Ellis has worked at National Lottery Heritage Fund (formerly the Heritage Lottery Fund) since 2015. As Policy Advisor Communities and Diversity she leads on promoting ambitious, inclusive practice across the heritage sector. This includes supporting staff in building skills and knowledge on inclusion, ensuring under represented communities are aware of Fund opportunities and working in partnership with wider sectors, including disability led organizations, race equality networks and LGBTQ leaders. Having trained as a mental health nurse, Liz studied Fine Art at St Martin's School of Art, London with subsequent national and international residencies and exhibitions. As Curator Community Learning at Tate Modern 2006 – 2014, Liz led high quality local, national and international partnerships. These included interdisciplinary programmes with NHS Trusts, mental health organizations, universities, and international artists. She is a member of the Wellcome Trust Diversity and Inclusion Steering Group. In 2012 she obtained an MA in Human Rights at UCL. A commitment to social justice and the power of cultural rights informs her practice.
Email: liz.ellis@heritagefund.og.uk

Christopher Howard Elmer is a Teaching Fellow in the Department of Archaeology, University of Southampton. He has worked for over three decades in the sphere of heritage education and archaeology and has spent many years developing, delivering, and evaluating innovative education programmes and community engagement projects within the formal and informal education spheres. Before completing his PhD in public engagement and archaeology, Chris worked as a field archaeologist, secondary school teacher, museum curator, and finally served in the position of Head of Education for Hampshire County Council Arts and Museums service (now Hampshire Cultural Trust). His work and research has enabled him to pursue interests in pedagogy and collaborative projects. Chris has an MA in Museums Studies, and is an Associate Member of the Museums Association.
Email: che1v17@soton.ac.uk

Mark Evans is CEO of Waterloo Uncovered, a charity he co-founded with friend and colleague Major Charlie Foinette. They both studied at the UCL Institute of Archaeology to Masters level, before joining the Coldstream Guards as officers. After serving in Afghanistan, Mark was diagnosed with PTSD and subsequently discharged from the army. His work with Waterloo Uncovered allows him to combine his past experience, with a project that undertakes valuable archaeology and helping others.
Email: mark@waterloouncovered.com

Stuart Eve is a Post-Doctoral Researcher at the University of Leicester, and a founding partner of L-P Archaeology. His research interests include virtual and augmented reality technology, and the exploration of the connections between archaeological method and theory. He is the joint director of excavations for the Waterloo Uncovered project. In addition, he is creating a multi-dimensional reconstruction of the landscape of Avebury, Wiltshire.
Email: se154@le.ac.uk

Lesley Hardy is Senior Lecturer in History at Canterbury Christ Church University. Her interests are in heritage, historiography, antiquarianism, and public and local history. She is Project Lead for the HLF-funded Finding Eanswythe: The Life and Afterlife of an Anglo-Saxon Saint project.
Email: lesley.hardy@canterbury.ac.uk

Vicki Haverkate-Emmerson is an experienced teacher, educational researcher, outreach professional and former archaeologist. At Waterloo Uncovered she combines these roles to enable the progress of student and veteran participants on the excavation to be recognized by the Utrecht University's Summer Schools program. During excavations seasons she also researches the project's impact on non-military participants.
Email: vicki@waterloouncovered.com

Rebecca L Hearne is a PhD researcher in the Department of Archaeology and School of English, University of Sheffield. She is interested in subjective experience of the past, radical pedagogy and alternative education, accessible research through the creative arts, and community engagement and development through heritage engagement.
Email: rlhearne1@sheffield.ac.uk

Vanessa Heaslip is Principal Academic and Deputy Head of Research in the Department of Nursing and Clinical Science at Bournemouth University. She has extensive experience in nursing, nurse education, and is an experienced qualitative researcher. Her general research interests are in the field of vulnerability and vulnerable groups in society whose voices are not traditionally heard in academic and professional discourse. As well as marginalized communities who experience inequity of opportunity in accessing health care services and education. Dr Vanessa Heaslip has numerous publications including book contributions, journal articles, editorials, and discussion papers.
Email: vheaslip@bournemouth.ac.uk

Andrew Hoaen is a Lecturer in Archaeology in the Department of Archaeology and Geography in the School of Science and the Environment at the University of Worcester.
Email: a.hoaen@worc.ac.uk

Helen Johnston is a Senior Community Archaeologist with the Thames Discovery Programme, supporting Foreshore Recording and Observation Group volunteers to monitor and record archaeology on the Thames foreshore. She worked on a three-year project funded by City Bridge Trust to run a programme of activities engaging with Londoners aged over 75 years. Helen studied archaeology at the University of York, and has an MA in Environment, Culture and Society from Lancaster University. She has experience of developing policies and procedures around participation and inclusion, and managing volunteer programmes at organizations including The Scout Association, Heritage Lottery Fund, Diabetes UK, and RNIB. She volunteered with the Thames Discovery Programme for eight years, coordinating the Greenwich Foreshore Recording and Observation Group.
Email: hjohnston@mola.org.uk

Zena Kamash is Senior Lecturer in Roman Art and Archaeology in the Department of Classics at Royal Holloway, University of London, and a Fellow of the Society of Antiquaries. She specializes in the Roman Middle East and Roman Britain, with wide-ranging interests including ancient technologies, memory, food, sensory understandings of the past, and religion. She is

particularly interested in how we present archaeology to the public, in museums and beyond, and how we interact with the past in the modern world. Her current research focuses on post-conflict cultural heritage in Syria and Iraq. She is British-Iraqi and finds that crafting helps relieve her PTSD.
Email: Zena.Kamash@rhul.ac.uk

Alice Kershaw is Head of Business Process Review at the National Lottery Heritage Fund (formerly the Heritage Lottery Fund) exploring how to improve the end to end grant management processes. Alice leads on developing and improving the grant-giving process at the Fund, supporting the practical side of implementing strategy and policy decisions. This can involve creating new processes, piloting new ideas, using customer and research insight to enhance aspects of the process, and developing new forms and technical infrastructure to underpin grant-giving. She was previously the Casework Manager, and prior to that a Senior Grants Officer in the London Team. Prior to her work with the Fund she was Heritage Regeneration Officer for Opportunity Peterborough and Peterborough City Council, working alongside a range of local partners to catalyse heritage activity across Peterborough Unitary Authority, and House Administrator and Operations Manager at Benjamin Franklin House. She lives in Leeds and enjoys running in the Yorkshire Dales in her spare time.
Twitter username @alicekershaw; Email: alice.kershaw@heritagefund.org.uk

Helen Loney is a Principal Lecturer in Archaeology in the Department of Archaeology and Geography in the School of Science and the Environment, at the University of Worcester.
Email: h.loney@worc.ac.uk

Sara Lunt is Chair of the Human Henge Project Board and a Trustee of the Restoration Trust. Trained as an archaeologist, she was Senior Curator for English Heritage, and responsible for the exhibition of objects in the new Visitor Centre at Stonehenge. She now works as an independent scholar, working on the pre-Spanish ceramics of the Peruvian Andes.
Email: saralunt13@gmail.com

Paul Murtagh is a Consultant Archaeologist at CFA Archaeology Ltd. He is an Affiliate Researcher at the University of Glasgow and holds a PhD on the Iron Age of Scotland from Durham University. He spends his summers volunteering on the Ardnamurchan Transitions Project and has interests in sports heritage and engaging non-traditional audiences in archaeology. Paul was the Heritage Project Officer for the Clyde and Avon Valley Landscape Partnership while at Northlight Heritage between 2015 and 2018..
Email: pmurtagh@cfa-archaeology.co.uk

Claire Nolan is an AHRC-funded doctoral researcher at the University of Reading. With training and a professional background in archaeology, psychotherapy, and community mental health, she has a special interest in the relationship between people, places, and the past. Her work focuses on the intrinsic value of heritage and its influence on individual lived experience, and it is particularly concerned with prehistoric archaeology and its relevance to modern society.
Email: Claire.Nolan@pgr.reading.ac.uk

Daniel O'Donoghue is Locality Manager for Richmond Fellowship Wiltshire. He has been working in voluntary sector mental health services in Wiltshire with Richmond Fellowship since 2004, focussing primarily on social inclusion, employment, and housing. Prior to this he

worked in Oxfordshire from 1996. The projects he has worked on have typically placed a strong emphasis on partnership working, practical activity, and client/service-user involvement in developing services.
Email: Daniel.ODonoghue@RichmondFellowship.org.uk

Tony Pollard is Professor of Conflict History and Archaeology at the University of Glasgow, and Director of the Centre for Battlefield Archaeology. Teaching responsibilities include convening the Masters course in Conflict Archaeology and Heritage, and his research interests range from the archaeology of medieval warfare to the cultural heritage of the Falklands War. He is the lead academic and joint director of excavations for the Waterloo Uncovered project.
Email: Tony.Pollard@glasgow.ac.uk

William Rathouse is a support officer and project coordinator for Mind Aberystwyth. He studied archaeology and anthropology at the University of Wales Lampeter, and went on to research a PhD examining the contestation of heritage in the UK at the University of Wales Trinity Saint David. Whilst engaged in this research he began working for the university's student support services, focussing on assistance for those with autism and mental health issues. On reading about Mind Herefordshire's Past in Mind project, and the MoD's Operation Nightingale, he set up a series of projects in Ceredigion that promoted mental health well-being through archaeology. He has also volunteered with Operation Nightingale, and has been working hard to extend mental health and well-being through archaeology projects in Wales and beyond. He has interests in promoting the inclusive management, presentation, and organization of heritage attractions.
Email: will.rathouse@gmail.com

Bob Ruffle is a former Chair of the Worcester Archaeological Society, and has a PhD in post-medieval Archaeology from the Department of Archaeology and Geography in the School of Science and the Environment at the University of Worcester.
Email: bob.ruffle@gmail.com

Yvette Staelens is a Visiting Research Fellow at Bournemouth University and a trained Natural Voice Practitioner. She currently leads community choirs in Somerset, and her career encompasses archaeology, museums, and performance. She is programme facilitator on the Human Henge project.
Email: ystaelens@bournemouth.ac.uk

Eleonora Steinberg is a neuroscientist, communicator and filmmaker. She co-ordinates research and publication at Waterloo Uncovered as part of their objective to study and understand war and its impact on people.
Email: elly.steinberg@gmail.com

Toby Sutcliffe is a consultant psychiatrist working within the North Wiltshire Community Mental Health Team. He has worked as a psychiatrist in Wiltshire for ten years and previously as Medical Lead, Postgraduate Tutor, and Clinical Director of Avon and Wiltshire Partnership Mental Health Services in Wiltshire. He is employed by Avon and Wiltshire Partnership Mental Health Trust, and holds an honorary teaching position at the University of Bristol.
Email: toby.sutcliffe@nhs.net

David Ulke is welfare lead for the Waterloo Uncovered project. He is a retired Royal Air Force Nursing Officer with an extensive background in mental health. He is an archaeology graduate from the University of Leicester, whose prize-winning research project examined the impact of participation in archaeology, on military veterans' mental well-being. His interests include conflict archaeology, and the recording and preservation of military cultural heritage.
Email: david@waterloouncovered.com

Ellie Williams is Lecturer in Archaeology at Canterbury Christ Church University. Her interests lie in the archaeology of death and burial, medieval archaeology, heritage, and community archaeology. She is a collaborator on Finding Easnwythe: the Life and Afterlife of an Anglo-Saxon Saint project.
Email: ellie.williams@canterbury.ac.uk

Foreword

Sara Lunt

Mental ill-health is a major problem of our time. Its impact is personal, social, and political. We cannot afford to ignore it, nor to depend on the conventional therapies offered to sufferers by over-stretched health and social care providers. To meet the crisis other pathways towards recovery are being explored and developed, amongst them the use of cultural resources. The therapeutic potential of culture in all its forms is being recognized and harnessed to alleviate mental ill-health and increase well-being.

Heritage resources represent a new category in this field. The Human Henge project operates under the auspices of the Restoration Trust, whose mission is to make 'culture therapy' an everyday part of mental health provision. The strategy is novel and innovative. Accompanied by archaeologists, singers, musicians, and craftspeople, our participants, all of whom live with long-term mental ill-health, journey through ancient landscapes. In doing so, they form a new community and connect with the people and places of the past. This is a healing experience and, based on the evaluation of our participants' reactions, we believe that the benefits can be life-changing and long-term.

Many months of discussion, planning, and fund-raising by the members of the Human Henge Project Board underpinned the outdoor sessions in the Stonehenge and Avebury World Heritage Site. Our continuing task is to research and assess the outcomes for mental health, to present and publicize our work, and to gain support for new programmes based on the accumulating experience of participants in this and other similar projects. Together we are building evidence to demonstrate the therapeutic value of ancient landscapes, and we sincerely believe that this evidence will be persuasive to National Health Service and social care commissioners and providers.

At the Theoretical Archaeology Group Annual Meeting in Cardiff in December 2017 and the Historic Landscapes and Mental Well-being conference at Bournemouth University in April 2018, the preliminary results of work on Human Henge were presented and discussed. A valuable wider context was provided by reports on other projects whose academic discourse or practical activities are also based on the therapeutic values of ancient and historic landscapes and places. We heard from representatives of funding bodies who generously supported the work of Human Henge and similar projects; from leaders in the field of culture and health; from mental health clinicians who have brought their skills to bear in evaluation and in providing expert advice; from archivists and archaeologists whose resources and expertise form the essential bedrock to heritage-based culture therapy; from practitioners and participants who have taken part in culture therapy projects; and from heritage managers who have promoted this kind of therapy in their organizations and facilitated access to the landscapes, monuments and collections in their care. It was exciting to hear just how much imaginative, inventive, and stimulating work is going on this field, much it now captured in the papers presented in this volume.

We would like to thank everyone who participated in the Cardiff and Bournemouth events, and all those who have contributed papers to this volume. It is a wonderful thing to see how the power of ancient places continues to resonate in the present day and how, used creatively, they can change lives for the better.

Without our partners and funders, Human Henge and its associated outreach activities could not have happened. We had funding from The Heritage Lottery Fund (now The National Lottery Heritage Fund), English Heritage, and Wiltshire County Council. The Restoration Trust, English Heritage, National Trust, Richmond Fellowship, Bournemouth University, and the Avon and Wiltshire Mental Health NHS Partnership Trust have made generous contributions of people, places, expertise, and help in kind. To all of these and the many other organizations that have helped in so many ways we extend our very grateful thanks. On a personal note, I would also like to take this opportunity to thank all the members of the Human Henge Project Board who generously gave their time to share their enthusiasm, devise our programmes, and assist in their implementation.

The Human Hengers themselves – the participants, facilitators, volunteers and staff – form the beating heart of Human Henge. They have struggled through wind and weather, listened, explored, sung and rejoiced, formed friendships, and created ceremonies. They have given us new insights into ancient places, and, in their frank responses to the very many variations on the theme of 'so how did that make you feel?' they have made a vital contribution to the future use of ancient landscapes to improve mental health and well-being. Several Human Hengers attended and contributed to the discussions in Cardiff and Bournemouth. Their voices were heard throughout the meetings and are represented in this volume, living proof of the success of our approach. We applaud their courage in making the Human Henge journey and hope that their achievements will be an inspiration to many others in years to come.

Chapter 1

Introduction: Heritage and well-being

Timothy Darvill, Kerry Barrass, Laura Drysdale, Vanessa Heaslip, and Yvette Staelens

Abstract

In introducing and contextualizing the papers in this volume attention is directed to the current prevalence and associated economic and social costs of mental health provision. The societal importance of finding non-medicalized approaches to the enhancement of mental health well-being is underlined, and it is argued that, as later chapters clearly show, cultural heritage has a lot to offer. Consideration is given to commonly used ways of defining 'well-being', and the scope and nature of cultural heritage represented as archaeological sites and ancient or historic landscapes. International, European Union, national, and regional treaties, agreements, legislation, strategies, and public policy in relation to heritage and well-being are reviewed, and attention given to the work of government agencies in the UK. The idea of therapeutic landscapes is evaluated as a starting point for thinking about cultural heritage therapy as a form of social prescribing and the wide range of case studies from Britain and the near continent included in this volume.

Keywords: Archaeology; Cultural heritage; Mental health; Social prescribing; Well-being

Introduction

Enhancing well-being in general, and mental health well-being in particular, is one of the most significant societal challenges currently facing communities across the world. Available statistics on the prevalence of mental illness make grim reading. The Adult Psychiatric Morbidity Survey conducted in 2014 suggests that around one in six (17%) of adults surveyed in England met the criteria for a common mental disorder (McManus *et al.* 2016), while National Health Service figures for the UK indicate that one in four adults (25%) experience at least one diagnosable mental health problem in any given year (NHS 2016a: 4). In Europe, more than one in three (38%) people suffer each year from a brain disorder such as depression, anxiety, insomnia, or dementia, according to a study carried out across 30 countries between 2008 and 2010 by the Institute of Clinical Psychology and Psychotherapy in Dresden University (Wittchen *et al.* 2011). Globally, the World Health Organization estimates that one in four people (25%) are affected by a mental health disorder at some point in their lives (WHO 2001: 20). The costs associated with these indispositions are eye-watering. In purely human terms, a low quality of life and premature mortality are significant, as too the social and emotional costs to individuals, families, and communities. Looked at in economic and monetary terms the total costs of mental ill-health across the 28 EU countries in 2018 have been estimated at over 600 billion Euros, more than 4 per cent of Gross Domestic Product (OECD and EU 2018: 26). The cost of mental health support and services in England alone equates to £34 billion each year, and this excludes dementia and substance abuse (NHS 2016a: 9), while the cost to the economy is estimated at £105 billion (NHS 2016a: 4). Unsurprisingly, international organizations, governments, and state agencies have now woken-up to the problem, begun examining its many dimensions, and are developing policies and strategies aimed at prevention as well as treatment. Some of these approaches extend well beyond traditional medical solutions by looking for remedies and therapies in new domains. As the papers in this volume clearly show, one such domain involves the innovative use of archaeological sites, ancient landscapes, and the wider historic environment for what can be called cultural heritage therapy.

Internationally, the overarching strategy on health and well-being is prominent on the list of 17 Sustainable Development Goals to be achieved by 2030 that were adopted at the seventieth session of the UN General Council in New York in September 2015 (UN 2016a; UNESCO 2015). Goal 3 is 'Good Health and Well-being' and includes the specific target of promoting mental health well-being (UN 2016b: Goal 3.4). One of the tools recognized by UNESCO for the attainment of the Sustainable Development Goals is 'culture', defined for this purpose as 'who we are and what shapes our identity'; as such it 'contributes to poverty reduction and paves the way for human-centred, inclusive and equitable development' (UNESCO 2016). According to UNESCO, 'no development can be sustainable without it' and 'placing culture at the heart of development policies constitutes an essential investment in the world's future and a pre-condition to successful globalization processes that take into account the principle of cultural diversity' (UNESCO 2016). Although not explicitly linked to Goal 3 in UNESCO's published texts, culture and the closely related notions of heritage and the historic environment have a potentially very significant role to play to promoting many aspects of good health and well-being, including mental health well-being that forms the focus of attention here. Indeed, as earlier overviews (Darvill *et al.* 2018; Reilly *et al.* 2018), ongoing projects (CHEurope 2019), and the papers in this volume clearly demonstrate, the potential enhancements to well-being that can be achieved through interdisciplinary teamwork combining insights from archaeology, anthropology, health-care, environmental therapy, and the creative arts are very considerable.

The origins of this volume lie in the contributions made to two related meetings, both arising out of the public outreach work associated with the HLF-supported Human Henge project. First, was a day-long session at the thirty-ninth annual meeting of the Theoretical Archaeology Group (TAG) held in the University of Cardiff, Wales, on the 18–20 December 2017. Entitled *Archaeology, Heritage, and Well-being* this well-attended session focused on using heritage resources of various kinds to promote well-being. It recognized such approaches as one of the most significant advances in archaeological resource management for many years, and provided an opportunity to share experiences and to discuss the outcomes, implications, and theoretical underpinnings of well-being projects. Second, was a whole-day multi-disciplinary conference held in Bournemouth University on the 13 April 2018 entitled *Historic landscapes and mental well-being*. More than 80 delegates from a wide range of backgrounds — including practitioners, experts by experience, heritage professionals, academics, and policy makers — discussed ways of using historic landscapes and heritage resources of various kinds to promote well-being and the boundless potential contribution that the historic environment can make to health-care and wellness initiatives. Some papers were presented at both events, some at only one, but all have been reconfigured and up-dated in the light of the discussions and subsequent work. One paper, included here as Chapter 4, was presented at a session entitled *Mental health in archaeology* at the thirty-eighth annual meeting of TAG in the University of Bradford on 15 December 2015.

Our aim in bringing these papers together is two-fold. First, is to illustrate how archaeological sites, ancient landscapes, and the historic environment more generally, are being used rather successfully as tools to enhance mental health well-being in a range of communities across Britain. The projects and approaches described here deserve wide recognition for their international levels of originality in terms of the deployment of aspects of the historic environment in novel ways, the significance of what is being achieved in changing people's lives for the better, and the rigour that has been applied in thinking through the underpinning logic and the practices themselves. Second, is to prompt further debate about the contribution that the historic environment can make to the attainment of Sustainable Development Goal 3 over the next decade or so, and to assess the contribution that this work can make to delivering public value from heritage assets.

Central to the thinking that underpins all the contributions in this volume is the idea that poor health and mental ill-health are not simply medical matters that can be solved by prescribing drugs and medication. Other factors are relevant and important, not least people's environment, and their identity, self-confidence, and relationships with others. Responding to the manifestations of poor mental health and treating symptoms is not the same as dealing with underlying causes. In words widely attributed to Bishop Desmond Tutu: there comes a point when we need to stop just pulling people out of the river; we need to go upstream and find out why they're falling in. One such journey upstream has been made by the controversial writer Johann Hari whose exploration of depression and anxiety revealed a range of disconnects between those living with such conditions and their wider personal, social, and environmental context. He suggests that for many people the drugs don't work, but that social prescribing which encourages reconnecting with one's self in new ways, with other people, with meaningful work and values, with the environment, and with a purposeful sense of the future can work wonders (Hari 2018). He is not the only one. Journalist Matthew Parris for example argues that it is wrong to spend so much money on talking therapies and medication when there is little evidence that they actually work (Parris 2018). Similarly, the DeStress Project set up to examine the impacts of austerity and welfare reform on mental health and well-being in low-income communities in England found widespread dissatisfaction with the current medical model for mental health amongst doctors and patients (Thomas et al. 2019: 13). However, it would be wrong to see social prescribing and other related approaches as 'cures' for mental illness, nor are they necessarily substitutes for properly administered medication. Integrated medical and social therapies are complementary actions, each supporting and enhancing the other, thereby offering what is known as integrated care as a robust and potentially sustainable way forward.

Axiomatic to such thinking is the recognition that mental illness is not a binary phenomenon. Whilst we recognize that there are severe and enduring diagnosed mental health conditions, we also know that, outside of clinical settings, each of us moves through sometimes acute variations in our mental health. In this context it useful to understand mental health in terms of a gradient or scale that everyone is on, and along which we move over time with varying degrees of susceptibility and resilience to internal and external influences. Rather than maintaining a strict focus on mental illness we prefer to explore the positive slope of the gradient and talk instead about mental health well-being that could, simplistically at least, be seen as ranging from very poor at one end of the gradient to very good at the other. Self-reflecting for a minute, where do you, the reader, feel you sit on the gradient right now? Where have you been, and which direction are you heading? And how might your story colour the way you explore the papers in this book?

In introducing the papers this volume, and setting the background for the book as a whole, we would like to explore four cross-cutting underlying themes. First, we unpack some of the essential terminology inherent to the title of the volume and the papers within. Second, we consider the strategic and policy context that folds around the UNESCO Sustainable Development Goals already mentioned, with a special emphasis on the situation in Britain and Europe. Third, we briefly explore the idea of therapeutic landscapes as natural, designed, or created places that promote health and well-being. And fourth, the natural extension of the first three, we outline the idea of what might be termed cultural heritage therapy.

Unpacking concepts and meanings

Two key terms deserving of attention and scoping run through the chapters of this volume and appear prominently in its title: historic landscapes and mental well-being. They are considered here in reverse order.

Despite its widespread use, mental well-being is hard to define, its content puzzling to unpack, and its existence or fulfilment tricky to measure. At a general and rather superficial level well-being, and also by implication mental well-being, refers to a state of being characterized by good (mental) health, contentedness, happiness, an assured quality of life, and a sense of positivity. But its meanings and implications run far deeper in technical and social spheres to embrace issues of morality, politics, law, and economics. Philosopher James Griffin usefully offers insights into understandings of well-being that apply to a multidimensional range of interconnected contexts including: mental well-being; physical well-being; social well-being; spiritual well-being; emotional well-being; economic well-being; and so on (Griffin 1986). The most common starting point is grounded in utilitarian thinking in which utility focuses on attaining the human experiences of pleasure and the absence of pain. Whether this occurs as a mental state fed by feelings and emotions, or is relational to the perceived state of the world and thus fed by actual or informed desires, is a matter of considerable debate, but for Griffin the approach is overly broad and generally inadequate (Griffin 1986: 7–20). By contrast there are objectivist understandings of well-being in which desires are replaced by an altogether more urgent and powerful feeling of 'need'. As he explains, 'desires have to do with how a subject of experience looks out on the world: needs have to do with whether one thing is in fact a necessary condition of another' (1986: 41). In this sense needs tend to be rather narrowly defined. While individuals and society as a whole may be flexible in how needs are described, understanding the extent to which needs are met becomes a moral judgement. However, better for the modern world than either utilitarian or objectivist perspectives are perfectionist accounts that are concerned with what a good life is for humanity in general. This approach, essentially Aristotelian in origin, proposes the existence of an ideal form for human life to take, a form in which human nature flourishes and reaches perfection. Thus the level of attainment of well-being for any individual is directly proportional to how near that person's life gets to the ideal (Griffin 1986: 56). Feelings of distance from perfection (alienation) are mainly negative and can be very damaging to mental well-being. So the trick, highly relevant to life in the twenty-first century, is to invert or flip Aristotle's vision of perfection grounded in the idea that very few people will ever achieve the high peaks (the 'Superman /

Superwoman Vision') and instead recognize that perfection is available to everyone. Looked at this way perfection is generated quite simply through the realization of what makes up human excellences and causes the human spirit to flourish, for example through: wisdom; courage; temperance; industry; humility; hope; charity; justice; creativity; engagement with others; respect; understanding; emotional enjoyment; and deep reciprocal personal relations (Griffin 1986: 63–67). In this view well-being does not involve a single universal 'right' balance of these things because the balance varies from person to person. As such, well-being is not so much about wellness *per* se as about a heightened sense of 'being', and an awareness of the continual process of 'becoming'. As Kathleen Galvin suggests in the introduction to the recently published *Routledge handbook of well-being*, well-being is intrinsically intertwined with the matter of 'how things are for you in the world' (Galvin 2018: 2). It is an idea grounded in phenomenology that she goes on to explore in detail with Les Todres in terms of a dialectic between dwelling and mobility (Galvin and Todres 2018; Todres and Galvin 2010). Thus well-being as they describe it is an existentialist account: 'a positive possibility that is independent of health and illness but is a resource for both ... an ontic everyday experience [that] is never complete' (Galvin and Todres 2018: 89).

The world as dwelling place for individuals and societies is itself a complex multidimensional space. Although it can only be experienced by any one person in the here and now, it encapsulates historic dimensions, and, like human experience itself, has a past, a present, and a future. As such the second of our key terms — historic landscape — could be seen as an allegory of human existence, representing the transience of life mapped against the physicality of the world. The historical or cultural dimensions of landscape represent where we have been, or where others have been, the pre-knowledge informing where we are now, as the starting point for an anticipated future. Traditional approaches to the study and analysis of historic landscapes have tended to be positivist or processual, emphasizing the relationships in time and space of the visible or reconstructable elements. The focus has been on creating the story of the landscape, a grand narrative outlining how it developed and changed over time (Darvill 2001: 36–38). More recently attention has turned towards relativist or post-processual ways of thinking that focus instead on relationships between people and the world they created for themselves (physically and conceptually) and in which they lived (Darvill 2001: 38–41). Experience, structuration, memory, and the cognitive creation of place are key themes of this new kind of landscape archaeology, and it is these approaches that the authors of the papers in this volume find appealing in relation to the promoting mental well-being. Modelling the way people perceive places as they move through them or around them, how cosmological beliefs were fixed in the landscape, and how people perceived and understood aspects of the physical world such as soil, water, rock, colour, plants, trees, animals, fire, and air have created numerous ways of interpreting and understanding landscapes past and present (David and Thomas 2008; Meier 2006). Moreover, such thinking connects terrestrial experiences with other important dimensions of the world as people experience it, including seascapes (Cooney 2003) and skyscapes (Silva 2019) to create the broader notion of the 'historic environment'.

A wide-ranging academic and public debate about Britain's historic environment under the title *Power of Place*, initiated in the early 2000s by English Heritage (EH) as the government agency responsible for the cultural heritage, opened up and exposed several broader visions (EH 2000a; 2000b; DCMS 2001). As a starting point it was felt that 'the historic environment is all around us: it is the map on which we write the future' (EH 2000a: 2). While the conclusions of the discussion went on to capture the duality and complexity of the historic environment noting that: 'at one level, it is made up entirely of places such as towns or villages, coast or hills, and things such as buildings, buried sites and deposits, fields and hedges; at another level it is something we inhabit, both physically and imaginatively. It is many faceted, relying on an engagement with physical remains but also on emotional and aesthetic responses and on the power of memory, history and association' (EH 2000a: 5).

Importantly, the *Power of Place* debate directed attention towards the need to integrate physical and emotional responses. It harked back to earlier thoughts about the iconography of landscape (Cosgrove and Daniels 1988) and the various ways of representing, structuring, and symbolizing our surroundings. It takes us into interesting territory in which the spirit of place can be conjured up through coupling engagement with imagination. More recently still, the intangible cultural heritage represented by words, poems, song, music, dance, beliefs, traditions, folklore, food, dress and many more things beside is being woven back into the fabric of the historic environment to give it a new richness and texture that enhances the somewhat traditional, some might even say rather 'dry', tangible heritage (Alves 2018; UNESCO 2003). There remains a long way to go in fusing these two strands of tangible and intangible cultural heritage, especially in the area of public policy and legislation. But the foundations have been laid and they provide an important base from which to animate the appreciation of archaeological sites and ancient landscapes as a means of enhancing health and mental well-being. Just as emotional and aesthetic responses can help people understand significant places, so, the other way round, significant places experienced in particular ways can stimulate the same kinds of feeling. With care and sensitivity these can be directed to positive benefit emphasizing human excellences and causing the human spirit to flourish.

Well-being, mental health and heritage in legislation, policy, and strategy

Mention has already been made of the Sustainable Development Goals approved by the United Nations that includes 'Good health and well-being' (UN 2016b). This international agreement, ratified by 193 countries, currently stands as the more comprehensive overarching statute and statement of global ambition to be pursued over the next decade or so. Both underpinning it and cascading from it are many layers of international, multi-national, national, regional, and local legislation, policy, and strategy that provide the legal frameworks and doctrinal context for organizational structures and roles, professional practice, research direction and support, and educational programmes and content. All embrace the concept of promoting well-being and good mental health as a desirable state for a population as a whole, although here it is only possible to touch on the content and implications of a few specific instruments at key scales of application, focusing on those that combine interests in mental health well-being and cultural heritage.

International

The World Health Organization (WHO) is the UN system agency responsible for the international agenda related to health issues. Their *Mental health action plan 2013-2020* published in 2013 has as its goal 'to promote mental well-being, prevent mental disorders, provide care, enhance recovery, promote human rights and reduce the mortality, morbidity and disability for persons with mental disorders' (WHO 2013a: 9). This is pursued through four main objectives: (1) to strengthen effective leadership and governance for mental health; (2)

to provide comprehensive, integrated and responsive mental health and social care services in community-based settings; (3) to implement strategies for promotion and prevention in mental health; and (4) to strengthen information systems, evidence and research for mental health (WHO 2013a: 10). The 2015 publication *Mental health, well-being and disability: A new global priority. Key United Nations resolutions and documents* affirms that 'mental and social well-being are the most fundamental and critical constituents of human life' (University of Tokyo 2015: 3) and provides a valuable set of reference materials and documents relating to the implementation of Sustainable Development Goal 3.

Developing the global *Mental Health Action Plan* in a European context, the WHO published *Health 2020: European policy framework and strategy for the 21st century* (WHO 2013b) and *The European mental health action plan 2013-2020* (WHO 2013c). The mental health plan gives four core objectives: (1) everyone has an equal opportunity to realize mental well-being throughout their lifespan, particularly those who are most vulnerable or at risk; (2) people with mental health problems are citizens whose human rights are fully valued, protected and promoted; (3) mental health services are accessible and affordable, available in the community according to need; and (4) people are entitled to respectful, safe and effective treatment (WHO 2013c: 4).

European

The European Union (EU) has a number of policies referring to well-being in general, headed by Article 3 of the *Treaty of the European Union* (also known as the *Treaty of Lisbon*) stating that 'The Union's aim is to promote peace, its values and the well-being of its peoples' (EU 2008: 21). The European Commission (the executive arm of the EU) has a well-developed mental health policy (EC 2016) building on an earlier joint publication with the WHO. The *European pact for mental health and well-being* states that mental health services should be developed '...which are well integrated in the society, put the individual at the centre and operate in a way which avoids stigmatization and exclusion' and which would also 'promote active inclusion of people with mental health problems in society' (EC and WHO 2008: 6).

Heritage and related matters are generally devolved from the European Union to the Council of Europe who have developed a series of relevant conventions and recommendations. Centre stage is the *Framework convention on the value of cultural heritage for society* (also known as the *Faro convention*) which emphasizes '...the value and potential of cultural heritage wisely used as a resource for sustainable development and quality of life in a constantly evolving society' and '... that the conservation of cultural heritage and its sustainable use have human development and quality of life as their goal' (COE 2005). This gave rise to the *Faro action plan* (COE 2016) which is still ongoing. Daniel Thérond (2009: 10) points out that the *Faro convention* provides a cohesive view of cultural heritage in that its protection and conservation is a means to an end, including the well-being of individuals, not an end in itself.

The Council of Europe's draft *Strategy 21* (COE 2015a) arose from the *Narmur declaration* (COE 2015b) and is based on a range of European conventions, including the *Faro convention* mentioned above. The *Narmur declaration* states that heritage should contribute to people's well-being (COE 2015b: 3) and promote public well-being (COE 2015b: 4). *Strategy 21* proposes a redefinition of the place and role of cultural heritage in Europe that includes its use to improve the quality of life (COE 2015a).

United Kingdom

Across the UK, well-being and mental health have become major areas of interest to legislators and policy makers. Central government has issued a series of strategy papers over recent years, all of which emphasize the need for, and benefits of, a population with good mental health and a strong sense of well-being. Examples include the 2010 White Paper for England *Healthy lives, healthy people* in which the coalition government of the day sought to devolve responsibility for public health to local and regional agencies, recognizing that mental health and well-being should be at the heart of a community-based strategy (DOH 2010a: 2). The accompanying Department of Health policy paper *Our health and wellbeing today*, again emphasizes the importance of a population's well-being for society as a whole (DOH 2010b: 6). It also points out that the term 'well-being' can have a wide range of interpretations, but adopts a fairly utilitarian definition used at that time by the Department for Environment, Food and Rural Affairs:

> '…a positive physical, social and mental state; it is not just the absence of pain, discomfort and incapacity. It requires that basic needs are met, that individuals have a sense of purpose, that they feel able to achieve important personal goals and participate in society. It is enhanced by conditions that include supportive personal relationships, strong and inclusive communities, good health, financial and personal security, rewarding employment, and a healthy and attractive environment.' (DOH 2010b: 13)

The paper also points out the difficulty of measuring well-being, and the central role played by mental health (DOH 2010b: 13).

In 2011 the Department of Health issued a paper outlining a new mental health policy for England, *No health without mental health* (DOH 2011). This stated that, whilst specific to England, devolved regional governments in the UK would also be addressing the issue (DOH 2011: 5). The cost of delivering mental health services is discussed, with two of the four ways of improving value for money given as: 'shifting the focus of services towards promotion of mental health, prevention of mental illness and early identification and intervention as soon as mental illness arises'; and 'broadening the approach taken to tackle the wider social determinants and consequences of mental health problems' (DOH 2011: 64). The paper also emphasizes the need to measure mental health and well-being through a series of key indicators in order to track the anticipated improvements (DOH 2011: 70–78). As a result, since 2012 well-being has been measured and tracked by the Office for National Statistics (ONS 2016). Four key measures are used — life satisfaction; worthwhile life; happiness; and anxiety — all of them scored by a sample population with reference to a gradient ranging from 0 (low) to 10 (high). Figure 1.1 shows the year-on-year pattern for all four measures. The three upper profiles are essentially positive measures that indicate generally high, and improving, levels of life satisfaction, worthwhile life, and happiness. The bottom profile is an essentially negative measure as it deals with anxiety; it indicates a generally low but decreasing level of anxiety over the period surveyed.

Building on an influential report published in 2008 entitled *Making recovery a reality* (Shepherd *et al.* 2008), the Sainsbury Centre for Mental Health looked at the delivery of mental health services in Britain and in 2012 started a campaign to promote organizational change (SCMH 2012). Importantly, they considered the question of mental health 'recovery' and noted that:

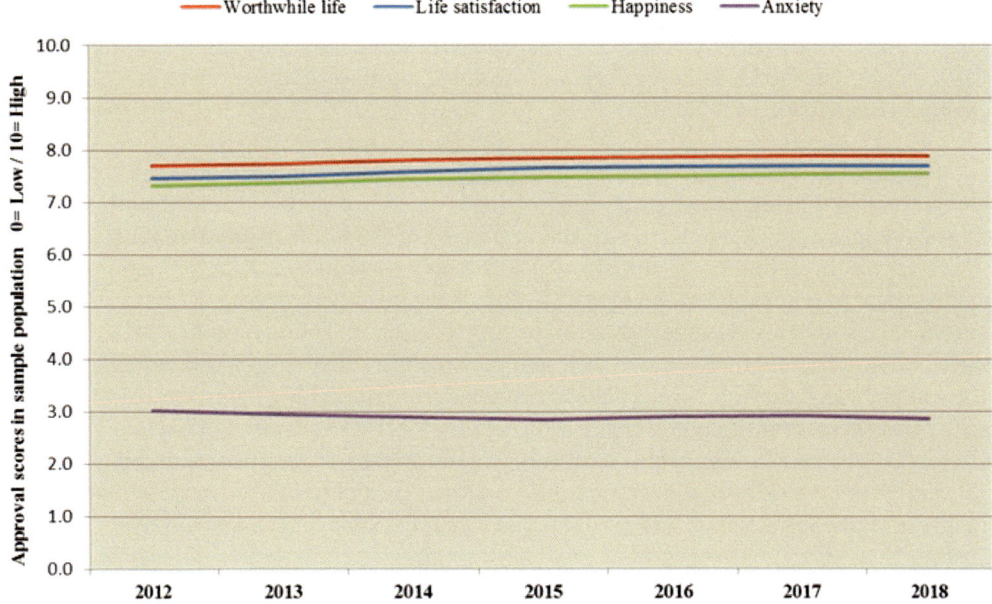

Figure 1.1. Line chart showing diachronic trends for four measures of well-being between 2012 and 2018 in the UK as recorded by the Office for National Statistics using sample populations. The left-hand scale shows mean average values based on approval ratings along a gradient ranging from low (0) to high (10). (Data from ONS 2019)

'at its heart is a set of values about a person's right to build a meaningful life for themselves, with or without the continuing presence of mental health symptoms. Recovery is based on ideas of self-determination and self-management. It emphasizes the importance of 'hope' in sustaining motivation and supporting expectations of an individually fulfilled life' (SCMH 2012: 1).

In this sense recovery can take place whilst symptoms persist, the aim of the initiative being to improve the quality of life for those with ongoing mental health conditions.

Spatial planning is recognized in government circles as another important tool for delivering well-being. In order to help inform policy in 2005 Tessa Jowell, then Culture Secretary, issued a personal essay entitled *Better places to live*. In it she discussed the role of the historic environment in building and maintaining identity, and how it might be managed by government agencies and other bodies (Jowell 2005). Responses were invited, paving the way for a conversation concerning heritage, culture, and their value to society. One output of this was the an annual 'Taking Part' survey, which aimed to measure levels of engagement with sport and culture and how this might impact on people's happiness (DCMS 2014). Bringing together the strands of culture and well-being, its conclusions included the finding that people who had visited a heritage site in the previous 12 months were significantly happier than those who had not, even when other factors are controlled for (DCMS 2014: 4). It provided powerful evidence that heritage can make a direct contribution to the well-being of individuals and, by extension, to society as a whole. When, in 2012, central government revised its guidance on town and country planning as the *National planning policy framework* these considerations come to the fore (DCLG 2012: 41) and this has been maintained and strengthened in later revisions (MHCLG 2019: 27–29). At a local level *The A-Z of planning and culture* issued by the Mayor of London's Office in 2015 embedded the concepts of heritage, culture, and well-being into London's planning framework (GLA 2015).

In 2007–08 the UK Government's futures think-tank known as Foresight ran a project on mental capital and well-being that created a set of evidence-based public mental health messages aimed at improving the mental health and well-being of the whole population (GOS 2008). One outcome was the definition of 'five ways to well-being' (GOS 2008: 21), simple actions that are summarized in graphic form as Figure 1.2. They have been widely used across many sectors and in 2011 a review was undertaken by the New Economics Foundation to look at how they have been used across the UK since their launch. Amongst other things, this work highlighted the ways in which the 'five ways' could be extended from something focused on by individuals to become themes for organizations to structure their activities around (Aked and Thompson 2011). Like the conclusions of the SCMH reports referred to above, the overarching theme of this initiative is the idea that everyone can fulfil their own potential, a conclusion very much in line with the perfectionist and existentialist ways of thinking discussed above.

The What Works Centre for Wellbeing (WWCW) was founded in 2014 and is funded jointly by the UK government, the Economic and Social Research Council (ESRC), and Public Health England. It was created in order to understand 'what national and local governments, along with voluntary and business partners, can do to increase wellbeing' (WWCW 2016a). In this context well-being is defined as 'about people, and creating the conditions for us all to thrive. It is quality of life and prosperity, positive physical and mental health, sustainable and thriving

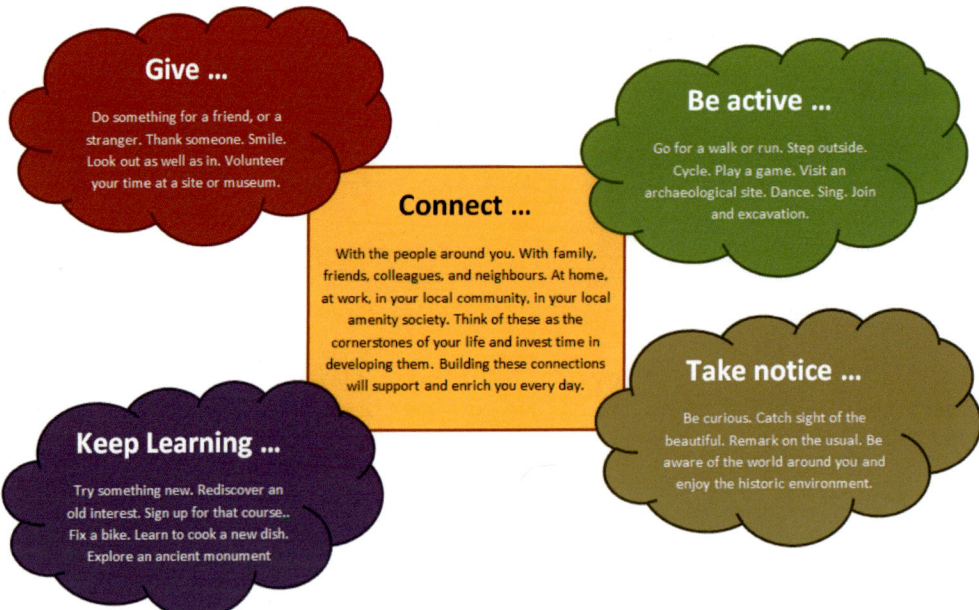

Figure 1.2. Five ways to well-being. (Based on GOS 2008: 21)

communities' (WWCW 2016b). The Centre published its first discussion paper on measuring well-being and cost effectiveness in December 2016 (Layard 2016).

The *Culture White Paper 2016* (DCMS 2016b) contained an undertaking that there would be an initiative to 'develop and promote the contribution of the cultural sectors to improving health and wellbeing' (DCMS 2016b: 9) with a key acknowledgement that 'we are beginning to understand better the profound relationship between culture, health, and wellbeing' (DCMS 2016b: 13). Throughout there was an emphasis on the role that culture plays in well-being, including the mental health aspect (DCMS 2016b: 15). Sadly, the White Paper was not taken further in its progress to becoming legislation, although it continues to provide a useful reference point summarizing thinking at the time of its creation and debate.

Mental health and well-being are also concerns of the UK's devolved governments. The Welsh Government maintains a dedicated website section on mental health (Welsh Government 2016a). It also issues updated delivery plans for its ten-year mental health strategy *Together for mental health* (Welsh Government 2012; 2016c). The concept of population well-being is linked to heritage and culture in the *Well-being of future generations (Wales) Act 2015*, that encourages 'a society that promotes and protects culture, heritage and the Welsh language' (Welsh Government 2015: 6). This link is continued in the *Taking Wales forward* strategy document (Welsh Government 2016b), where the promotion and encouragement of Welsh heritage and culture form one of the key objectives (Welsh Government 2016b: 8). It is explained that 'culture and heritage are a source of identity and distinctiveness as a nation and there is growing evidence on the wider benefits culture can bring to society. Culture supports our economy and international profile, contributes to health and wellbeing, promotes diversity and innovation and helps educate our young people' (Welsh Government 2016b: 20).

The Northern Ireland Executive Department of Health hosts an active suite of web information with strategy and action documents (NIEDOH 2016a) and has a long-term strategy set out in *Health and wellbeing 2026* (NIEDOH 2016b). The Northern Ireland Environment Agency is tasked with creating prosperity and well-being through effective environment and heritage management and regulation (NIEA 2016), again linking well-being with heritage as a key part of a strategic governmental objective. The Historic Environment Fund is a Northern Ireland Executive initiative that seeks, amongst other things, to fund community heritage projects which 'promote the social value of our historic environment and the innate contribution this can make to wellbeing and sustainable employment' (NIE 2016).

Similarly, the Scottish Government focuses on mental health and well-being across many sectors (Scottish Government 2016a; 2016b). Its strategy document *Our place in time* lays out plans for Scotland's historic environment and gives its objective as being 'to ensure that the cultural, social, environmental and economic value of Scotland's heritage makes a strong contribution to the wellbeing of the nation and its people' (Scottish Government 2014).

Government agencies and other related bodies have important roles in delivering health and well-being strategies linked to heritage and culture. The key provider of mental health services in the UK is the National Health Service (NHS). Here the NHS Choices website is designed to be a first contact point for people requiring basic health information. Building on the work of Foresight already referred to, the webpage on mental well-being proposes a view that well-being is the responsibility of the individual, who can take positive steps to acquire and maintain it (NHS 2016a). The five suggested steps (see Figure 1.2) are: connecting with other people; being active; learning new skills; giving to others; and being mindful.

Natural England, the government's statutory advisor on countryside, wildlife, nature, and the natural environment looked at the therapeutic potential of these things in its 2009 report *Experiencing landscapes: Capturing the cultural services and experiential qualities of landscape* (Natural England 2009). The report states that engaging with the outdoor environment and landscape can bring considerable mental health benefits, and recommends further study around this aspect (Natural England 2009: 111).

Historic England (formerly English Heritage), the government's statutory advisor on the historic environment, has long been interested in the relationship between cultural heritage and well-being, and in 2014 published a detailed report on the topic as *Heritage and wellbeing* (Fujiwara *et al.* 2014a; 2014b). This explored how to measure improvements to well-being as a result of engagements with cultural heritage. It developed and explained a Wellbeing Valuation approach as an attempt to monetarize the benefits. In this way the well-being value of visiting heritage sites was calculated as equivalent to £1,646 per person year, the amount of money that would have to be taken away from a person to restore them to their level of well-being had they not visited a heritage site (Futiwara *et al.* 2014b: 6). Since 2016 measures relating to the wider issue of heritage and society have been included as a separate component within the annual *Heritage counts* report prepared and published by Historic England on behalf of the Historic Environment Forum (HE 2016; 2017; 2018). Although only concerned with the situation in England, it usefully brings together data from a range of sources, including the results of the Taking Part survey referred to above (and see DCMS 2016a). Most recently a review of well-being and the historic environment advocates a framework to help Historic England develop further contributions to the agenda in which six key relationships were identified: heritage as process (e.g. volunteering); heritage as participation (e.g. visiting); heritage as mechanism (e.g. sharing); heritage as healing (e.g. therapy); heritage as place (e.g. belonging); and heritage as environment (e.g. experiencing). Operationalized through a logic model, the strategic objectives are then taken from the five ways to well-being summarized in Figure 1.2 (Reilly *et al.* 2018; Monckton and Reilly 2019; and see NLHF 2019).

Taking a slightly wider view, an inquiry by the All-Party Parliamentary Group on Arts, Health and Wellbeing (APPGAHW) concluded that it was time to recognize the powerful contribution the arts can make to health and wellbeing, noting three key areas of beneficial impact: keeping us well, aiding recovery and supporting longer lives; helping to meet major challenges facing health and social care in relation to ageing, long-term conditions, loneliness and mental health; and helping to save money in the health service and social care (APPGAHW 2017: 4). One area highlighted for praise in their report was the success achieved by museums and galleries that offer non-clinical, non-stigmatizing, environments in which people can undertake journeys of self-exploration. In support, it is claimed that more than 600 museum-based programmes targeting health and well-being outcomes had been identified in a recent study (APPGAHW 2017: 76). The creation in 2018 of the Culture, Health and Wellbeing Alliance to connect and support everyone who believes that creative and cultural engagement can transform health and wellbeing provides a useful network through which to share experiences (CHWA 2018).

Overall, the message communicated through legislation, strategy, and policy at all levels from the international down to the local is clear: cultural heritage has an important role to play in promoting people's well-being and the enhancement of their mental health. The challenge for academics, practitioners, and professionals working in the field is turning those good intentions into meaningful actions with positive outcomes. But how should we do it? What tools and approaches do we have? And how can we show our projects deliver? These are questions that will be returned to later in this introduction, and answered by examples in later chapters. First though, it is relevant to tease out two important strands of underpinning thinking: the idea of therapeutic landscapes and its natural development the notion of cultural heritage therapy.

Therapeutic landscapes

Special places, whether single sites, monuments, townscapes, or landscapes feature prominently in much of the policy and strategy relating to the perceived positive benefits between heritage and well-being. It is in fact a relationship that goes back deep into the ancient world and one that prompted the American cultural geographer Will Gesler to develop the idea of 'therapeutic landscapes' in the early 1990s (Gesler 1992; 1993; 1996; 1998). What underpinned the concept was the simple recognition that certain places or situations are perceived to be therapeutic by those that experience them, places that have achieved lasting reputations for providing physical, mental, and spiritual healing (Gesler 1992; Kearns and

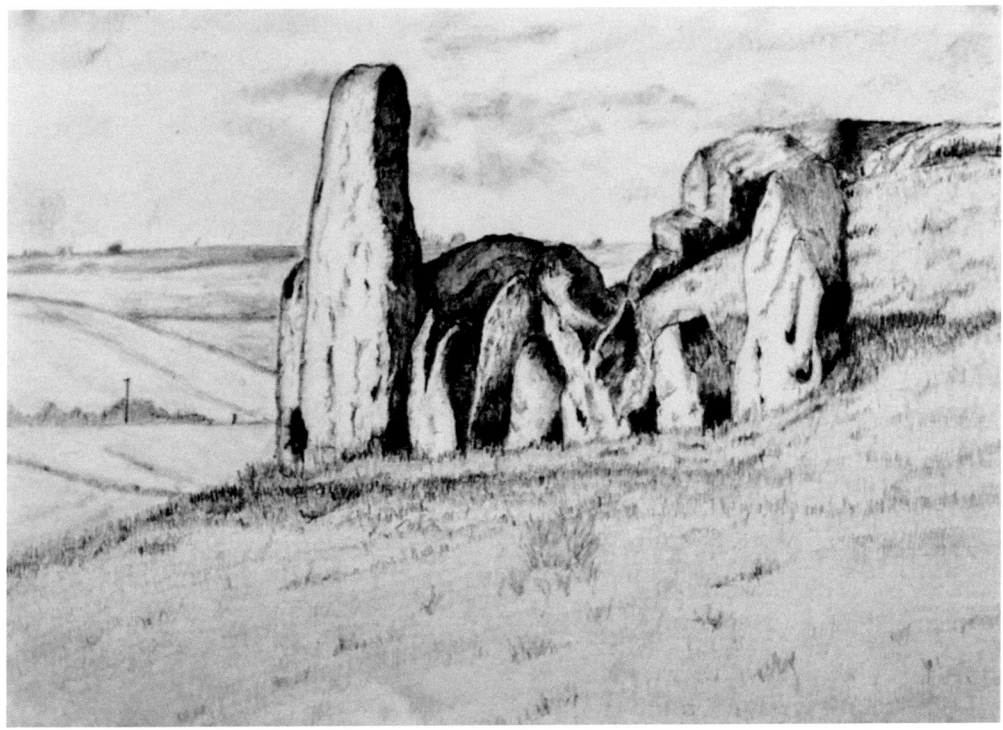

Figure 1.3. A powerful landscape: West Kennet Long Barrow, near Avebury, Wiltshire. (Drawing by Donna Songhurst. Copyright reserved)

Gesler 1998: 8). The power of place is the important thing here (Figure 1.3) The story of the subsequent maturation and expansion of the concept has been well told by Allison Williams in her introduction to a wide-ranging volume essays covering natural and built environments of many different kinds (Williams 2007), and the several later chapters in this volume explore core aspects of the idea in a variety of ways (e.g. Chapters 6, 12, and 13).

Beyond its initial formulation, the concept of therapeutic landscapes have been widely used as an analytical tool through which to explore relationships between people, land, and well-being across time and space. Clare Hickman (2005; 2013) for example uses it for her historical analysis of hospital gardens in England during the nineteenth and early twentieth centuries. Clare Madge (1998) applies it to an examination of indigenous human and ethnoveterinary medical beliefs and practices of the Jola, The Gambia, documenting and focusing in particular on the role of herbal medicine to discusses interactions between indigenous medicine and biomedicine. While Kathleen Wilson (2003) looks at the relationships between land, place, culture, and well-being amongst First Nation communities in Ontario, Canada. The list of examples is long but, more recently, several books have focused particularly on therapeutic landscapes in relation to mental health, notably Ezra Griffith's volume *Belonging, therapeutic landscapes, and networks: Implications for mental health practice* (2018) in which he explores environmental, individual, societal, and attachment factors that come together in the healing process in both traditional and non-traditional landscapes.

Recognizing, documenting, and trying to understand established therapeutic landscapes is part of the picture, and mainly passive in its intent. Set against it is the more active dimension of creating therapeutic landscapes and embedding the idea of well-being in the design and construction of places and spaces along the lines that were discussed by Tessa Jowell in her paper *Better places to live* (2005) touched on above. Although they were not the first in the field, Robin Kearns and Wil Gesler brought much-needed theory and structure to such thinking in their book *Putting health into place: Landscape, identity, and well-being* published in 1998. Drawing heavily on post-structuralist thinking, they recognized the agency embedded in both the physical qualities of certain places and the emotional charge that results from being immersed in such worlds and decoding, both consciously and sub-consciously, the culturally specific meanings and attributes all around (Kearns and Gesler 1998: 8–9). Place-making and place-production has become a significant element in designing urban and rural environments (Andrews 2004; Conradson 2005; Harmanşahe 2015; Morse Dunkley 2009; Rose 2012; Schneekloth and Shibley 1995) and in bridging cultures (Nasser 2015). Cultural heritage can play a key part in this (Darvill 2014; 2015; Schifferes 2015), enhancing well-being and in some cases providing therapeutic experiences. Landscape architect Martha Tyson looks at how to plan, design, construct and evaluate gardens that best serve healing needs and can also ease the work of care-givers (Tyson 1998). Similarly, Clare Cooper Marcus and Naomi Sachs developed an evidence-based approach to designing and building healing gardens and restorative outdoor spaces for different kinds of therapeutic needs, for example cancer patients, frail elderly people, those with Alzheimer's and dementia, and those with mental and behavioural health issues (Marcus and Sachs 2014).

How exactly therapeutic landscapes work, how they actually make a difference to people's well-being, is an area of neuroscience that is still in its infancy. One promising field of inquiry is that of brain plasticity, also known as neuroplasticity, which refers to the brain's ability to grow, change, and adapt as a result of physical, mental, and emotional experiences throughout a person's life (Costandi 2016; Wexler 2011). In Britain, studies undertaken for the National Trust and reported in *Places that makes us* (NT 2017) point the way forward, and provide some interesting preliminary results. The research was carried out by the Department of Psychology in the University of Surrey and market research group Walnut Unlimited, and was based on a sample of 2000 participants. Interviews showed that visits to meaningful places evoked feelings of calm, joy and contentment, energy, discovery, identity, and belonging (NT 2017: 23–25). Focusing on mental well-being when visiting their meaningful place, 53 per cent of those interviewed said it was my escape from everyday life, 41 per cent said it gave time to be myself, 39 per cent said they felt rejuvenated, 35 per cent said it refocused my mind, 34 per cent said it gave them perspective, and 33 per cent said it gave them headspace (NT 2017: fig. 4). A smaller sample of 20 individuals were examined in greater detail, and were subject to functional magnetic resonance imaging (FMRI) of their brains to explore how they felt and behaved when faced with favourite places. The pilot study concluded that engagement with meaningful places generated a significant response in areas of the brain most commonly associated with positive emotions, clearly demonstrating a strong emotional connection between people and places (NT 2017: 5).

Cultural heritage therapy

Using aspects of cultural heritage to enhance well-being is not new, although full recognition of its power and potential, and its use to target mental health well-being, is recent and timely. For decades public participation in excavations, surveys, and just exploring sites and monuments in the landscape has been a mainstay of local societies and community groups across Britain. A survey by the Council for British Archaeology in 1986 found that there were nearly 200 amenity societies with a combined membership of over 40,000 (CBA 1987). A more recent survey focusing on the activities of local history and archaeology between 2010 and 2015 suggested a headline figure of about 2,400 projects a year across all areas of interest (Hedge and Nash 2016: 10). The Archaeological Investigations Project recorded about 600 specifically archaeological projects undertaken by amenity societies and local groups in England between 1990 and 2010 (Darvill *et al.* 2019: 134 and tab. 6.1).

Two main reasons lie behind these developments. One is the supportive and facilitative nature of ancient monuments legislation in England, Wales, and Scotland. Access to sites and monuments is relatively easy, work at those sites not protected as Scheduled Monuments is unconstrained by licensing (although does require permission from the landowner), and the British landscape is bristling with upstanding and hidden remains. As a result it is very easy for individuals and groups to get involved in viewing or exploring aspects of the historic environment in a way that is simply not possible in most other countries of the world. A second reason is undoubtedly the influence of strategic guidance and policy frameworks at international, national, regional, and local level that, as reviewed above, embed the need to address issues of well-being and create public value out of what we do. The rapid growth of Community Archaeology in recent years, much of it supported through Heritage Lottery Fund awards, underlines the attractiveness of such activities to wide sections of the population (Applejuice Consultants 2008; BOP 2009; 2010; 2011; Ellis 2015; HLF 2011; 2012). Moreover, heritage-based initiatives have the ability to reach marginalized communities and those with traditionally low participation rates.

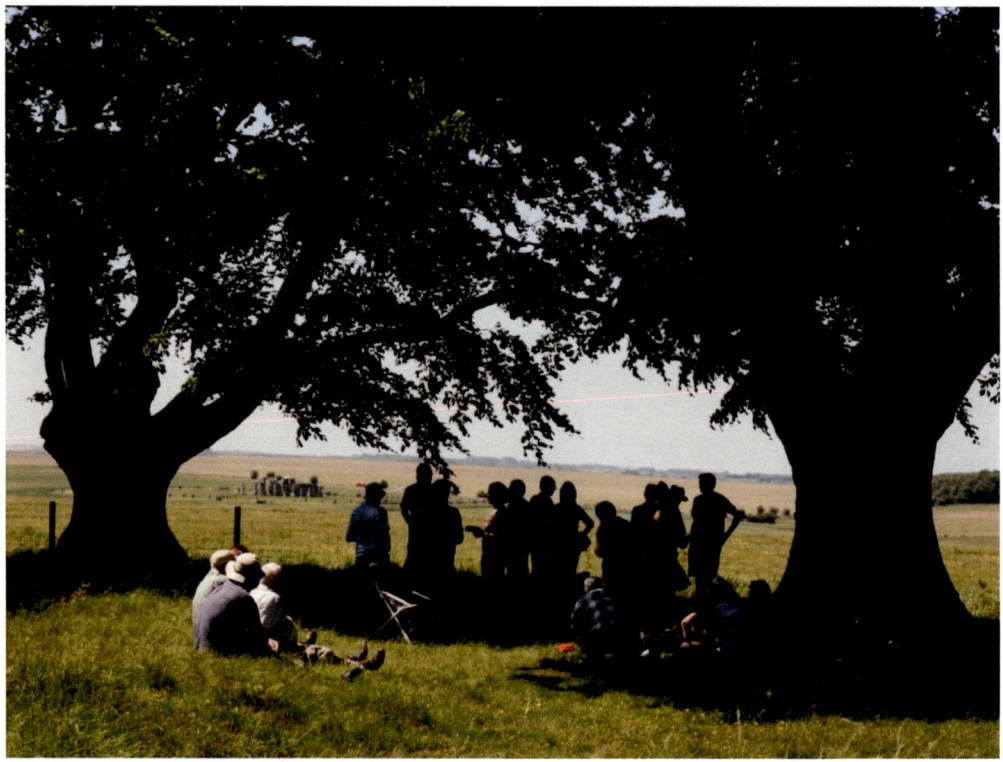

Figure 1.4. Being in the landscape: Participants and facilitators of the Human Henge project on King Barrow Ridge overlooking Stonehenge Wiltshire. (Photograph by Timothy Darvill, Human Henge project. Copyright reserved)

A wide range of creative archaeological and heritage projects include therapeutic activities amongst their aims and objectives; a summary account published in 2018 listed more than twenty cases (Darvill *et al.* 2018: 115–119) and there are more in this volume. Some build out from what are described above as therapeutic landscapes by linking directly to parks and gardens (Hartig and Marcus 2006; Thrive 2006), woods and forests (NHS 2016b), coastlines (Bell *et al.* 2015a), good views (Ulrich 1984; Ulrich *et al.* 1991), or simply being outside (Bell *et al.* 2015b; Cleary *et al.* 2017; Doughty 2013; Edensor 2000; Kaplan 1995). A variation on this is illustrated by Human Henge (Chapters 5 to 11) where specific selected sites provide arenas for structured immersive experiences, some creative and some performative (Figure 1.4).

Surveys and non-interventional projects are common, including work along the Thames foreshore (Chapter 14), a graveyard in Folkestone town centre (Chapter 17), St Wulstan's local nature reserve at Malvern (Chapter 18), and the war memorials of Ceredigion (Chapter 19). Others involve direct interventions through excavation, conservation work and restoration, as at Harmony Woods near Andover (Chapter 15), Roman baths near Glasgow (Chapter 16), and the battlefield at Waterloo in Belgium (Chapter 20). Mention may also be made here of the Past in Mind project that brought together a group of volunteers to investigate the history and archaeology of Studmarsh, a rural area in Herefordshire (Lack 2014), and also the Breaking Ground Heritage project set up in 2015 and now working in partnership with Operation Nightingale (Wessex Archaeology 2019) to provide opportunities for injured veterans from the armed forces to engage with heritage-based projects that promote physical and psychological well-being (Bennett 2018; and see also Finnegan 2016). Whether digging makes you happy or not is a more moot point, and one explored recently by Faye Sayer (2015). But not all projects are based out-doors, museums and museum collections taken to other venues are also important (Ander *et al.* 2011; 2013; Camic and Chatterjee 2013; Chatterjee and Noble 2009; Cutler *et al.* 2016; Solway *et al.* 2015; Thomson and Chatterjee 2015; Thomson *et al.* 2012) as the work at the Petrie Museum in London and other venues across the country very well illustrates (Chapter 21).

The variety of endeavours to connect heritage with well-being indicates the strength of the movement and the wealth of experimentation now underway. Improving mental health well-being is not just a matter of belief, and what is emerging are interdisciplinary initiatives that can have positive impacts on health by combining contributions from suitably aware archaeologists and heritage practitioners, experts from the health-care sector, and communities themselves. Legislation, strategic guidance, and public policy provide the framework, organizations, groups and individuals provide the impetus. While some of what is being done does genuinely contribute to the creation of new knowledge about the past (narrative knowledge), the aims of many programmes are not archaeological but social; they generate other equally valid but different kinds of knowledge, for example connective knowledge grounded in emotion and experience (Darvill 2015). It is an exciting time to be involved in this field of endeavour as the contributions to this volume so eloquently illustrate.

Overview of the book

The 20 chapters forming the core of this book unfold and expand upon the core themes discussed above in various ways and in a wide range of voices. They offer many different perspectives and provide a spectrum of case studies some of which are very practical in outlook while others dip into a variety of post-processualist theory. Sidelights are thrown on what has been achieved, and where this work might take us next, in the Foreword by Sara Lunt and the Afterword by Alex Coulter that bookend the volume.

Although not formally divided into sections, the book falls into three parts or movements. First, Chapters 2 to 4 set the scene by providing context and background. In Chapter 2 Liz Ellis and Alice Kershaw explain something of the background to National Lottery Heritage Fund support for work in this field and some of the projects supported. They look forward to the development of new initiatives through simplified application processes and greater emphasis on public value. Chapter 3 takes a different track as Toby Sutcliffe provides an overview of mental health-care arrangements in England today, and reflects back on how we got to where we are now with a brief history of mental health intervention. Chapter 4 builds on that experience with a contribution from William Rathouse that focuses on how people with mental health problems can engage effectively with archaeological and heritage projects, and how, in turn, those projects can adjust their operations to be more inclusive.

The second movement, Chapters 5 to 11, unfolds the work of the Human Henge project from a range of quite different contrasting perspectives, supported by words from participants and a handful of beautifully crafted original illustrations by Donna Songhurst who was a participant in the Avebury iteration of Human Henge. Her work can also be seen on the front cover and as our frontispiece. In Chapter 5 Laura Drysdale sets the scene from the viewpoint of the Restoration Trust as an organization that provides culture therapy of various kinds for those with mental health issues. She explains how Human Henge got off the ground and its wider aims and objectives, and ends with a plea to expand such opportunities as a standard part of health-care prescribing. In Chapter 6 Timothy Darvill takes a closer look at the two ideas upon which the Human Henge project was built: the recognition that healing ceremonies were key reasons for the construction and use of many sites across Britain during the Neolithic and early Bronze Age (4000 to 2000 BC); and developments in the field of archaeological resource management that encourage appropriate innovative and sustainable uses of ancient sites and landscapes to fulfil societal needs today. Yvette Staelens, the co-ordinator and main facilitator of Human Henge, follows this up in Chapter 7 with an overview of the way the project developed and how it unfolded in the Stonehenge landscape and then around Avebury. Illuminated with words from participants, this chapter is supported by two sound files available to listen to on the website associated with this publication. What comes across is the way participants and facilitators alike made new connections: with the land, with sites, with each other, and with themselves. It is a theme taken further but from a different angle in Chapter 8 where Daniel O'Donoghue describes his experiences on Human Henge as a mental health and social inclusion practitioner, along the way drawing on his own thoughts and memories, and also those of the participants. The emphasis is on practical considerations and what can be learnt from the project. Chapter 9 looks in from another quite different direction as Vanessa Heaslip considers the impact of the Human Henge programme on the mental health and well-being of the participants as she measured and assessed it before, during, and after the sessions. Both qualitative and quantitative measures reveal how the creative exploration of these ancient landscapes provide an uplift in overall mental health well-being. In Chapter 10, Martin Allfrey of English Heritage considers earlier ways in which heritage properties in State care have been used to promote mental health and well-being initiatives over the past century or so, and looks forward to how the success of Human Henge at Stonehenge can be used to encourage similar programmes at other sites in the portfolio of English Heritage properties. Briony Clifton of the National Trust builds the picture further in Chapter 11, with a consideration of how a balance can be struck between using internationally important landscapes such as that around Avebury for a range of different interests at the same time. Clear analogies between the work of Human Henge and the wider remit of the National Trust are identified, especially in relation to access, inclusion, and understanding the spirit of place.

In the third movement, Chapters 12 to 21, attention shifts towards the wider domain of innovative heritage related mental-health and well-being projects across Britain and beyond. Together they illustrate the breadth, depth, and original nature of what is currently in train. The journey starts in Chapter 12 with Rebecca Hearne's analysis of why and how archaeological sites and ancient landscapes can be made to work in the context of mental health recovery. Building on Michael Shank's idea of the 'Archaeological Imagination' she explores how encountering the 'magic of the past' can catalyse emotional and intellectual processes. Her plea to win recognition of such work as a new direction for traditional practices echoes calls in other chapters and underlines the sense of urgency in making archaeological evidence relevant to communities in the twenty-first century. Chapter 13 helps build the case as Claire Nolan introduces the idea of 'transitional space' as a framework though which to develop imaginative engagements with the historic environment that she illustrates with a case study drawing on qualitative research amongst visitors to Stonehenge, Avebury, and the

Vale of Pewsey in Wiltshire. Volunteering as a means of engagement is explored in Chapter 14 where Helen Johnston takes us to the Thames foreshore in London to ask the question 'is volunteering in archaeology good for you?' and show how volunteer management practices create new ways of working with communities. A similar theme is explored in a terrestrial landscape in Chapter 15 where Christopher Elmer describes how concepts such as 'gifts' 'sense of place' and 'spirit of place' can be used within the framework of agency theory to create networks linking people, places, and things that can bring disparate communities together around better understandings and appreciation of the natural and historic environment. His case study at Harmony Woods near Andover in Hampshire illustrates the problems as well as the achievements of such an approach. Paul Murtagh's account in Chapter 16 of the Recovery Through Heritage project deals with rather different communities, those with drug and alcohol problems, who were brought together to create a heritage trail and restore a Roman bath-house in North Lanarkshire, Scotland. Like Elmer, he draws on assemblage theory to understand how the heritage trail that was built emerged from a series of relationships between people, places, objects, and landscapes. At the other end of the county Chapter 17 introduces the work of Lesley Hardy and Eleanor Williams in the sea-side town of Folkstone on the south coast of England where a community-based survey of graveyard at the Church of St Mary and St Eanswythe worked because the project immersed itself in the local community rather than imposing on it. And in Wales, Chapter 19 outlines work by William Rathouse for Mind Aberystwyth that systematically recoded war memorials in Ceredigion both as a means of providing a record of these vulnerable elements of the historic environment and as a means of enhancing self-confidence, promoting well-being, and assisting recovery amongst participants that were drawn from mental health service users.

In Chapter 20, Mark Evans and colleagues takes us across the English Channel to the site of Waterloo in Belgium where a collaborative team of professional archaeologists and volunteers work with serving military personnel and veterans to assist them in their recovery from mental and physical injuries and the transition to civilian life. The work has enhanced understandings of how the Battle of Waterloo unfolded on the 18 June 1815, and provides a new approach to the way support is provided to the armed forces. Finally, in Chapter 21, Zena Kamash introduces two museum-based public engagement projects that connected with people of Middle Eastern and North African background living in Britain. Remembering the Romans in the Middle East and North Africa involved the use of objects from museum collections to stimulate create activities such as drawing, writing, and photography, while Rematerialising Mosul Museum recreated objects that had once been in Mosul Museum or monuments in the city through making wet-felted panels.

Acknowledgements

In addition to all the contributors to this volume we would also like to thank the audiences at both the Cardiff and Bournemouth meetings for their illuminating contributions to the discussion of matters considered here, and the open way in which they shared their experiences. Likewise, all the participants in the Human Henge project as well as the helpers, volunteers, and members of the project steering committee that contributed their thoughts so freely. Donna Songhurst kindly allowed us to reproduce some of the pencil drawings she made during the Human Henge project at Avebury. We would particularly like to thank David Davison and colleagues at Archaeopress for their patience and guidance in producing this volume.

Bibliography

Aked, J. and S. Thompson 2011. *Five ways to well-being. New approaches, new ways of thinking* [Online document]. London: New Economic Foundation. Viewed 23 May 2019, < https://neweconomics.org/uploads/files/d80eba95560c09605d_uzm6b1n6a.pdf>.

Alves, S. 2018. Understanding intangible aspects of cultural heritage: The role of active imagination. *The Historic Environment: Policy and Practice* 9(3–4): 207–228.

Ander, E., L. Thomson, G. Noble, A. Lanceley, U. Menon and H. Chatterjee 2011. Generic well-being outcomes: Towards a conceptual framework for well-being outcomes in museums. *Museum Management and Curatorship* 26(3): 237–259.

Ander. E., L. Thomson, G. Noble, A. Lanceley, U. Menon and H. Chatterjee 2013. Heritage, health and well-being: Assessing the impact of a heritage focused intervention on health and well-being. *International Journal of Heritage Studies* 19(3): 229–242.

Andrews, G. 2004. (Re)thinking the dynamics between healthcare and place: Therapeutic geographies in treatment and care practices. *Area* 36(3): 307–318.

APPGAHW 2017. *Creative health: The arts for health and wellbeing* (Second edition) [Online document]. London: APPGAHW. Viewed 29 May 2019, < https://www.culturehealthandwellbeing.org.uk/appg-inquiry/Publications/Creative_Health_Inquiry_Report_2017_-_Second_Edition.pdf>.

Applejuice Consultants 2008. *Social impact of Heritage Lottery Funded projects. Evaluation report on research conducted for Heritage Lottery Fund during 2006-2007* [Online document]. London: Heritage Lottery Fund. Viewed 16 December 2016, <https://www.hlf.org.uk/file/13050/download?token= XG2vjlut_NYfe2VzPcSKf3X-dv195-5vt2WEQzFUoMw>.

Bell, S., C. Phoenix, R. Lovell and B. Wheeler 2015a. Seeking everyday wellbeing: The coast as a therapeutic landscape. *Social Science and Medicine* 142: 56–67.

Bell, S., C. Phoenix, R. Lovell and B. Wheeler 2015b. Using GPS and geo-narratives: A methodological approach for understanding and situating everyday green space encounters. *Area* 47: 88–96.

Bennett, R. 2018. Saving lives: Breaking Ground Heritage. *British Archaeology* 161 (July-August 2018): 50–55.

BOP Consulting 2009. *Assessment of the social impact of volunteering in HLF-funded projects: Final report June 2009* [Online document]. London: Heritage Lottery Fund. Viewed 16 December 2016, <https://www.hlf.org.uk/file/11534/ download?token=0lTSl2-qW4_RTA2mu9TuRyFDBQmZH cF4Udx24axC4g>.

BOP Consulting 2010. *Assessment of the social impact of volunteering in HLF-funded projects: Year 2* [Online document]. London: Heritage Lottery Fund. Viewed 16 December 2016, <https://www.hlf.org.uk/file/11533/download? token=3lI97GMGCOGkylj7MNoPlx7heDzi wo2T5FgC038GwSk>.

BOP Consulting 2011. *Assessment of the social impact of volunteering in HLF-funded projects: Year 3* [Online document]. London: Heritage Lottery Fund. Viewed 16 December 2016, <https://www.hlf.org.uk/ file/11531/download?token= DUL4N7q04g7BrSPuqTVuVSRru3fVhhQOuGboWs9VHA4>.

Camic, P. and H. Chatterjee 2013. Museums and art galleries as partners for public health interventions. *Perspectives in Public Health* 133(66): 66–71.

CBA 1987. Archaeological societies in the UK. *British Archaeological News* 2(3): 29–30.

Chatterjee, H. and G. Noble 2009. Object therapy: A student-selected component exploring the potential of museum object handling as an enrichment activity for patients in hospital. *Global Journal of Health Science* 1(2): 42–49.

CHEurope 2019. Work Package 4: Heritage and wellbeing. [Project website]. Viewed 21 May 2019, <https://ich.unesco.org/en/convention>.

CHWA 2018. About the alliance [Webpage]. Viewed 29 May 2019, < https://www.culturehealthandwellbeing.org.uk/who-we-are/about-alliance>.

Cleary, A., K. Fielding, S. Bell, Z. Murray and A. Roiko 2017. Exploring potential mechanisms involved in the relationship between eudaimonic wellbeing and nature connection. *Landscape and Urban Planning* 158: 119–128.

COE 2005. *Council of Europe Framework convention on the value of cultural heritage for society* (Council of Europe Treaty Series – No. 199) [Online document]. Strasbourg: Council of Europe. Viewed 12 December 2016, <http://www.coe.int/en/web/ conventions/full-list/-/conventions/ rms/0900001680083746>.

COE 2015a. *Strategy 21: European cultural heritage strategy for the 21st century* [Online document]. Strasbourg: Council of Europe. Viewed 25 November 2016, <http://www.coe.int/en/web/culture-and-heritage/strategy-21>.

COE 2015b. *The Namur Declaration* [Online document]. Strasbourg: Council of Europe. Viewed 12 December 2016, <https://rm.coe.int/CoERMPublicCommonSearchServices/DisplayDCTMContent?documentId=09000016806a89ae>.

COE 2016. *Faro Action Plan* [Online document]. Strasbourg: Council of Europe. Viewed 12 December 2016, <http://www.coe.int/en/web/culture-and-heritage/faro-action-plan>.

Conradson, D. 2005. Landscape, care and the relational self: Therapeutic encounters in rural England. *Health and Place* 11: 337–348.

Cooney, G. (ed.) 2003. *Seascapes* (World Archaeology 35 (3)). London: Routledge.

Cosgrove, D. and S. Daniels (eds.) 1988. *The iconography of landscape*. Cambridge: Cambridge University Press.

Costandi, M. 2016. *Neuroplasticity*. Cambridge (MA): Massachusetts Institute of Technology Press.

Cutler, C., P. Palma and A. Innes 2016. Tales of the sea: Connecting people with dementia to the UK heritage through maritime archaeology. *Dementia: The International Journal of Social Research and Practice* [Online document]. Viewed 15 November 2016, <http://dem.sagepub.com/content/early/2016/09/20/1471301216666171.full.pdf+html>.

Darvill, T. 2001. Traditions of landscape archaeology in British: Issues of time and scale, in T. Darvill and M. Gojda (eds.) *One land, many landscapes. Papers from a session held at the European Association of Archaeologists Fifth Annual Meeting in Bournemouth 1999* (BAR International Series 987): 33–46. Oxford: Archaeopress.

Darvill, T. 2014. Rock and soul: Humanizing heritage, memorializing music and producing places. *World Archaeology* 46(3): 462–476.

Darvill, T. 2015. Making futures from the remains of the distant past. Archaeological heritage, connective knowledge, and the promotion of well-being, in M. van den Dries, S. van der Linde and A. Strecker (eds.) *Fernweh: Crossing borders and connecting people in archaeological heritage management. Essays in honour of Prof. Willem J.H. Willems*: 42–46. Leiden: Sidestone Press.

Darvill, T., K. Barrass, V. Constant, E. Milner and B. Russell 2019. *Archaeology in the PPG16 Era. Investigations in England 1990-2010*. Oxford: Oxbow Books.

Darvill, T., V. Heaslip and K. Barrass 2018. Heritage and well-being: Therapeutic places, past and present, in K.T. Galvin (ed.) *Routledge handbook of well-being*: 112–123. Abingdon: Routledge.

David, B. and J. Thomas (eds.) 2008. *Handbook of landscape archaeology*. Walnut Creek (CA): Left Coast Books.

DCLG 2012. *National planning policy framework* [Online document]. London: Department for Communities and Local Government. Viewed 15 December 2016, <https://www.gov.uk/government/uploads/system/uploads/attachment_data/file/6077/ 2116950.pdf>.

DCMS 2001. *The historic environment: A force for the future*. London: Department for Culture, Media and Sport.

DCMS 2014. *Culture, sport and wellbeing: An analysis of the Taking Part Survey* [Online document]. London: Department for Culture, Media and Sport. Viewed 15 December 2016, <https://www.gov.uk/government/uploads/system/uploads/attachment_data/file/476322/Culture_Sport_and_Wellbeing_-_An_analysis_of_the_Taking_Part_Survey.pdf>.

DCMS 2016a. *Taking Part Survey* [Online document]. London: Department for Culture, Media and Sport. Viewed 25 January 2017, <https://www.gov.uk/guidance/ taking-part-survey>.

DCMS 2016b. *The Culture White Paper* [Online document]. London: Department for Culture, Media and Sport. Viewed 25 November 2016, <https://assets.publishing.service.gov.uk/government/uploads/system/uploads/attachment_data/file/510798/DCMS_The_Culture_White_Paper__3_.pdf >.

DOH 2010a. *Healthy lives, healthy people* [Online document]. London: Department of Health. Viewed 14 December 2016, <https://www.gov.uk/government/uploads/system/uploads/attachment _data/file/216096/dh_127424.pdf>.

DOH 2010b. *Our health and wellbeing today* [Online document]. London: Department of Health. Viewed 12 December 2016, <https://www.gov.uk/government/uploads/ system/uploads/attachment_data/file/215911/dh_122238.pdf>.

DOH 2011. *No health without mental health* [Online document]. London: Department of Health. Viewed 14 December 2016, <https://www.gov.uk/government/uploads/system/uploads/attachment_data/file/213761/dh_124058.pdf >.

Doughty, K. 2013. Walking together: The embodied and mobile production of a therapeutic landscape. *Health and Place* 24: 140–146.

EC 2016. *Mental health policy* [Online document]. Brussels: European Commission. Viewed 25 November 2016, <http://ec.europa.eu/health/mental_health/policy/index_en.htm>.

EC and WHO 2008. *European pact for mental health and well-being* [Online document]. Brussels: European Commission. Viewed 25 November 2016, <http://ec.europa.eu/health/mental_health/docs/mhpact_en.pdf>.

Edensor, T. 2000. Walking in the British countryside: Reflexivity, embodied practices, and ways to escape. *Body and Society* 6(3–4): 81–106.

EH 2000a. *Review of policies relating to the historic environment. Discussion paper 1: Understanding*. London: English Heritage.

EH 2000b. *The power of place. The future of the historic environment*. London: English Heritage.

Ellis, L. 2015. *Heritage and positive mental health* [Online document]. London: Heritage Lottery Fund. Viewed 16 December 2016, <https://www.hlf.org.uk/about-us/news-features/heritage-and-positive-mental-health>.

EU 2008. *Consolidated versions of the Treaty on European Union and the Treaty on the functioning of the European Union* [Online document]. Brussels: Council of the European Union. Viewed 12 December 2016, <http://register.consilium.europa.eu/doc/ srv?l=EN&f=ST%206655%20 2008%20INIT>.

Finnegan, A. 2016. The biopsychosocial benefits and shortfalls for armed forces veterans engaged in archaeological activities. *Nurse Education Today* 47: 15–22.

Fujiwara, D., L. Kudrna and P. Dolan 2014b. *Quantifying and valuing the wellbeing impacts of culture and sport* [Online document]. London: Department for Culture, Media and Sport. Viewed 14 December 2016, <https://www.gov.uk/government/uploads/system/uploads/attachment_data/ file/304899/Quantifying_and_valuing_the_wellbeing_impacts_of_sport_and_culture.pdf>.

Fujiwara, D., T. Cornwall and P. Dolan 2014a. *Heritage and wellbeing* [Online document]. London: English Heritage. Viewed 16 December 2016, <https://content.historicengland.org.uk/content/heritage-counts/ pub/2190644/heritage-and-wellbeing.pdf>.

Galvin, K.T. 2018. Introduction, in K.T. Galvin (ed.), *Routledge handbook of well-being*: 1–13. Abingdon: Routledge.

Galvin, K.T. and L. Todres 2018. Dwelling-mobility: An existential theory of well-being, in K.T. Galvin (ed.), *Routledge handbook of well-being*: 84–90. Abingdon: Routledge.

Gesler, W. 1992. Therapeutic landscapes: Medical issues in light of the new cultural geography. *Social Science and Medicine* 34(7): 735–746.

Gesler, W. 1993. Therapeutic landscapes: Theory and a case study of Epidauros, Greece. *Environment and Planning D: Society and Space* 11: 171–189.

Gesler, W.M. 1996. Lourdes: Healing in a place of pilgrimage. *Health and Place* 2: 95–105.

Gesler, W.M. 1998. Bath's reputation as a healing place, in R.A. Kearns and W.M. Gesler (eds.) *Putting Health into Place*: 17–35. Syracuse: Syracuse University Press.

GLA 2015. *An A-Z of planning and culture* [Online publication]. London: Greater London Authority. Viewed 15 December 2016, <https://www.london.gov.uk/sites/default/ files/an_a-z_of_planning_and_culture.pdf>.

GOS, 2008. *Foresight Mental Capital and Wellbeing Project (2008). Final project report* [Online document]. London: Government Office for Science. Viewed 23April 2019, < https://assets.publishing.service.gov.uk/government/uploads/system/uploads/attachment_data/file/292450/mental-capital-wellbeing-report.pdf >.

Griffin, J. 1986. *Well-being. Its meaning, measurement and moral importance*. Oxford: Clarendon Press.

Griffith, E. 2018. *Belonging, therapeutic landscapes and networks. Implications for mental health practice*. Abingdon: Routledge.

Hari, J. 2018. *Lost connections. Uncovering the real causes of depression and the unexpected solutions*. London: Bloomsbury.

Harmanşahe, O. 2015. *Place, memory and healing*. Abingdon: Routledge.

Hartig, T. and C.C. Marcus 2006. Essay: Healing gardens – places for nature in healthcare. *The Lancet* 368 (Supplement 1): S36–S37.

Hedge, R. and A. Nash 2016. *Assessing the value of community-generated historic environment research*. Worcester: Worcester County Council (Historic Environment Project Report 7178).

Hickman, C. 2005. The picturesque at Brislington House, Bristol: The role of landscape in relation to the treatment of mental illness in the early nineteenth-century asylum. *Garden History* 33: 47–60.

Hickman, C. 2013. *Therapeutic landscapes. A history of English hospital gardens since 1800*. Manchester and New York: Manchester University Press.

Historic England 2016. *Heritage counts: Heritage and society 2016*. Swindon: Historic England.

Historic England 2017. *Heritage counts: Heritage and society 2017*. Swindon: Historic England.

Historic England 2018. *Heritage counts: Heritage and society 2018* [Online document]. Swindon: Historic England. Viewed 23 May 2019, < https://historicengland.org.uk/content/heritage-counts/pub/2018/heritage-and-society-2018-pdf/>.

HLF 2011. *The social benefits of involvement in heritage projects* [Online document]. London: Heritage Lottery Fund. Viewed 16 December 2016, <https://www.hlf.org.uk/social-benefits-involvement-heritage-projects>.

HLF 2012. *A lasting difference for heritage and people: Heritage Lottery Fund strategic framework 2013-2018* [Online document]. London: Heritage Lottery Fund. Viewed 16 December 2016, https://www.hlf.org.uk/file/10986/download?token=BJttfffDJPhI_k9dFFHvadQWaERndkeS0xnfoHjj7B0>.

Jowell, T. 2005. *Better places to live. Government, identity, and the value of the historic and built environment.* London: Department for Culture, Media and Sport.

Kaplan, S. 1995. The restorative benefits of nature: Toward an integrative framework. *Journal of Environmental Psychology* 15(3): 169–182.

Kearns, R.A. and W.M. Gesler 1998. Introduction, in R.A. Kearns and W.M. Gesler (eds.), *Putting health into place. Landsape, identity, and well-being*: 1–17. New York: Syracus University Press.

Lack, K. 2014. *Past in mind. A heritage project and mental health recovery.* Leominster: Privately published.

Layard, R. 2016. *Measuring wellbeing and cost-effectiveness analysis using subjective wellbeing* [Online document]. London: What Works Centre for Wellbeing. Viewed 14 December 2016, <https//whatworkswellbeing.files.wordpress.com/2016/08/common-currency-measuring-wellbeing-series-1-dec-2016.pdf>.

Madge, C. 1998. Therapeutic landscapes on the Jola, The Gambia, West Africa. *Health and Place* 4(4): 293–311.

Marcus, C.C. and N.A. Sachs 2014. *Therapeutic landscapes. An evidence-based approach to designing healing gardens and restorative outdoor spaces.* New Jersey: Wiley.

McManus S., P. Bebbington, R. Jenkins and T. Brugha (eds.) 2016. *Mental health and wellbeing in England: Adult psychiatric morbidity survey 2014* [Online document]. Leeds: NHS digital. Viewed 23 May 2019, < https://digital.nhs.uk/data-and-information/publications/statistical/adult-psychiatric-morbidity-survey/adult-psychiatric-morbidity-survey-survey-of-mental-health-and-wellbeing-england-2014>.

Meier, T. (ed.), 2006. *Landscape ideologies.* Budapest: Archaeolingua.

MHCLG 2019. *National planning policy framework* (Revised) [Online document]. London: Ministry of Housing, Communities, and Local Government . Viewed 23 May 2019, < https://assets.publishing.service.gov.uk/government/uploads/system/uploads/attachment_data/file/779771/NPPF_Feb_2019_print.pdf>.

Monckton, L. and S. Reilly 2019. Wellbeing and historic environment: Why bother? *Historic England Research* 11: 8–17. [Online publication]. Viewed 12 April 2019, <https://historicengland.org.uk/images-books/publications/historic-england-research-11/he-research-11/>.

Morse Dunkley, C. 2009. A therapeutic taskscape: Theorizing place-making, discipline and care at a camp for troubled youth. *Health and Place* 15: 88–96.

Nasser, N. 2015. *Bridging cultures. The guide to social innovation in cosmopolitan cities.* Markham (ON): 10-10-10 Publishing.

Natural England 2009. *Experiencing landscapes: Capturing the cultural services and experiential qualities of landscape* [Online document]. Cheltenham: Natural England. Viewed 16 December 2016, <http://publications.naturalengland.org.uk/file/70035>.

NHS 2016a. *The five year forward view for mental health*. [Online document]. Viewed 12 November 2018, <https://www.england.nhs.uk/wp-content/uploads/2016/02/Mental-Health-Taskforce-FYFV-final.pdf> .

NHS 2016b. NHS Choices: Five steps to mental wellbeing [Webpage]. Viewed 15 December 2016, http://www.nhs.uk/Conditions/stress-anxiety-depression/Pages/improve-mental-wellbeing.aspx.

NHS 2016c. NHS forest: Growing forests for health [Webpage]. Viewed 15 December 2016, <http://nhsforest.org/>.

NIE 2016. Givan launches funding scheme to help realise the value of our Heritage [Webpage]. Viewed 19 December 2016, <https://www.northernireland.gov.uk/news/givan-launches-funding-scheme-help-realise-value-our-heritage>.

NIEA 2016. Northern Ireland Environment Agency [Webpage]. Viewed 19 December 2016, <https://www.daera-ni.gov.uk/northern-ireland-environment-agency>.

NIEDOH 2016a. Mental health and learning disabilities [Webpage]. Viewed 15 December 2016, <https://www.health-ni.gov.uk/topics/mental-health-and-learning-disabilities>.

NIEDOH 2016b. *Health and wellbeing 2026* [Online document]. Belfast: Northern Ireland Executive. Viewed 15 December 2016, <https://www.health-ni.gov.uk/ sites/default/files/ publications/health/health-and-wellbeing-2026-delivering-together.pdf >.

NLHF 2019. *Wellbeing guidance* [Online document]. London: NLHF. Viewed 29 May 2019, < https://www.heritagefund.org.uk/sites/default/files/media/attachments/Wellbeing%20guidance.pdf>.

NT 2017. *Places that make us. Research Report* [Online document]. Swindon: National Trust. Viewed 21 May 2019, <https://nt.global.ssl.fastly.net/documents/places-that-make-us-research-report.pdf>

OECD and EU 2018. *Health at a Glance: Europe 2018: State of Health in the EU Cycle* [Online document]. Paris: OECD Publishing Paris. Viewed 29 May 2019, https://doi.org/10.1787/health_glance_eur-2018-en.

ONS 2016. Well-being [Webpage]. Viewed 14 December 2016, <https://www.ons.gov.uk/peoplepopulationandcommunity/wellbeing>.

ONS 2019. Personal well-being datasets [Webpage]. Viewed on the 23 May 2019, <https://www.ons.gov.uk/peoplepopulationandcommunity/wellbeing/datasets/headlineestimatesofpersonalwellbeing>.

Parr, H. 2007. Mental health, nature work, and social inclusion. *Environment and Planning D: Society and Space* 25(3): 537–561.

Parris, M. 2018. Pouring billions into treating mental illness doesn't add up. *The Times* 26 November 2018.

Reilly, S., C. Nolan and L. Monckton 2018. *Wellbeing and the historic environment* [Online document]. London: Historic England. Viewed 21 May 2019, <https://historicengland.org.uk/images-books/publications/wellbeing-and-the-historic-environment/>.

Rose, E. 2012. Encountering place: A psychoanalytic approach for understanding how therapeutic landscapes benefit health and well-being. *Health and Place* 18(6): 1381–1387.

Rountree, K. 2006. Performing the divine: Neo-pagan pilgrimages and embodiment at sacred sites. *Body and Society* 12(4): 95–115.

Sayer, F. 2015. Can digging make you happy? Archaeological excavations, happiness and heritage. *Arts and Health* 7: 247–260.

Schifferes, P. 2015. *Heritage, identity and place: Seven themes from the heritage index* [Online publication]. London: RSA. Viewed 16 December 2016, < https://www.thersa.org/discover/publications-and-articles/reports/seven-themes-from-the-heritage-index >.

Schneekloth, L.H. and R.G. Shibley 1995. *Placemaking. The art and practice of building communities.* New York: John Wiley.

SCMH 2012. *Implementing recovery through organisational change* [Online document]. London: Sainsbury Centre for Mental Health. Viewed 23 May 2019, < http://imroc.org/wp-content/uploads/2016/09/implementing_recovery_paper.pdf>.

Scottish Government 2014. *Our place in time: the historic environment strategy for Scotland* [Online document]. Viewed 19 December 2016, <http://www.gov.scot/Resource/0044/00445046.pdf>.

Scottish Government 2016a. *Mental health in Scotland* [Online document]. Edinburgh: Scottish Government. Viewed 15 December 2016, <http://www.gov.scot/Topics/Health/Services/Mental-Health>.

Scottish Government 2016b. *Mental health in Scotland - a 10 year vision* [Online document]. Edinburgh: Scottish Government. Viewed 15 December 2016, <https://consult.scotland.gov.uk/mental-health-unit/mental-health-in-scotland-a-10-year-vision/>.

Shepherd, G., J. Boardman and M. Slade 2008. *Making recovery a reality* [Online document]. London: Salisbury Centre for Mental Health. Viewed 23 May 2019, < https://www.centreformentalhealth.org.uk/sites/default/files/2018-09/Making%20recovery%20a%20reality%20policy%20paper.pdf>.

Silva, F. 2019. *Towards skyscape archaeology.* Oxford: Oxbow Books.

Solway, R., L. Thomson, P. Camic and H. Chatterjee 2015. Museum object handling groups in older adult mental health inpatient care. *International Journal of Mental Health Promotion*, 17 (4), 201–214.

Thérond, D. 2009. Benefits and innovations of the Council of Europe Framework Convention on the Value of Cultural Heritage for Society, in Council of Europe, in Anon. (ed.) *Heritage and beyond*: 9–12. Strasbourg: Council of Europe Publishing [Online document]. Viewed 22 May 2019, <https://rm.coe.int/16806abdea>.

Thomas, F., L. Hansford, J. Ford, S. Hughes, K. Wyatt, R. McCabe and R. Byng 2019. *Poverty, pathology and pills. DeStress Project final report* [Online document]. Exeter, Plymouth and London: DeStress Project. Viewed 29 May 2019, < http://destressproject.org.uk/wp-content/uploads/2019/05/Final-report-8-May-2019-FT.pdf>.

Thomson, L. and H. Chatterjee 2015. Measuring the impact of museum activities on well-being: Developing the museum well-being measures toolkit. *Museum Management and Curatorship* 30(1): 44–62.

Thomson, L., E. Ander, U. Menon, A. Lanceley and H. Chatterjee 2012. Quantitative evidence for wellbeing benefits from a heritage-in-health intervention with hospital patients. *International Journal of Art Therapy* 17(2): 63–79.

Thrive 2016. Thrive: What is social and therapeutic horticulture? [Project website]. Viewed 22 May 2019, < https://www.thrive.org.uk/what-is-social-and-therapeutic-horticulture.aspx>.

Todres, L. and K. Galvin 2010. 'Dwelling-mobility': An existential theory of well-being. *International Journal of Qualitative Studies on Health and Well-Being* 5(3): 1–6.

Tyson, M.M., 1998. *The healing landscape. Therapeutic outdoor environments.* New York: McGraw-Hill.

Ulrich, R. 1984. View through a window may influence recovery from surgery. *Science* 224 (4647): 420–421.

Ulrich, R. R. Simons, B. Losito, E. Fiorito, M. Miles and M. Zelson 1991. Stress recovery during exposure to natural and urban environments. *Journal of Environmental Psychology* 11(3): 201–230.

UN 2016a. Sustainable development goals [Webpage]. Viewed 21 May 2019, <http://www.un.org/sustainabledevelopment/sustainable-development-goals/>.

UN 2016b. Sustainable Development Goal 3 [Webpage]. Viewed 22 May 2019, <https://sustainabledevelopment.un.org/sdg3>.

UNESCO 2003. *International convention for safeguarding of the intangible cultural heritage* [Online document]. Paris: UNESCO. Viewed 21 May 2019, <https://ich.unesco.org/en/convention>.

UNESCO 2015. UNESCO and the Sustainable Development Goals [Webpage]. Viewed 21 May 2019, <https://en.unesco.org/sdgs>.

UNESCO 2016. Sustainable Development Goals for Culture on the 2030 Agenda [Webpage]. Viewed 22 May 2019, <https://en.unesco.org/sdgs/clt>.

University of Tokyo 2015. *Mental health, well-being and disability: A new global priority. Key United Nations resolutions and documents* [Online document]. Tokyo: UN, UN University, World Bank Group and University of Tokyo. Viewed 23 May 2019, < http://pubdocs.worldbank.org/en/619761454942779225/Mental-Health-Well-being-Disability-A-New-Global-Priority.pdf>.

Welsh Government 2012. *Together for mental health* [Online document]. Cardiff: National Assembly for Wales. Viewed 15 December 2016, <http://gov.wales/docs/dhss/publications/121031tmhfinalen.pdf >.

Welsh Government 2015. *Well-being of future generations (Wales) Act 2015. The essentials* [Online document]. Cardiff: National Assembly for Wales. Viewed 19 December 2016, <http://www.cynnalcymru.com/wp-content/uploads/2016/08/Guide-to-the-WFGAct.pdf >.

Welsh Government 2016a. Mental health [Webpage]. Viewed 15 December 2016, <http://gov.wales/topics/health/nhswales/ mental-health-services/?lang=en>.

Welsh Government 2016b. *Taking Wales forward. Welsh government's well-being objectives (2016)* [Online document]. Cardiff: National Assembly for Wales. Viewed 19 December 2016, <http://avow.org/wp-content/uploads/2016/11/Taking-Wales-Forward_-The-Welsh-Governments-well-being-objectuves-2016....pdf >.

Welsh Government 2016c. *Together for mental health. Delivery plan: 2016-19* [Online document]. Cardiff: National Assembly for Wales. Viewed 15 December 2016, <http://gov.wales/docs/dhss/publications/ 161010deliveryen.pdf>.

Wessex Archaeology 2019. Operation Nightingale [Project website]. Viewed 23 May 2019, < https://www.wessexarch.co.uk/our-work/operation-nightingale#main-content>.

Wexler, B.E. 2011. Neuroplasticity, culture and society, in J. Illes and B.J. Sahakian (eds.), *Oxford handbook of neuroethics*. Oxford: Oxford University Press.

WHO 2001. *The World Health Report 2001: New understanding, new hope* [Online document]. WHO: Geneva. Viewed 23 May 2019, <https://www.who.int/whr/2001/en/whr01_en.pdf?ua=1>.

WHO 2013a. *Mental health action plan 2013-2020* [Online document]. Geneva: World Health Organization. Viewed 22 May 2019, < https://www.who.int/mental_health/publications/action_plan/en/>.

WHO 2013b. *Health 2020: A European policy framework and strategy for the 21st century* [Online document]. Copenhagen: World Health Organization Regional Office for Europe. Viewed 12 December 2016, <http://www.euro.who.int/ __data/assets/pdf_file/0011/199532/Health2020-Long.pdf?ua=>.

WHO 2013c. *The European mental health action plan 2013-2020* [Online document]. Copenhagen: World Health Organization Regional Office for Europe. Viewed 12 December 2016, <http://www.euro.who.int/__data/assets/pdf_file/0004/ 194107/63wd11e_MentalHealth-3.pdf?ua=1>.

Williams, A. (ed.) 2007. *Therapeutic landscapes.* Aldershot: Ashgate Publishing.

Wilson, K. 2003. Therapeutic landscapes and First Nations peoples: An exploration of culture, health and place. *Health and Place* 9: 83–93.

Wittchen, H.U., F. Jacobi, J. Rehm, A Gustavsson, M. Svensson, B. Jönsson, J. Olesen, C. Allqulander, J. Alonso, C. Faravelli, L. Fratiglioni, P. Jennum, R. Lieb, A. Maercker, J. van Os, M. Preisig, L. Salvador-Carulla, R. Simon, and H.C. Steinhausen 2011. The size and burden of mental disorders and other disoders of the brain in Europe 2010. *Journal of European Neuropsychopharmacology* 21(9): 655–679.

WWCW 2016a. What Works Centre for Wellbeing. About the Centre [Webpage]. Viewed 23 May 2019, <https://whatworkswellbeing.org/about/about-the-centre/>.

WWCW 2016b. What is well-being? [Webpage]. Viewed 23 May 2019, <https://whatworkswellbeing.org/about/what-is-wellbeing/>.

Chapter 2

Mental well-being and historic landscapes: The heritage context

Liz Ellis and Alice Kershaw

Abstract

National Lottery Heritage Fund staff Liz Ellis and Alice Kershaw discuss the rising interest in mental well-being within historic landscapes, looking at the outcomes of the Fund (prior to January 2019 known as Heritage Lottery Fund or HLF) support for projects, and also at ways in which the Fund aims to support mental well-being through its processes. They describe projects and partnerships which exemplify this work, delivering the Fund's aim to benefit communities and marginalized individuals, and ensuring that participation in, and access to, heritage, is widened. They explain the ways in which funding has been made more accessible by altering the Fund application process successfully piloted through a project run in Barrow-in-Furness, Cumbria. They highlight the well-being of project grantees and organizers, explaining how this must be taken into consideration as an integral part of such projects. Finally, they look to the future for Fund projects, emphasizing the desire to bring lasting positive change.

Keywords: Communities; Funding outcomes; Heritage; Inclusion; Well-being

Introduction

The Heritage Lottery Fund was established in 1994 as one of the 'good causes' benefitting from the National Lottery. Since then, HLF has distributed over £7.9 billion through grants made to organizations across the United Kingdom, and has worked with a very wide range of heritage bodies, site owners, and communities. In January 2019 HLF was renamed the National Lottery Heritage Fund.

It is core to the purpose of the National Lottery Heritage Fund (hereafter the 'Fund') that people seeking funding should self-define what heritage means with reference to the specific local and national context of their application. Over the last 25 years this has led to a wonderfully rich and broad-ranging scale and type of heritage being represented and funded. As a snapshot, funded projects include: capital investment in Gressenhall Farm, Museum of Norfolk Life (Bartlett 2014); Welsh Caribbean elders sharing within intergenerational settings the experiences of arriving in the 1950s to work in the UK (HLF 2016); learning disabled people in Glasgow leading an oral history project into the lived experiences of a long stay hospital (Ladysbridge Stories 2017); and the prize-winning major refurbishment of Victorian hothouse The Tropical Ravine in Belfast (BBC News 2018).

In order to deliver UK-wide heritage support, the Fund has national and country offices in Scotland, Wales, and Northern Ireland, together with area teams in England. Fund colleagues work closely together to inspire, lead, and resource UK heritage in order to create positive and lasting change for people and communities, both now and in the future.

The Fund uses an outcomes framework that enables grantees to achieve positive change through their projects; involving 'a wider range of people' in heritage is the one mandatory outcome for the Fund set out in the Strategic Funding Framework in 2019–24 (NLHF 2019) and has been increasingly significant for the work of the Fund over many years. As a non-departmental public body, the Fund is answerable to Department of Digital Culture Media and Sport (DDCMS), and every few years it undergoes a review. Following the DDCMS Tailored Review of HLF in 2017 (DDCMS 2017), the Fund has been focussing efforts on promoting inclusion and diversity, with the development of an inclusion strategy. Recognizing the integration of process, policy, and practice as vital to embedding the values, processes, and systems necessary in resourcing an inclusive heritage sector, the authors co-delivered a presentation on the subject to the 'Historic Landscapes and Mental Well-Being Conference' in Bournemouth in April 2018, and also co-wrote this paper by drawing on their differing roles in relation to the Fund.

National Lottery Heritage Fund, heritage and well-being

Through their daily work at the Fund, the authors recognize the natural fit that exists between heritage and well-being, including the role that the 'big landscapes' of Stonehenge or Avebury have in connecting us with each other across time and place. Exploring these landscapes, and learning more about the people who made these wonderful and extraordinary places, offers us all powerful and enjoyable opportunities.

In particular, the Fund is very conscious of the crucial role heritage has to play in connecting people with each other in their daily lives. As a UK-wide funder, the Fund believes these connections between people are vital for all of us within the broader context of a thriving, democratic society, and in promoting the mental health of individuals. Since 1994, research on heritage volunteering and participation (BOP Consulting 2012), as well as the lived experience of the tens of thousands of people enjoying heritage sites, has demonstrated the role of heritage in helping to build strong relationships and extensive networks with each other. BOP's research for the Fund on the social impact of volunteering found that levels of mental health and well-being are higher for those who volunteer in heritage projects than for the general population. It has also shown that heritage is a successful vehicle for promoting social cohesion and cultural understanding. Over £50 million of National Lottery funding has supported 858 community archaeology projects across the UK. These projects have encouraged a wider range of people to enjoy archaeology, with the added benefit of enabling a more contemporary representation of UK people and communities in the heritage sector. This benefits all of us and makes heritage more sustainable for everyone.

Within a current context involving many national, local, social, and political divisions across the UK, in addition to many international conflicts, learning more about our connections through easy access to heritage offers us all unlimited and creative opportunities to learn more about each other, both in the past and present. In addition, the Fund is aware of the current high levels of mental ill-health in the UK, the relationship between inequality and poor health, and the uneven and unequal access to heritage. Through an evidence-based approach using national data and research, the Fund aims to lead the heritage sector in enabling a wider range of people to access the heritage that belongs to us all.

Heritage projects and well-being: Three case studies

Enjoying historic landscapes and connecting with local archaeology groups, are two of the many ways in which we can experience the impact of time, learning more about the past, and experiencing a wider range of opportunities. With the right kind of welcome, and structured, flexible help, these landscapes can also enable new life experiences, increased confidence, and improved skills. This is particularly important when considering the range of barriers that exist and which can prevent access to heritage. These include structural inequalities, attitudinal barriers, and personal circumstances. We know that many people are currently unable to access UK cultural assets and the cultural rights to which all citizens are entitled within a functioning democratic society. Access to historic landscapes — and heritage more broadly — is not a luxury or a 'nice to have', but a right as articulated in Article 27 of the UN *Universal Declaration of Human Rights 1948*. The heritage sector can lead in delivering this in order that everyone can flourish and that society can truly reflect everyone's experience. The following case studies demonstrate how new ways of exploring heritage enable learning and provide access to cultural rights for everyone involved

Digability

First, the Workers' Education Association (WEA) in Yorkshire and Humber led a three year inclusive archaeology project, 'Digability', that aimed to widen participation in archaeology for those often blocked from equal access.

By listening to what people with learning disabilities said about their preferred learning styles, and making reasonable adjustments to planned activities, the project provides an excellent model of co-production. These reasonable adjustments included using sensory materials as opposed to providing lengthy texts or small labels. In providing engagement opportunities for people from minority ethnic communities whose first language was not English, WEA tutors worked collaboratively with English for speakers of other languages (ESOL) tutors and community networks, thus attracting a wider range of people to engage with community archaeology.

WEA tutors learned about how to make adjustments in teaching, including integrating mixed learning styles into standard teaching plans, providing object handling sessions, and practical site surveys. Key archaeology skills, including mapping and finds processing, were then shared in group activities and presentations that were led by a wider range of people. These participants included people of many ages and those from minority ethnic communities who had been previously unaware of the local history and wider archaeological context of the Yorkshire area.

Involving more than 300 people over the course of three-year project, partnerships were formed between many individuals and groups, including the participants, care and community organizations, voluntary groups, heritage groups, community archaeologists, and WEA staff and tutors. All of these contributed to a rich process of shared learning. Specialist expertise took many forms within this context; there was wider sharing of practical skills and knowledge, including the lived experience of disability or discrimination. Using these experiences to learn more about each other, as well as about historic landscapes and archaeology, enriched and connected everyone involved. As an example, WEA staff gained wider experience of how many disabled people prefer to learn through the everyday relationships of working together. The evaluation of this project found that the majority of participants gained knowledge and confidence in accessing historical sites and heritage organizations that had previously been experienced as exclusionary or unwelcoming. These shared opportunities influenced everyone's experience, leading to positive relationships and improved interest in taking part in heritage by a wider range of people.

Yorkshire history was learnt from archaeologists and other colleagues, who framed these narratives within enjoyable and flexible learning methods, including creative outdoor activities. This resulted in high quality project outcomes for heritage, people, and communities. Unexpected positive outcomes included improved disability awareness for many academic staff involved, and opportunities for challenges to unconscious bias and stigma for many involved in the project, regardless of their role. These were informal, enjoyable opportunities for shared learning about the capabilities we all possess, and such activities strengthen civic life for us all. By becoming more representative of local communities, the involvement of a wider range of people also strengthens and supports the heritage sector in becoming more sustainable in the future. Heritage participation can bring people together in new ways, contributing to stronger social connections between groups of people who might not meet in other contexts. This is achieved whilst contributing to a wider appreciation of what is around us all in our daily lives, framed by history, and enabling us to move ahead with new skills and increased confidence too.

The Croome Landscape

A very different example of how equal access to historic landscapes benefits us all comes from Croome, Worcestershire, the surroundings of Croome Court country house. The landscape was designed by Capability Brown, and the property is now owned by the National Trust. As part of activities to celebrate the 300th anniversary of Brown's birth in 2016 the National Trust undertook major landscape improvements, partly funded by HLF (HLF 2017). This work included investment in widening access for people who had traditionally not visited Croome.

Garden and Outdoors Manager Katharine Alker and Creative Partnerships Manager for South Worcestershire Rachel Sharpe, were keen to listen to the experiences of profoundly disabled children and young people, who had previously never been actively encouraged to visit the site. They did this by initiating contact with neighbouring special schools, and sharing the desire to welcome a wider range of people with local families including profoundly disabled children. They sought the experience of these schools and families on how they could improve Croome together and to identify favourite areas. In particular, Katherine and Rachel invited the children and young people to explore what gave them pleasure. These explorations 'mapping joy' at Croome were then used to fundamentally inform the development of a sensory trail. This trail was subsequently designed using co-production methods with the young disabled people, many of whom do not use language. By highlighting the sensory pleasures of making sounds that echo under a bridge, the feeling of grass under the feet, or mapping favourite spaces to rest and relax, all of us can enjoy this beautiful and extraordinary historic landscape using the trail. The 'Potter and Ponder' sensory trail is freely available (NT 2016) at Croome for all visitors. It provides high quality opportunities for us all to connect with each other, and with our own senses by indicating points in the Croome landscape where we might breathe, slow down and notice what is around us.

Katherine and Rachel have shared the impact and legacy of this project widely since launching the trail in 2017. More than eighteen months on from launching the free trail, they explained these, not only for staff, volunteers and visitors at Croome, but more widely as learning experiences for the National Trust that will help them contribute to a more equal society:

> 'We've recognized that vulnerability has a voice and a power- and we are all vulnerable. ... [Co-producing the trail] has made us bolder!'
> 'We have seen what people power can do and we love it!!! We are forever changed, in a good way.'

Both Digibility and the Croome Landscape project provide snap-shots of major, complex, heritage projects that demonstrate the impact on everyone involved in making beautiful historic sites and landscapes more widely accessible and inclusive. They demonstrate how much we can learn about ourselves and each other through co-production and collaborative partnerships and processes.

Restoration Trust projects

Our third case study that the Fund has been proud to support relates to two projects led by the Restoration Trust: one focussing on a Norfolk archive and the second known as Human Henge. At the Historic Landscapes and Mental Well-being conference in Bournemouth in April 2018, the long term impact and success of the Human Henge creative experiences were presented. The benefits for everyone involved in Human Henge, through engagement with the historic landscapes of Stonehenge and Avebury were very evident, these are fully discussed by colleagues in later chapters. The authors were especially impressed by the consistently high-quality outcomes that resulted from the considerable care and time spent by the Restoration Trust in developing trusted partnership models for these two projects, including working with the Richmond Fellowship, the National Trust, English Heritage, and Bournemouth University. Within the Fund we know that such partnership work is highly skilled, and that it is reliant on adequate funding that recognizes the true costs of high-quality partnership work.

The Fund also recognizes that for heritage to truly be inclusive, project budgets need to reflect necessary adjustments in order to reach beyond traditional audiences and participants. The budgets should include funding for sufficient planning time, flexible timetables, and small group sizes within participant cohorts where people may be vulnerable. Ensuring that robust evaluation is built in to the process is vital too, not least in order to assess the impact of engagement with historic landscapes for everyone involved. Human Henge was exemplary in planning, evaluation, and research methods that asked participants to provide their reflections both during and after the experience. Follow-up work included collecting participant feedback one year on from involvement in their Human Henge programme that related to personal levels of well-being. The evaluation of Human Henge, and the impressive outcomes it achieved, reflect the need for sustainable partnerships across the heritage sector. These are especially needed in order to continue the delivery of high-quality engagement with vulnerable people who may experience fluctuating levels of physical and mental health during their heritage experiences.

National Lottery Heritage Fund and the well-being of project planners / facilitators

The projects the Fund supports through its grant programmes can lead to positive well-being outcomes for participants and others too. However, the way funders expect projects to be delivered can also have an impact on grantee well-being. Projects are often well-advanced in their planning within groups and organizations long before they are submitted to the Fund or other funders. They can have project lifecycles of up to eight years, so projects cover a significant portion of people's lives, and deal with heritage that is often highly significant and valuable to individuals and their communities. This can put a huge amount of pressure on those applying for and delivering projects. They invest personally in the success of projects, and successful delivery of these projects can be linked to both professional reputation and personal pride. The Fund process aims to support this by building in aspects that support good project management, such as regular and frequent communication, regular projects reviews, the use of risk tables, and ways in which grantees are advised on how to manage the inevitable changes occurring during the delivery of a project. The Fund is also able to appoint external professionals to act as project mentors to provide additional support.

In order to identify when in particular the process is beneficial to both applicants and grantees the Fund conducted some Key Driver Analysis research in 2017. This is an analytical technique designed to understand the inferred influences on an overarching area, calculating which of the specific elements of the grant-giving process have the greatest influence on overall satisfaction scores. It was implemented using data from the Customer Care survey that covered a significant portion of work within the last strategic funding framework (2014 to 2016). The results highlighted that in terms of areas that make grantees more satisfied about the process there is a clear correlation between Fund staff helpfulness and overall satisfaction; this was highest amongst single-round projects under £100,000, and projects from church congregations and religious organizations.

There is a general correlation between the level of contact with a grants officer and overall satisfaction levels. This is a potential proxy for perceptions of stress and pressure, so those who are more satisfied overall may experience less stress in their project. This finding was particularly relevant for commercially focused organizations, and those applying for less than £10,000. In terms of the advice given by staff that is most beneficial to grantees, the research showed that the smallest award band of grants, under £10,000, have grantees who require the widest range of support to ensure satisfaction.

Widening access to National Lottery Heritage Fund funding

Recently, the Fund has been exploring different ways of delivering grants, in order to remove some of the barriers to access, especially for smaller first-time applicants. This 'micro-grants' experiment was conducted from late 2017 to early 2018 in Barrow-in-Furness, Cumbria. Barrow was at the time one of a small number of Priority Development Areas for the Fund; this means that to date it had received a lower than average amount of National Lottery funding per capita. The local Fund team had met groups who felt that the online part of the process was too daunting, or that the minimum grant of £3000 was too large for a novice or small organization. The idea of smaller grant awards was not an aspect that the Fund had previously explored, and staff worked hard to streamline the process in order to make smaller grant awards for this pilot initiative.

Those attending our initial events in Barrow, told us they had a need for smaller grants and a faster process. Some had harboured project ideas for years, but did not know how to test them out and take them forward. Some had felt that the online nature of the application form and the perceived effort of filling it in were barriers. They were excited to share project ideas, and appreciated the fact that we were trialing this new approach with them. There was clearly enormous value for people in being able to discuss their project and have someone 'demystify' the process for them. Being able to explain a project, then seeing how it fitted into the application form, helped to make the process less daunting.

The projects that came out of the pilot project were hugely diverse and exciting ones. They included 'virtual reality' bell-ringing, Viking heritage, the history of local shops, Industrial Folk Art, women in First World War (WWI), and the history of shipyards. It led to a significant increase in the number of Fund projects in Barrow. In the preceding five years, only six projects had been funded in the area; the pilot funded twenty new ones. It has resulted in new applicants approaching the Fund. Fourteen of the 18 organizations who applied had not applied to the Fund before, with six having never applied to any funder before. Applicants have increased in confidence, with 15 of 18 survey respondents stating that they were now more confident to apply to the Fund. This increased confidence shows the value of reviewing the process in order to enhance the experience for those who have to work within it.

National Lottery Heritage Fund and the future

The Fund is now operating within the Strategic Funding Framework for 2019–2024, listening to and learning from the experience of all those who contribute, and whom it seeks to continue supporting: grant applicants, National Lottery players, participants, volunteers, and heritage stake-holders continue to be vital. These learning opportunities for the Fund have helped inform a strategy that aims to be ambitious and inclusive.

In representing the diverse communities of the UK today, it is essential that heritage is relevant and responsive. It must work with wider sector partners, including voluntary and community organizations, health and research colleagues. The Fund is proud to work in partnership with these allies and many more, to inspire, lead, and resource UK heritage. In this way, the Fund can create positive and lasting change for people and communities, now and in the future.

Bibliography

Bartlett, L. 2014. Gressenhall Farm and Workhouse: Adventures of a visitor services trainee [Blog]. Viewed 5 December 2018, <https://gressenhallfw.wordpress.com/tag/heritage-lottery-fund/page/3/>.
BBC News 2018. Belfast's tropical ravine wins major award [Webpage]. Viewed 5 December 2018, <https://www.bbc.co.uk/news/uk-northern-ireland-44254929>.
BOP Consulting and HLF 2012. Social impact research — summary analysis [Webpage]. Viewed 5 December 2018, <https://www.hlf.org.uk/social-impact-research---summary-analysis>.
DDCMS 2017. Tailored review of the Heritage Lottery Fund [Webpage]. Viewed 5 December 2018, <https://www.hlf.org.uk/about-us/our-strategy/tailored-review-heritage-lottery-fund>.
HLF 2016. The Windrush Intergenerational Project case study [Webpage]. Viewed 5 December 2018, <https://www.hlf.org.uk/our-projects/windrush-intergenerational-project>.

HLF 2017. Capability Brown festival puts grandfather of landscape architecture on the map [Webpage]. Viewed 5 December 2018, <https://cymraeg.hlf.org.uk/about-us/news-features/capability-brown-festival-puts-grandfather-landscape-architecture-map>.
Ladysbridge Stories 2017. Ladysbridge Stories [Website]. Viewed 5 December 2018, <https://www.ladysbridgestories.com/>.
NLHF 2019. Strategic Funding Framework 2019–2024 [Webpage]. Viewed 12 February 2019, <https://www.heritagefund.org.uk/publications/strategic-funding-framework-2019-2024>.
NT 2016. *Potter & ponder: Sensory experiences at Croome, map of sensory experiences on site* [Online document]. Swindon: National Trust. Viewed 5 December 2018, <https://www.nationaltrust.org.uk/croome/documents/potter-and-ponder-map.pdf >.
UN 1948. Universal Declaration of Human Rights [Webpage]. Viewed 5 December 2018, <http://www.un.org/en/universal-declaration-human-rights/>.

Chapter 3

Therapeutic landscapes past and present: The mental health context

Toby Sutcliffe

Abstract

This paper is written from the perspective of a senior consultant psychiatrist working within the NHS. It considers mental health provision and the development of the treatments and services offered in Britain through time. It outlines the position in the present day, describing the various approaches used to improve mental well-being, and the ways in which these are organized and accessed. It then gives a brief background history of mental health provision, from its early recognition and the rudimentary ways in which British society first dealt with mental health issues, through the eighteenth and nineteenth century asylum system and its developing rationales. The author's interest in his working county of Wiltshire is reflected in the discussion. This contribution aims to provide a context for other papers in this volume, by presenting wider contexts, historic and current, within which mental well-being provision sits.

Keywords: Context; Medical practice; Recovery; Treatment history; Wiltshire

Introduction

The purpose of this paper is primarily to describe current mental health service provision in order to contextualize these activities within the wider landscape of mental health interventions. Whilst much of what I consider here may appear to have little connection to later chapters, I hope it adds to the multidisciplinary feel of this volume and illustrates some of the many dimensions of mental health care. Working in a county such as Wiltshire, where history is so clearly evident, I will describe something of the development of mental health services and treatments. I consider the concepts of illness and recovery in the light of developing cultural heritage therapy interventions, and suggest that these might be at the vanguard of a new generation of bespoke, small-scale, user-led interventions.

It should be borne in mind that in describing the development of mental ill-health concepts, a number of out-dated and stigmatized terms are used. I make no apology for this, but the reader should be aware that these are purely historic; they are not used within modern mental health services and would now be considered highly inappropriate. It also should be noted that there is a current debate around the term 'mental illness' itself, and whether this is unhelpful in potentially over-medicalizing a human response to circumstances past and present. The language of the field is constantly evolving; the content of this paper reflects that continuous search for improvement and clarity.

Mental health provision today

When seeking to understand the current service provision, it is still the case that the family doctor or General Practitioner (GP) remains the gatekeeper to many available resources.

However, there are a number of non-statutory provisions accessible directly by individuals. These organizations vary between areas depending on what has been commissioned and paid for locally, and the hope is that these will reflect the particular needs of the local population. For example, the support for carers would usually be provided by this sector, as would support for a return to employment.

The Improving Access to Psychological Therapies (IAPT) services again have some local variation, but are commissioned within a centrally mandated template to provide a variety of simple, rather than complex, psychological therapies. These talking therapies are usually accessible directly by individuals, that is without the need for referral by a GP or other medical professional. The development of the IAPT programme has indeed widened the availability of simpler, evidence-based psychological therapies. This has somewhat displaced the previously available 'practice counsellors' who had been able to provide longer term interventions than is possible within the IAPT model.

GPs offer a number of interventions, some formal others less so. Particularly where they have had a longer-term professional relationship with their patient, they are well-placed to offer tailored lifestyle advice and psychoeducation, as well as the prescription of some medications such as antidepressants. GPs are key in filtering and managing the many situations in which physical conditions such as infection and hormone or chemical disturbance first present as an apparently unconnected distress or confusion.

Where the degree of complexity or risk appears to be higher, the GP is able to consider a referral into the 'secondary' care services (as opposed to 'primary' care, which relates to activities in and around the GP surgery). These comprise the elements that people would most readily think of when considering mental health services. In-patient hospital provision, Home Treatment Teams, and Community Mental Health Teams (CMHTs) would be the most significant services, but there are often numerous additional services, again reflecting the needs of the population.

There is, of course, a huge spectrum of mental distress that is seen collectively within these services. The psychotic illnesses, principally schizophrenia, but also bipolar affective disorder, can present with disturbance of perceived reality such as delusions (fixed false beliefs) and hallucinations (visual or auditory perceptions in the absence of stimuli). The 'affective' (mood) disorders such as depression and anxiety can be managed in either primary or secondary care settings. A relatively poorly understood entity is described as 'personality disorders'. These can be rather difficult to quantify, but essentially comprise a collection of coping strategies that are unhelpful to an individual or to society. These include repetitive self-injurious behaviour, difficulty functioning independently and persistent suspicion of others. The key element in personality disorders is that the specific difficulties have been, and are, persistent throughout an individual's lifetime. In the past, this has been a 'diagnosis of exclusion' (i.e. no other diagnosis could be made to 'fit') with the patient's presenting difficulties. However, with improved understanding and the development of some effective treatments (notably talking therapies), it is now a more helpful diagnosis.

It is nowadays the case that diagnosis and support for individuals with the various dementias, usually in older age, are carried out by GPs and third sector (voluntary and/or charitable) organizations. The secondary care services only tend to become involved in situations of complexity or risk. There would be an expectation that reactions to 'normal human experience', for example bereavement, ill-health or unemployment, would be managed where possible within primary care or non-statutory settings, rather than secondary care mental health services.

Current mental health treatment is described as the 'biopsychosocial model', or biological, psychological and social interventions. Biological treatments largely comprise the wide spectrum of medications available (antidepressants, antipsychotics, anxiolytics, and mood stabilizers being the major classes), but there are some, less commonly used, treatments such as electroconvulsive therapy (ECT).

Psychological treatments comprise the various talking therapies. These include psychodynamic therapies (loosely speaking based around a Freudian model of the mind) which tend to be less available within publicly funded services. Cognitive Behavioural Therapy (CBT) is often favoured by commissioners because of the time-limited nature of the intervention and its amenability to measurement (i.e. its effectiveness can be clearly demonstrated in research studies). There are usually a number of arts-therapies — such as art, dance and movement, music or drama therapy — available within statutory services to a limited degree.

The social interventions are perhaps less easy to define, and involve paying attention to an individual's place in the world, their family, and the community. Social interventions could include providing assistance with engagement in occupation, a move to more appropriate accommodation, or links to likeminded individuals. Small changes in these realms can of course have a profound impact on an individual's mental well-being. It would probably be most accurate to consider the Human Henge project as a 'social intervention.'

It is important to remember that although used relatively rarely, secondary care services are legally permitted to treat people against their wishes under various sections of the *Mental Health Act 1983*. This legislation does provide for the treatment of some individuals who would be otherwise unwilling to accept help. However, it should also be remembered that there may be unintended consequences to this course of action. The knowledge that this is a possibility can at times mean that people are more wary of speaking openly with health professionals about their concerns for fear that they may be sectioned as a result.

Having described the present provision, it is interesting to think about the development of mental health treatment over time in order to better understand how he have arrived at our current situation. When I say 'over time', I refer to the blink of an eye compared to the archaeological timescales.

A brief history of mental health intervention

Very little is known about views and treatments for mental illness in prehistoric times, and necessarily this will be largely speculative. Evidence of trepanation is found on some human skulls from prehistoric contexts. This process involved making a hole in the skull of a living person, and may have been a response intended to relieve symptoms of mental illness amongst other possible medical conditions (Gross 2003: 313). There is some interesting work examining current beliefs in shamanism around the world and its use in dealing with mental illness (e.g.

Heinz and Pankow 2017; Kottler *et al.* 2004; Mayer 2013). Non-western approaches are varied and can offer valuable alternative methods (Fernando 2014: 23–27), although it is important not to idealize these. There can certainly be significant stigmatization of affected individuals, and discrimination against them, in cultures and countries where limited or no formal services exist (e.g. Poreddi *et al.* 2013: 121–122).

In pre-Enlightenment Britain, the management of people in poor mental health consisted of little more than accommodation in church institutions, prisons, or, latterly, workhouses (Stainton 2001), with many cared for by struggling families or by living on the street (HE 2019). There were a number of private 'mad houses', with some hospital and patient records for Wiltshire surviving today (Moles 2017). Wiltshire had a relatively large provision (Historic Hospitals 2018), perhaps as a result of the transport links between London and Bristol; they thrived by importing patients from the capital. Right across the county the buildings constructed for these institutions remain, although most have been repurposed or redeveloped.

The first formal statute law that mandated the management of people with mental health difficulties was the *Vagrancy Act 1744*. This allowed magistrates to order the detention of the 'furiously mad' where they were seen as posing a danger (Hamilton 1983: 1720). To our eyes, this does not appear enlightened or sensitive, but it did allow for individuals to be detained and conveyed to whichever institution was felt to be most appropriate. It is interesting that to this day, we as a society can have difficulty separating the symptoms of mental illness from criminal behaviour; the use of the police in these circumstances remains a very live issue (College of Policing 2017; The Guardian 2018; Independent 2018).

As we enter the period of the Enlightenment there is a slight shift in view whereby an individual's choices or behaviours were considered to impact on their mental health, although the mechanisms remained unknown and were still considered by some to involve the supernatural. This is well illustrated in the widely reproduced series of cartoons engraved by William Hogarth, distributed in the 1730s and currently displayed at the Sir John Soane's Museum, London. They were intended both as entertainment and a morality tale. They describe how 'Tom Rake' progresses following the inheritance of his father's fortune. Despite the attempts of others to guide him he repeatedly chooses unwise paths: debauchery, gambling, and alcohol which initially lead first to prison then to incarceration in Bedlam, or the Bethlem Hospital as it was properly called (Sir John Soane's Museum 2018). There is an intricacy of diverting detail contained in the pictures, but the message was and remains a clear one: Tom, through foolish choices, had engineered his own financial and social downfall and that he therefore bore sole responsibility for his mental illness and sorry state.

The 'madhouses' of the eighteenth and nineteenth centuries were by most accounts unpleasant and often cruel environments (Jones 1955; Sir John Soane's Museum, London 2018). In England, it took an individual, William Tuke, a Quaker, to consider the benefits of 'moral treatment' (Kibria and Metcalfe 2016). He founded the 'York Retreat' — which remains in use today as The Retreat, York (The Retreat 2018) — and famously released 'inmates' (it is notable that they were not yet referred to as 'patients') from mechanical restraints (Borthwick *et al.* 2001: 428–430). He then helped to forge the *County Asylum Act 1808*, requiring each county in England to provide an asylum, many of which remain in use today in one form or another (Jones 1955).

During the nineteenth century, Philippe Pinel, who has been considered the father of psychiatry, noticed particular patterns of symptoms associated with certain physical illnesses (Charland 2008: 20; Suzuki 2006: 115) and thus began the transition from considering residents as inmates, to being patients. A multitude of helpful and unhelpful treatments have fallen in and out of favour over the years. However, the principle has remained that these symptoms represent an illness and that there exist treatments delivered by doctors and nurses that will be of benefit. This approach is now seeing further development into a more empowering model.

It is interesting to reflect that the Wiltshire County Lunatic Asylum, later Wiltshire County Mental Hospital and then Roundway Hospital — a stone's throw from the office in Green Lane Hospital in which I am writing this —at its peak in the 1940s housed more than 1500 patients (Devizes Heritage 2018). Green Lane Hospital, its successor, opened in 1995, now has 20 beds. There are a multitude of reasons for this, and for the greater part, this deinstitutionalization has been a positive move.

Conclusion

Since the latter part of the twentieth century, we have been developing a greater awareness of the value of diversity, from which has arisen the recovery movement. This in turn developed from the disability rights movement, together with some principles of Alcoholics Anonymous (Jensen 2000: 62). In essence, the core concept of mental health recovery is that we, as individuals, should aim for an optimization of our potential, rather than an absence of symptoms. This can be seen as empowering for individuals, who then have choices rather than deficits.

It is in this frame that visionary projects such as the Human Henge can be seen less as 'treatments' provided to unfortunate 'patients', and more as empowering projects in which individuals can choose to participate so that they can actively maximize their own fulfilment. The establishment of a connection with others in their community, and with local environments treasured by our ancestors, are critical elements of Human Henge. Whilst the project carries echoes of earlier benign interventions intended to improve mental well-being, it brings fresh perspectives and new approaches that no doubt help to progress mental health provision into the twenty-first century.

Acknowledgments

As a psychiatrist working in Wiltshire I am proud of my association with the Human Henge project, having had a role on the project board. I was also thrilled to have been asked to participate in the Historic Landscapes and Mental Well-being Conference at Bournemouth University in April 2018. However, my presentation there was notable in that it was not based on primary research but rather a description and explanation of the then current mental health service provision. Its inclusion here, alongside accounts of the innovative interventions described in other chapters, provides an indication of the assistance that people are likely to find within their local services.

Bibliography

Borthwick, A., C. Holman, D. Kennard, M. McFetridge, K. Messruther and J. Wilkes 2001. The relevance of moral treatment to contemporary mental health care. *Journal of Mental Health* 10(4): 427–439.

Charland, L.C. 2008. A moral line in the sand: Alexander Crichton and Philippe Pinel on the psychopathology of the passions, in L.C. Charland and P. Zachar (eds.) *Fact and Value in Emotion*: 15–34. Amsterdam and Philadelphia: John Benjamins Publishing Company.

College of Policing 2017. *Memorandum of Understanding — The police use of restraint in mental health and learning disability settings* [Online document]. Ryton-on-Dunsmore, Coventry: College of Policing. Viewed 7 January 2019, <https://www.college.police.uk/What-we-do/Support/.../ERG_Final_Copy.pdf>.

Devizes Heritage 2018. Wiltshire County Asylum for Insane – Roundway Hospital [Website]. Viewed 10 January 2019, <https://web.archive.org/web/20130420193634/http://www.devizesheritage.org.uk/roundway_hospital.html>.

Fernando, S. 2014. *Mental health worldwide: Culture, globalization and development*. Basingstoke: Palgrave Macmillan.

Gross, C.C. 2003. Trepanation from the Palaeolithic to the internet, in R. Arnott, S. Finger and C.U.M. Smith (eds.) *Trepanation: History, discovery, theory*: 307–322. Lisse, Netherlands: Swets & Zeitlinger B.V.

Hamilton, J.R. 1983. Contemporary themes: Mental Health Act 1983. *British Medical Journal* 286 (6379): 1720–1725.

HE 2019. Disability history: Mental illness in the 16th and 17th centuries [Webpage]. Viewed 30 January 2019, <https://historicengland.org.uk/research/inclusive-heritage/disability-history/1485-1660/mental-illness-in-the-16th-and-17th-centuries/>.

Heinz, A. and A. Pankow 2017. Return of the religious: Good shamanism and bad exorcism, in H. Basu, R. Littlewood and A. S. Steinforth (eds.) *Spirit and mind: Mental health at the intersection of religion and psychiatry*: 57–66. Berlin: LIT Verlag.

Historic Hospitals 2018. English hospitals (RCHME survey): Wiltshire [Webpage]. Viewed 30 January 2019, <https://historic-hospitals.com/english-hospitals-rchme-survey/wiltshire/>.

Independent 2018. NHS failings 'forcing police to respond to mental health incidents rather than crimes', report finds [Webpage]. Viewed 7 January 2019, <https://www.independent.co.uk/news/uk/crime/nhs-mental-health-police-crime-uk-failings-funding-government-a8653121.html>.

Jensen, G.H. 2000. *Storytelling in alcoholics anonymous: A rhetorical analysis*. Carbondale, IL: Southern Illinois University Press.

Jones, K. 1955. *Lunacy, law and conscience 1744-1845. The social history of the care of the insane*. Abingdon: Routledge.

Kibria, A.A. and N.H. Metcalfe 2016. A biography of William Tuke (1732–1822): Founder of the modern mental asylum. *Journal of Medical Biography* 24(3): 384–388.

Kottler, J.A., J. Carlson and B. Keeney 2004. *American shaman: An Odyssey of global healing traditions*. New York and Hove: Brunner Routledge.

Mayer, G.A. 2013. Spirituality and extraordinary experiences: Methodological remarks and some empirical findings. *Journal of Empirical Theology* 26: 188–206.

Moles, M. 2017. Wiltshire and Swindon History Centre. Pauper and private: Early mental health care in Wiltshire [Webpage]. Viewed 30 January 2019, <http://www.wshc.eu/blog/item/early-mental-health-care.html>.

Pinel, P. 1806. *A treatise on insanity*. London: Cadell and Davies.

Poreddi, V., Ramachandra, K. Reddemma and S.B. Math 2013. People with mental illness – a developing countries [sic] perspective. *Indian Journal of Psychiatry* 55(2): 117–124.

Sir John Soane's Museum 2018. 'A Rake's Progress' [Webpage]. Viewed 7 January 2019, <https://www.soane.org/collections-research/key-stories/rakes-progress>.

Stainton, T. 2001. Medieval charitable institutions and intellectual impairment c.1066–1600. *Journal on Developmental Disabilities* 8(2): 19–30.

Suzuki, A. 2006. *Madness at home: The psychiatrist, the patient, and the family in England, 1820-1860* (Medicine and Society 13). Berkeley: University of California Press.

The Guardian 2018. Police 'Picking up pieces of mental health system', says watchdog [Webpage]. Viewed 7 January 2019, <https://www.theguardian.com/society/2018/nov/27/police-mental-health-system-patients>.

The Retreat 2018. The Retreat, York [Website]. Viewed 7 January 2019, <https://www.theretreatyork.org.uk/about-us/>.

Chapter 4

Inclusion and recovery: Archaeology and heritage for people with mental health problems and/or autism

William Rathouse

Abstract

This chapter introduces two distinct but interrelated areas: the inclusion of people with autistic spectrum conditions (ASCs) and mental health problems (MHPs) in archaeological heritage; and the use of archaeological heritage to promote good mental health. Having examined the nature of ASCs and MHPs, and the ways in which general exclusion from heritage may occur, examples are given of the ways in which the design and operation of heritage attractions have served to exclude people affected by these conditions. Means of ameliorating or removing these obstacles to inclusion are discussed, and compromises with competing needs evaluated. The chapter then explores the rationale for undertaking archaeology in order to promote good mental health, identifying reasons for the anticipation of improved outcomes. It then describes some of the earliest projects in this field, discussing the challenges experienced and those that might be anticipated. Finally, key elements of best practice in this field are presented.

Keywords: Archaeology; Autism; Heritage; Mental health; Mind

Introduction

This chapter provides an introduction to the development of two distinct but closely related issues in archaeology and heritage and presents a case for further research. Archaeological fieldwork involves a range of activity beyond excavation. These include surveying, measuring, recording, and reporting surface features, architecture, and portable antiquities. 'Heritage' for the purpose of this chapter, refers to historical sites and buildings, museums and their collections, as well as other locations and items of archaeological and historical significance.

The United Nations (UN) World Health Organization (WHO) includes mental health in the definition of health used in its constitution: 'Health is a state of complete physical, mental and social well-being and not merely the absence of disease or infirmity' (WHO 2006: 1). The UK Governmental organization Public Health England states that:

> 'Being in good mental health brings resilience to cope with difficulties, have good relationships with others and an ability to think clearly, participate in decision making, and have optimism, sense of control and self efficacy. These are important for staying healthy.' (Public Health England 2018)

Thus, mental health problems (hereinafter referred to as MHPs) are conditions which compromise this emotional resilience, impacting physical, social, and mental well-being. Examples include: depression, which is not merely unshakeable sadness but generally combines it with despair, self-doubt, self-loathing, and emotional numbness; Generalized anxiety disorder (GAD), which can make a person so fearful that to leave their own home can induce a panic attack, which may feel like a heart attack; psychotic disorders in which a person's beliefs or ideas become problematic or their perceptions of reality become unreliable with visual, olfactory, and especially auditory hallucinations occurring. MHPs are therefore profoundly limiting, distressing to experience, and difficult to live with. An American study suggested that 90 per cent of suicides are associated with a psychiatric condition (Conwell *et al.* 1996). The effects of MHPs are further exacerbated by public ignorance of the seriousness of these ailments. This can result in judgemental reactions to crises and distress accompanied by a general sense of stigma towards the mentally unwell (McNair *et al.* 2002).

Autistic spectrum conditions (ASCs) are not MHPs, although people who have an ASC may be more at risk of developing a MHP. ASCs are defined as developmental disorders although autistic people with whom the author has worked have argued that they are variations in the neural architecture of the brain and ought not to be seen as disorders. Some prefer to describe themselves as 'neurodivergent'. As the term 'spectrum' implies, there are a range of presentations of autism. These were formerly defined as one of two main conditions: the milder Asperger's Syndrome and the much more life-limiting Kenner's Autism. The latter can imply such severe symptoms (in some cases inability to communicate verbally) that many sufferers require residential care and constant one-to-one support. People with such conditions may find that participation in archaeological field projects would require a very high degree of disability adaptation, and their involvement may be somewhat limited in scope because of health and safety considerations.

Other heritage focused projects involving site visits and handling displays similar to that described by Lilla Vonk (2016) may have value for people with these diagnoses. The British Museum has been running a series of events aimed at people with developmental disorders including autism. The session observed by the author on the 17 July 2018 featured a storyteller. It was very well received by an audience with a range of conditions, including ASDs towards the Kanner syndrome end of the spectrum.

Asperger Syndrome, sometimes described as high-functioning autism, is characterized by problems with social interaction. People with this condition sometimes struggle to understand subtleties of communication such as body language and allegory. They may be very literal in their understanding of language. They often find interacting with non-autistic (neurotypical) people stressful, and may prefer to avoid interpersonal interaction (Stanford 2015: 26–27). People with this kind of autism have benefited from archaeological projects as we shall see later in this chapter.

Exclusion from heritage

Inclusion is a prominent watchword in heritage discourse. It refers to the intention to make heritage relevant to the widest possible audience and to encourage the sense that all individuals are stakeholders. Smith & Waterton (2009: 11) emphasize the importance of inclusion, in that those with an interest in the past are more than just stakeholders. The authors argue that these people should have an equal say in how heritage is managed and presented.

It can be argued that heritage exclusion is part of a broader social malaise of cultural disconnection, which may be associated with poor mental health, crime, poverty, addiction, and xenophobia. Johann Hari (2018) suggests that disconnection is a key issue in conditions such as depression and anxiety.

It may be hoped that heritage could serve to focus people's tribal instinct away from group identities, such as gang membership and racial supremacist ideas, and towards more positive affiliations such as city, community, or neighbourhood by giving a greater appreciation and understanding of these larger affiliations. Through engagement with heritage, it may be possible to help people who feel disconnection. Economic and vocational hopelessness may be avoided, addiction and crime averted, and MHPs relieved. Heritage has the potential to give people the experience of health, well-being, and membership of a cohesive and supportive community.

If we accept that heritage is beneficial, it is important to establish what prevents people from engaging with it. The means by which people may be excluded from archaeological heritage can be divided into three categories: physical, financial, and psychological. Perhaps the most obvious, and the most thoughtfully addressed form of exclusion, is the physical. This is particularly relevant to those with mobility problems, whether resulting from an inherited or acquired condition, injury, or age. Access to heritage sites may be obstructed by steps, staircases, narrow corridors, or stiles, many of which are hard to overcome without transforming the character of the site to the detriment of its sense of authenticity. Manually-opened doors may be a problem, and rough uneven ground may also impose difficulties.

Complaints have been made about being priced out of heritage. This was a recurring theme in the campaign for access to Stonehenge by contemporary Druids (Rathouse 2015: 105). It is particularly relevant in this context, as people with physical disabilities or mental health problems are statistically more likely than most to experience poverty (Tinson *et al.* 2016). They are therefore often limited in their ability to access sufficient disposable income to allow easy access to heritage. Disability and MHPs may also carry additional costs which are not always met by the welfare state. Examples might include the need for an escort to provide assistance, or difficulties in using cheaper forms of public transport leading to the use of taxis instead.

People who are physically and financially able to engage with heritage may be prevented from doing so by factors associated with their state of mind. They may feel no connection (no sense of being a stakeholder) with some or all cultural heritage. However, there are also instances where aspects of the way a heritage attraction is presented might exacerbate or trigger psychiatric distress. One of the effects of autism, for example, is a reduction in the ability to filter inputs to the brain (National Autistic Society 2018). People with ASCs can lack the instincts underpinning social interaction and find it hard to read body language and facial expressions. They tend to lack the ability to filter out sensory inputs and therefore find that noisy environments (especially with lots of people), strong smells, and bright busy decorative patterns can cause a sensory overload. This can result in severe distress and, sometimes, in extreme cases, a fight or flight response. In the professional experience of this author, several clients with ASCs have displayed stronger than usual abjective responses to heritage attractions. Whilst a few lived in some squalor, others responded to lack of order and cleanliness with anxiety and avoidance. One person displayed an obsessive compulsion to wash his hands or use hand sanitizer when he had witnessed dirty environments. Williams (2015) explains that his daughter (diagnosed with Asperger Syndrome) finds crowds at heritage attractions a problem. Noise is another issue, especially hand dryers in bathrooms. He explains that she has a strong aversion to animal faeces, including that from sheep and rabbits, and to out of control vegetation. Enclosed spaces and spiral staircases are also sources of stress.

Noise and crowds are often problems for people with anxiety disorders. Post-traumatic stress disorder (PTSD) is a kind of anxiety disorder usually resulting from an experience or experiences associated with extreme danger and/or severe suffering. People affected by generalized anxiety disorder (GAD), and especially those with PTSD, may find that severe stress or panic ensues from triggers such as unexpected loud noises, certain smells (e.g. burning), or imagery depicting suffering, violence, death, or decay.

Inclusion in heritage

Bearing in mind the problems listed above, there are a number of adaptations that site managers can put in place in order to reduce exclusion and facilitate participation in heritage for people with ASCs and those experiencing MHPs. Williams describes the way in which queuing at Stonehenge was a problem for his daughter (2015). By contrast, when asked how they facilitated access for visitors with ASCs, staff at the British Museum explained that a fast track entry with priority security checks could be arranged. However, it appears this provision could be better advertised. For people who find that dirt and rubbish induce anxiety, regular cleaning is essential. Rubbish, and spillages, especially those involving strong smells, need to be cleaned up or removed quickly. Good maintenance of lighting to avoid flickering strip-lights and malfunctioning exhibition equipment, will also reduce the risk of sensory overload. Lighting should be designed to avoid excessively bright illumination, especially sudden transitions between dark and light areas. Visual design and decoration ought to be carefully planned, avoiding loud colours and busy intricate patterns that can sometimes cause sensory overload. Galleries, displays, and attractions relating to death, injury, violence, or other traumatic experiences, should be signalled by advanced warnings for people affected by anxiety disorders.

Madge (2016) highlights 'unsupportive and judgmental front of house staff that have no autism awareness' as being a particular problem. Ideally, all front of house staff should have training in autism, and in recognizing and assisting people in psychiatric distress. If this is not possible then staff responsible for maximizing accessibility need training in autism awareness and mental health first aid. All staff should be encouraged to take a non-judgemental stance on unusual behaviour and even on mildly antisocial behaviour such as rudeness or intolerance.

People with ASCs can be very uncomfortable going to new and unfamiliar places, especially if they are unsure about what to expect. One solution to this problem might be to take exhibits out of the museum building and into the community, as has been done with projects such as that described by Lilla Vonk (2016). Similarly, the Museum of London Archaeology's Thames Discovery Programme has a handling display that is taken to people who are unable to visit sites or museums.

Archaeological fieldwork in support of mental health

Projects including people with social disadvantages — including mental health problems — had been conducted previously, but this field really took off in 2012 when two projects were launched that specifically sought to use archaeological fieldwork to promote mental health. Past in Mind (Past in Mind 2014) was conceived and directed by Jenny Macmillan and Ian Bapty for Mind Herefordshire. It was a one-off project investigating a mediaeval village at Studmarsh. Mental Health service users were involved in the whole process, from planning, through data collection, to interpretation and dissemination of findings. The project is well recorded in Kate Lack's excellent book (Lack 2014). Also in 2012, Sergeant Diarmaid Walshe of the Royal Army Medical Corps, and Richard Osgood of the Defence Infrastructure Organization, launched Operation Nightingale (DAG 2018; MOD & DIO 2019). The aim of this project was to support the recovery of wounded, injured, and sick service personnel by using archaeological fieldwork, and to introduce those leaving the forces to archaeology and heritage as a potential post-service career.

Following these, Mind Aberystwyth began to offer archaeological volunteering opportunities to its members. Small numbers were taken on digs at Llanllyr near Talsarn, Ceredigion, in 2014 and 2015, and in 2015 at Strata Florida Abbey near Pontrydfendigaid. The members involved had a variety of diagnoses and included people with ASCs, depression, and psychosis. Feedback was very positive and led to a further project examining war memorials which is fully described in Chapter 19.

Why use archaeological fieldwork to promote mental health and well-being?

The rationale for exploring archaeological fieldwork as a beneficial activity for people suffering difficulties as a result of MHPs and ASCs, is supported by the following seven factors:

1. It is a real task with an output that is desirable to people, rather than merely something to keep someone occupied and out of trouble. That is what Creek (2002: 75) describes as 'purposeful activity and meaningful occupation'. Archaeological fieldwork provides a product in the form of information about the past, which is much sought after by institutions and members of the public.
2. The processes of trowelling back archaeological layers and producing plans and section drawings, all of which take up much archaeological fieldwork time, require a degree of concentration and focus. In some ways this mirror the techniques of distraction and mindfulness employed to prevent people suffering depression and anxiety from dwelling on distressing thoughts.
3. Physical exercise provided by shifting soil, mattocking, barrowing, and moving around sites has been shown to alleviate anxiety and depression (Harvey *et al.* 2018)
4. Sunlight and fresh air of the kind provided by archaeology as a largely out-of-doors activity have been shown to improve mental health (Harvard Medical School 2010).
5. Archaeology is a teamwork activity providing practice in social interactions, and, if properly managed, can help build friendships and thus bolster self-confidence and self-esteem.
6. A University of Bristol (2007) study has suggested that the *Mycobacterium vaccae* bacteria, which is often present in the soil, secretes a chemical which helps to fight depression.
7. Archaeology and heritage give an understanding of the past of a place and the development of its cultures. This in turn may provide a sense of connection and belonging.

Potential pitfalls

The clinical practice and profession of using work and recreational activity to promote independence and overcome or prevent disability is referred to as occupational therapy (OT). The World Federation of Occupational Therapists (2017: 66) explains that OT in Britain is a client-centred health profession that 'enables people to achieve health, well being and life satisfaction through participation in occupation', where occupation is defined as 'daily activities that reflect cultural values, provide structure and meaning to individuals' and which 'meet human needs for self-care, enjoyment and participation in society'. We might therefore consider that archaeological activity for people with mental health problems or autism comes within this definition. However, care must be taken, since the use of the term 'therapy' can be taken to imply clinically proven outcomes. At present, evidence demonstrating such outcomes is still being gathered and is considered by some to be somewhat anecdotal. It would be neither safe, appropriate, nor ethical, for archaeologists, heritage professionals and others lacking appropriate professional training to present themselves as carrying out OT. Nevertheless, the field of OT has a great deal to offer archaeologists and heritage professionals who seek to use their skills and resources to promote and enhance mental health well-being.

One of the primary considerations when working with people experiencing MHPs, is to safeguard their personal information. In a society which still stigmatizes MHPs, and which contains individuals who are liable to take advantage of associated vulnerabilities, a desire for privacy should always be assumed. MacMillan and Bapty's 'Past in Mind' project specifically avoided differentiating between mental health service users and other volunteers on the dig. This served to make mental health status less obvious unless or until participants chose to disclose that information to others.

One potential problem requiring advance planning is the possibility that a participant experiences a meltdown or mental health crisis. This is defined as an incident often, but not exclusively, triggered by an external stimulus, that results in an inability to cope with sensory input or emotions. This in turn brings about behaviours which may include, but are not limited to, disengagement, absences, avoidant behaviour, and in more serious cases, angry outbursts or self-harm. If such situations escalate, physical violence or attempts at suicide are not impossible. It is therefore of great importance to respond to such events quickly and appropriately, to ensure de-escalation and a return to a situation of safety. These incidents are characterized by adrenaline-fuelled 'fight or flight' reactions. It should be borne in mind that adrenaline can take between 20 and 90 minutes to be reabsorbed from the bloodstream, and thus such situations do not resolve quickly. Responses need to be person-centred and results focused. Urging someone in such a situation to 'get a grip', or instructing them to 'calm down', with a threat of sanctions if they do not is unlikely to produce the desired effect and will most likely escalate the situation. A person in distress is more likely to respond positively to reassurance. When calm has been restored, a non-judgemental approach should be used to establish which of their needs are not being met so that these may be addressed.

Creek (2002: 74) states that the aim of OT is for 'the client to be able to meet his own needs, as far as possible, and to have the motivation to continue working towards fulfilling his full potential'. It would be neither helpful nor ethical to create or maintain dependence on services for an individual who could manage a higher degree of independence. Walshe (pers. comm.) has therefore emphasized the need for mental health archaeology projects to avoid creating dependence.

A comparison of two pioneering projects

The Past in Mind project was a one-off initiative carried out in Herefordshire in 2012. In her book, Lack (2014: 4–5) emphasizes that there was no template in place for such a project. However, common ground between the archaeological process and the mental health recovery processes suggested the use of narrative and analysis in association with past traumas, and a combination of peer support and social inclusion with people whose mental health was stronger. She also underlined the importance of a sense of shared ownership for the project. This could be fostered by participants being engaged from the earliest planning stages, and a blurring of lines between staff, volunteers, and service-users.

By contrast, Operation Nightingale has run a series of 'exercises' in which serving and former service personnel, assisted by professional and trainee archaeologists, have undertaken a series of excavations across the UK and beyond (BBC 2012; BBC News 2012a, 2012b, 2013; DAG 2018). It has not exclusively been a mental health project, but emphasizes recovery from physical injury and illness, as well as suggesting possible career paths for those leaving the forces. Typical 'exercises' involve a set up phase, during which staff set up the facilities. Topsoil may be removed mechanically and equipment put in place. Participants then arrive and are allocated accommodation, usually provided by the Ministry of Defence (MoD) or service charities. Trained and trainee archaeologists are integrated with participants, to oversee, guide, and facilitate learning for those new to the discipline. Food is generally provided by the MoD at discounted rates. Medical staff trained in mental health needs are also on site and usually participate in the work. There may be several digs each year, and participants are welcome to join as many or as few as they wish to.

Inspired by these projects, Mind Aberystwyth began to offer archaeological participation on digs run by Dyfed Archaeology Trust and the University of Wales Trinity Saint David. In 2014, one member volunteered on a dig near Talsarn, and in 2015, members returned and volunteered at Strata Florida Abbey. During each of these events, mental health cover and transport were provided by a single support officer, who also guided the members in their archaeological work. With a maximum of three members present at any one time, this was manageable but not ideal. Subsequent projects have added to the corpus of experience and will be expanded upon in Chapter 19.

Towards best practice

Archaeology for the benefit of mental health is still at an early stage in its development. More study is needed, preferably led by psychologists and psychiatrists rather than archaeologists. One important question is: how, and to what extent, should participants be selected for involvement in archaeology projects aimed at improving mental health? Needs and capabilities may require some consideration, but care must be taken to avoid exclusion. Adjustments should be made to ensure access and inclusion wherever possible, taking account of both physical and psychological issues. Existing support systems and networks may need to be discussed and, if a participant is separated from them (e.g. by participating in a dig away from home), then substitute arrangements may be required. If a treatment plan or contract is in place, it should be consulted upon. Participants' goals and expectations, and the reasons for wanting to participate, may also need to be discussed in advance. By avoiding unrealistic expectations, it is more likely that participants will feel more positive about their experiences, and experience lower stress levels. Indeed, for participants who have an ASC and/or an anxiety related condition, it may be essential for their well-being to have detailed explanations in advance of all aspects of the project.

The Past in Mind project involved participants with mental health problems not only in the fieldwork, but also in prior planning, and subsequently in presentation of the excavation results. This project and Operation Nightingale both ensured the presence of trained mental health professionals during archaeological activities.

The vulnerability conferred by, and contributing to, mental health problems, makes it a priority to ensure the privacy of participants. Thus all involved in mental health archaeology projects should treat disclosed and observed personal information as confidential. However, in situations where non-disclosure is likely to result in danger to anyone, confidentiality may have to be set aside and information disclosed to an appropriate authority. Permission for disclosure should always be sought in such circumstances and, if refused, a warning issued that information may have to be disclosed nevertheless. It is important to remember that data protection is regulated by law, and the current data protection guidelines can be found on the UK Government website (HMG 2018).

Any outbursts or meltdowns need to be addressed quickly, calmly, reassuringly, and non-judgementally. Creek (2002: 79–81) describes an ongoing process or cycle used in occupational therapy, of Assessment => Treatment => Evaluation. It is important for such a process that regular and detailed records of kept of work undertaken and that outcomes are recorded and monitored. These then need to be reviewed for opportunities to develop practice to optimize effectiveness and outcomes.

A key caveat expressed by Walshe (pers. comm.) concerns what happened to participants at the end of a project. A situation was described where participants might have had a very positive experience during the project, but would then find themselves returned to the same difficulties they faced before participating. Care must be taken to avoid building dependence. Archaeological projects supporting mental health, especially in the absence of strong clinical evidence, should never present themselves as providing a 'cure' for MHPs. Experience suggests that it is unlikely that an archaeological research project would result in complete recovery, and it should be borne in mind that an activity which assists one person may have little effect on another.

Conclusion

It is becoming increasingly apparent that archaeology and heritage can provide assistance in promoting and maintaining cultural connections, exercise, fresh air, and positive social experiences, and hence good mental health. In order to do this effectively, heritage attractions need to be as accessible as possible to people at risk of, or experiencing, MHPs. Two key approaches to maintaining accessibility are: avoiding situations likely to cause distress (e.g. dirt, smells, confined spaces and bright lighting); and training staff to recognize and respond appropriately when someone is in distress.

Evidence has been described as largely anecdotal in relation to the efficacy of engagement in archaeological activities to safeguard or improve mental health and to support coping with or recovery from psychiatric conditions. Other chapters in this volume demonstrate that some recent projects included systematic data collection that should in due course provide qualitative and quantitative evidence of the effectiveness of ideas pioneered by Bapty, MacMillan, Osgood, Walshe and others described here.

Acknowledgements

This paper is based on a presentation to a session on mental health in archaeology organized by Sarah Brockmeyer and Lewis Colau at the Theoretical Archaeology Group meeting in Bradford on 15 December 2015.

Bibliography

BBC 2012. All in the mind: Preventing PTSD; Archaeology and mental health; Organophosphates [Webpage]. Viewed 26 November 2018, <http://www.bbc.co.uk/programmes/b01p71gx>.

BBC News 2012a. Celtic history: Injured soldiers learn new skills on warrior dig [Webpage]. Viewed 26 November 2018, <http://www.bbc.co.uk/news/uk-wales-20172872>.

BBC News 2012b. Soldiers uncover 27 ancient bodies on Salisbury Plain [Webpage]. Viewed 26 November 2018, <http://www.bbc.co.uk/news/uk-england-wiltshire-19147035>.

BBC News 2013. Crashed WWII Spitfire being dug up on Salisbury Plain [Webpage]. Viewed 26 November 2018, <http://www.bbc.co.uk/news/uk-england-wiltshire-23942610>.

Conwell, Y., P.R. Duberstein, C. Cox, J.H. Herrmann, N.T. Forbes and E.D. Caine 1996. Relationships of age and axis I diagnoses in victims of completed suicide: A psychological autopsy study. *The American Journal of Psychiatry* 153(8): 1001–1008.

Creek, J. 2002. Treatment, planning and implementation, in J. Creek (ed.) *Occupational therapy and mental health* (Third edition): 119–139. Edinburgh and London: Churchill Livingstone.

DAG 2018. Defence Archaeology Group [Website]. Viewed 26 November 2018, <http://www.dag.org.uk/page2.html>.

Finlay, L. 2002. Groupwork, in J. Creek (ed.) *Occupational therapy and mental health* (Third edition): 245–264. Edinburgh and London: Churchill Livingstone.

Goodman, J., J. Hurst and C. Locke (eds.) 2008. *Occupational therapy for people with learning disabilities: A practical guide* (First edition). Edinburgh and London: Churchill Livingstone.

Gutman, S.A., E.I. Raphael, L.M. Ceder, A. Khan, K.M. Timp and S. Salvant 2010. The effect of a motor-based, social skills intervention for adolescents with high-functioning autism: Two single-subject design cases. *Occupational Therapy International* 17(4): 188–197.

Hari, J. 2018. *Lost connections: Uncovering the real causes of depression, and the unexpected solutions.* London: Bloomsbury Circus.

Harvard Medical School 2010. Harvard Health Letter: A prescription for better health: Go alfresco [Webpage]. Viewed 26 November 2018, <https://www.health.harvard.edu/newsletter_article/a-prescription-for-better-health-go-alfresco>.

Harvey, S.B., S. Overland, S.L. Hatch, S. Wessely, M. Arnstein and M. Hotopf 2018. Exercise and the prevention of depression: Results of the HUNT Cohort Study. *American Journal of Psychiatry* 175(1): 28–36.

HMG, 2018. Guide to the General Data Protection Regulation [Webpage]. Viewed 25 November 2018, <https://www.gov.uk/government/publications/guide-to-the-general-data-protection-regulation>.

Kiddey, R. 2014. Homeless heritage: Collaborative social archaeology as therapeutic practice. Unpublished PhD dissertation, University of York.

Lack, K. 2014. *Past in mind: A heritage project and mental health recovery*. Bromyard, Herefordshire: Privately published.

Madge, C. 2016. Autism in museums [Webpage]. Viewed 26 November 2018, <https://network.autism.org.uk/good-practice/case-studies/autism-museums>.

McNair, B.G., N.J. Higher, I.E. Hickie and T.A. Davenport 2002. Exploring the perspectives of people whose lives have been affected by depression. *Medical Journal of Australia*, 176 (Supplement), S69–76.

Mind Aberystwyth 2015. Therapeutic archaeology dig @ Mind Aberystwyth [Webpage]. Viewed 26 November 2018, <http://mindaberystwyth.org/therapeutic-archeology-dig-mind-aberystwyth/>.

MOD and DIO 2019. Operation Nightingale [Webpage]. Viewed 6 February 2019, <https://www.gov.uk/guidance/operation-nightingale>.

National Autistic Society 2018. Meltdowns [Webpage]. Viewed 26 November 2018, <https://www.autism.org.uk/about/behaviour/meltdowns.aspx>.

Past in Mind 2014. Blog from the bog: The official blog for the Herefordshire Past in Mind project [Blog]. Viewed 26 November 2018, <https://pastinmindproject.wordpress.com/>.

Public Health England, 2018. Guidance: Wellbeing and mental health: Applying all our health [Webpage]. Viewed 26 November 2018, <https://www.gov.uk/government/publications/wellbeing-in-mental-health-applying-all-our-health/wellbeing-in-mental-health-applying-all-our-health>.

Rathouse, W. 2015. Contested heritage: Examining relations between contemporary pagan groups and the archaeological and heritage professions in Britain. Unpublished PhD dissertation, University of Wales Trinity Saint David.

Smith, L. and E. Waterton 2009. *Heritage, communities and archaeology*. London: Duckworth.

Stanford, A. 2015. *Asperger Syndrome (Autism Spectrum Disorder) and long-term relationships* (Second edition). London and Philadelphia: Jessica Kingsley Publishers.

Tinson, A., H. Aldridge, T.B. Born and C. Hughes 2016. *Disability and poverty: Why disability must be at the centre of poverty reduction* [Online document]. London: New Policy Institute. Viewed 26 November 2018, <https://www.npi.org.uk/files/3414/7087/2429/Disability_and_poverty_MAIN_REPORT_FINAL.pdf>.

University of Bristol 2007. Getting dirty may lift your mood [Webpage]. Viewed 26 November 2018, <http://www.bristol.ac.uk/news/2007/5384.html>.

Vonk, L. 2016. Archaeology as activity in dementia: A presentation of the potential effects of an active engagement in archaeology on the wellbeing of people living with dementia. Unpublished MA dissertation, Leiden University.

WHO 2006. *Constitution of the World Health Organization. Basic documents* (Forty-fifth edition, Supplement, October 2006). Geneva: World Health Organization.

Williams, H. 2015. Asperger, heritage and archaeodeath [Blog]. Viewed 26 November 2018, <https://howardwilliamsblog.wordpress.com/2015/08/09/aspergers-heritage-and-archaeodeath/>.

World Federation of Occupational Therapists 2017. Definitions of occupational therapy from member organizations, revised June 2017 [Webpage]. Viewed 26 November 2018, <http://www.wfot.org/ResourceCentre>.

Chapter 5

Walking with intent:
Culture therapy in ancient landscapes

Laura Drysdale

Abstract

The Restoration Trust is an organization that offers culture therapy for those with mental health issues. The paper describes the ways in which interacting with ancient monuments and landscapes can be therapeutic, and how this relates to current mental health practice in the UK. It explains the Trust's pivotal role in the Human Henge project and how its activities satisfy both well-being requirements and the Trust's own success criteria. It presents a call to action, a plea for this type of culture therapy to become a standard part of health prescribing. The paper concludes with poems from a Human Henge volunteer that give an insight into the impressions that the project can make.

Keywords: Access; Human Henge; Inclusion; Restoration Trust; Well-being

'I like the walking and talking and learning all at the same time, and being a human being rather than, as ***** said, an illness or a condition, or a client or an end-user; y'know, I've actually been a human being for three months.' (Participant, Human Henge focus group)

Restoration Trust and mental well-being

Founded in 2014, the Restoration Trust promotes the use of heritage, art, and culture to assist people with mental health issues to improve their mental health; we call this 'culture therapy'. We are producers and facilitators of culture therapy in the sense that we initiate and develop projects, broker partnerships, source funding, and project-manage the resulting programmes. We also act as consultants to others who want to create similar experiences.

Since 2014 we have engaged more than 400 people with serious mental health problems in around 250 sessions, mainly focusing on work connected with archives, museums, and historic landscapes. Archives and archaeology in particular materialize an interesting creative tension between the quest for knowledge and the impossibility of total success in that quest; it is there, in the space between knowing and not knowing, that our projects make the most difference, for that is where imagination lives. Accessibility and inclusion are fundamental precepts for everything we do. Good-quality research is a hallmark of our projects, and their impact on mental health and well-being is an important focus for us throughout.

Human Henge is discussed in detail in later chapters. Here I would like to reflect on how it relates to the wider context of new approaches to heritage and mental health that both underpin and are informed by our work.

Henges and humans: Human Henge

Human Henge involved programmes of facilitated events for groups of around a dozen people who live with mental health challenges. Managed by the Restoration Trust, it ran in partnership with Bournemouth University, Richmond Fellowship, English Heritage, and the National Trust, and in association with many organizations including the Avon and Wiltshire Mental Health NHS Partnership Trust. It was funded by the Heritage Lottery Fund (now National Lottery Heritage Fund), Wiltshire County Council, and English Heritage. Three cycles were completed, two at Stonehenge from October to December 2016 and from January to March 2017, and one at Avebury from January to March 2018.

The name 'Human Henge' captures the essence of a therapeutic relationship between people and ancient places. As humans, we reach back through thousands of years to connect with other humans who used these sites over generations. Participants, support workers, volunteers, board members, funders, partners, experts, musicians, researchers and staff all do what humans have always done in ancient places. We scan the horizon from the vantage point of our upright posture and move through the landscape, walking with intent. We warm our hands, create sounds, and weave common narratives. We are sociable. We eat and laugh together. We explore our spirituality, our history, our geography. We trade, experiment, learn, share, dispute, and (sometimes) agree. Perhaps we are pilgrims; certainly, we are travellers.

In Human Henge we connected with each other through the henges and associated monuments at Stonehenge and Avebury, an area inscribed on the World Heritage List in 1986 because of its recognized Outstanding Universal Value. These are extraordinary places. They are also places where humans do ordinary things: they drive, shop, work, farm, wander about, use mobile phone. They are places where people are humans — whatever that means for the time in which they live. The combination of extraordinary and ordinary in the interaction between people and place creates the Human Henge experience.

Heritage and mental health

When considering the ways in which Human Henge affects mental health, we must remind ourselves of how devastating mental illness can be. People with serious mental health problems often die before their time; they have a 10- to 25-year reduction in life expectancy (Mental Health Foundation 2015: 89). This is partly due to suicide, as well as the impact on mental health of chronic physical illness. Social and economic factors such as poverty and poor housing also play their part. It seems that there are insufficient funds, specialists, and treatments to make any significant impact on this global crisis. Lack of social or political will may be an issue. Despite parity of esteem with physical health having been enshrined in UK law in 2012, mental health accounts for 28 per cent of the overall UK disease burden but receives only 13 per cent of NHS funding (Centre for Mental Health 2018).

While the demand for treatment is rising, provision is shrinking. National and local governments need new ways to help people with their mental health. Treatments such as medication, talking therapies, and hospitalization are being supplemented by other kinds of interventions. Activities such as walking and outdoor exercise, spending time in green spaces, music, and community involvement, can all make a positive difference. Human Henge delivers all of these and more with its additional heritage element. It counters the high well-being inequality (or lower well-being) associated with deprivation and rurality by offering better access to, and higher levels of engagement with, heritage activities and use of green space. Studies show that greater engagement with heritage and green spaces benefits people with lower life satisfaction. (Abdallah *et al.* 2017).

Heritage, in the sense of archaeology, ancient landscapes, and historic buildings, has been underused for mental health when compared to art, music, drama, and museums. It does not feature in the aims of the new Culture, Health and Wellbeing Alliance (CHWA 2018), and was barely mentioned in the All-Party Parliamentary Group on Arts, Health and Wellbeing report *Creative Health: The Arts for Health and Wellbeing* (APPGAHW 2017). Yet we have so much of it. It is all around us, visible and hidden, tangible and intangible. There are 1,302 Scheduled Monuments in Wiltshire alone. The National Trust owns 400 square miles of open access land. And 33 million people — over 74 per cent of all adults in England — visited a heritage site in 2016–17. The idea of the therapeutic landscape lies deep within us.

We have a duty, and an economic imperative, to make these assets work for mental health. Using the HACT social value calculator (HACT 2018), by relieving anxiety and depression Human Henge has a 1:9 social value ratio. Monetarized, this means that every £1 spent has had £9 of impact. According to the much-quoted 'statistic', one in four people in the UK experience a mental health problem each year (Mind 2017). This implies that each year potentially 395,000 of the 1.58 million visitors to Stonehenge (2016–17) will be affected by mental health problems. Therefore, we can assume that there is already significant mental health engagement with heritage, although it is not declared as such. And why should it be? A person's mental health status is not their whole identity.

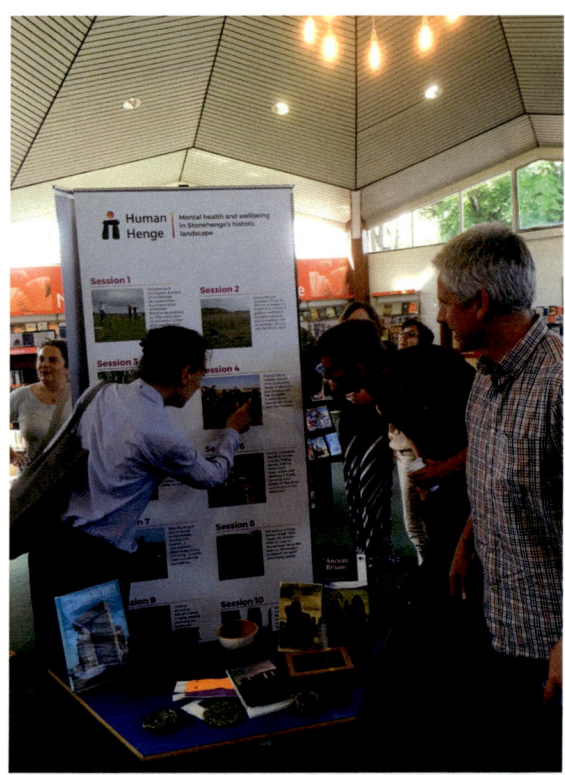

It is curious to me that, again and again, I encounter mental health and social care commissioners, and senior professionals, who talk about their own engagement with heritage at a personal level but do not connect it to the practice of their specialisms. They speak with nostalgia about their student holidays on an archaeological dig, or tell me about visiting National Trust properties to relieve stress; these are ordinary ways for ordinary people to feel well — to feel human as the words cited at the head of this chapter reveal. But why do these

Figure 5.1 The Human Henge travelling exhibition at Amesbury Town Library, May 2017. (Photograph by Timothy Darvill, Human Henge project. Copyright reserved)

health professionals not support the people they serve by encouraging them to do the same to assist their recovery, as an ordinary part of provision?

There is clearly a need to promote projects that use cultural heritage to enhance mental health and well-being to wider audiences, to increase public awareness of what is possible. Accordingly, we included an outreach and communication programme within the Human Henge project. Table 5.A summarizes the numerous events undertaken. Picking a few highlights, we were

Table 5.A A Summary of the outreach activities and media coverage relating to the Human Henge project 2017-2019

Activity	Details
Conferences and conference sessions	'Being human: Walking and well-being in ancient landscapes' paper at the *Archaeology in Wiltshire Conference*, Devizes, 23 March 2019
	Presentation of Human Henge at the *National Womens' Register* regional conference, Salisbury, 6 October 2018
	Full day conference *Historic Landscapes and Mental Wellbeing*, Bournemouth University, 13 April 2018
	Presentation of Human Henge at the *West of England Learning Symposium Conference*, 6 March 2018
	Half-day session entitled 'Archaeology, Heritage and Well-being' Building 'Brickhenge' at the *Theoretical Archaeology Group (TAG) Annual Meeting*, Cardiff University, 19 December 2017
	'Human Henge: Cultural heritage therapy and its impact upon mental health and well-being' paper at the *Humanising Conference*, Bournemouth University, 29–30 June 2017
	'Human Henge: Cultural heritage therapy in action' paper at the *Culture, Health and Well-being Conference*, Bristol University, 19 June 2017
Lectures, seminars, and presentations	Heritage and Wellbeing Workshop, University of Canterbury, Human Henge presentation, 7–8 June 2018.
	'Human Henge and Heritage Well-being.' Lecture to the Stonehenge and Avebury History and Archaeology Research Group Meeting, Devizes Museum, 2 June 2017.
	Cultural heritage and therapy in action.' Public lecture in the Stonehenge Education Room, Stonehenge, 27 March 2017
Participation in festivals and open days	Wiltshire Farm Open Day, Temple Farm, Marlborough, Wiltshire, Human Henge exhibition, 10 June 2018
	World Heritage Day Human Henge walk at Avebury, 20 April 2018
	Trowbridge Users Group Human Henge discussion, 12 March 2018
	University of the Third Age lecture at Bournemouth University, 11 September 2017
	Heritage Open Day, Stonehenge, 8 September 2017
	Festival of Archaeology, Salisbury Museum. Human Henge Exhibition, building Brickhenge activity, and Human Henge workshop. 22–23 July 2017
	Human Henge Sharing Event, Wiltshire Museum, Devizes, 25 May 2017

Activity	Details
Human Henge mobile exhibition	Wiltshire Museum, Devizes, July 2018
	Marlborough Library, 14 – 29 June 2018
	National Trust Avebury Visitor Centre, 17 May – 10 June 2018
	Devizes Library, 6 – 17 November 2017
	Chippenham Library, 16 October – 30 October 2017
	Melksham Library, 2 October – 16 October 2017
	Salisbury Library, 18 September – 2 October 2017
	English Heritage Stonehenge Visitor Centre 24 July – 3 September 2017
	Green Lane Hospital, Devizes, 20 June – 20 July 2017
	Amesbury Library, 25 May – 6 June 2017
Magazine articles, reviews, case studies, blogs, internet presence	Human Henge Twitter feed: https://twitter.com/humanhenge 2019
	Human Henge Facebook page: https://www.facebook.com/humanhenge/ 2018
	Heritage and Health, Heritage Alliance report (forthcoming late 2018) Case Study
	Heritage Lottery Fund, Human Henge Stonehenge case study, 2018
	Case Study: Restoration Trust – Human Henge. In: *Museums as Spaces for Wellbeing. A second report by the Alliance for Museums, Health and Wellbeing*, 2018: 37
	How Stonehenge can improve mental health and well-being. *HLF Website: News Features and blogs.* Posted: 21 June 2018
	The Guardian Website, 21 December 2017
	Creative Arty Facts from the Human Henge project. Guest blog by Mr BPD, *Arts in Wiltshire website.* Posted 1 September 2017
	The People I Meet: Human Henge. *My Weekly*, Summer Special, 2017
	Human Henge: Cultural heritage therapy in action. *Megalith*, 6 (Summer 2017): 20–21
	Human Henge. *Current Archaeology*, 329 (July 2017): 44–46
	Stonehenge visits can be 'cultural therapy'. *English Heritage Members Magazine*, May 2017: 12
	Human Henge: How can historic landscapes be good for you? *English Heritage website: Your stories.* Posted: 21 April 2017
	English Heritage Staff Newsletter, March 2017
Radio and television reports	BBC Radio Wiltshire. News item, May 2017
	BBC Breakfast News, 22 March 2017
	BBC1 Points West. News item, first screened 27 March 2017
	BBC Radio 4. Open Country. Interview and commentary, first broadcast 21 April 2017

Activity	Details
Publications and reports	Heaslip, V., Mahdaninia, M. Hind, T. Darvill, Y. Staelens, D. O'Donoghue, L. Drysdale, S. Lunt, C. Hogg, M. Allfrey, B.Clifton and T. Sutcliffe, Forthcoming. Locating oneself in the past to influence the present: Impacts of Neolithic landscapes on mental health well-being. *Health and Place*
	Heaslip, V. and T. Darvill, 2019. *Human Henge Wellbeing Research: Findings Group 3. 1 Year post involvement* [Unpublished printed report. 34pp]
	Heaslip, V. and T. Darvill, 2018. *Human Henge Wellbeing Research: Final Report* [Online document]. Viewed 4 February 2019, <http://eprints.bournemouth.ac.uk/31571/> .
	Drysdale, L., 2018. *Human Henge Evaluation Report for the Heritage Lottery Fund* [Online document]. Viewed 4 February 2019, <https://humanhenge.org/2019/01/30/human-henge-evaluation-report/>.
	Darvill, T. and V. Heaslip, 2017. *Human Henge Wellbeing Research: First report*. Bournemouth: Bournemouth University and Human Henge project. [Unpublished printed report. 20pp]
	Darvill, T., V. Heaslip and K. Barrass, 2018. Heritage and wellbeing: therapeutic places, past and present. In. K. Galvin (ed.) *Handbook of Well-being*. Abingdon: Routledge. 112–123

Heaslip, V., Mahdaninia, M. Hind, T. Darvill, Y. Staelens, D. O'Donoghue, L. Drysdale, S. Lunt, C. Hogg, M. Allfrey, B.Clifton, T. Sutcliffe Forthcoming. Locating oneself in the past to influence the present: Impacts of Neolithic landscapes on mental health well-being. *Health and Place*

the subject of a BBC Radio 4 'Open Country' broadcast in April 2017 that reached 1.27 million listeners (BBC 2017). The project featured on local TV and radio, and on the websites run by *The Guardian* (2017), English Heritage (EH 2017), and the Heritage Lottery Fund (HFL 2018). A small but powerful exhibition toured sites, events, and public libraries across Wiltshire, and was seen by around 44,000 people (Figure 5.1). And we also took a stand at the Festival of Archaeology in Salisbury in July 2017 where with the help of visitors we built a 'Brickhenge' to promote the project (Figure 5.2). Overall, we estimate that some 2.3 million people have heard about the project through the media.

Human Henge and Mental Well-being

Our grant applications to the Heritage Lottery Fund stated that Human Henge would develop upon the Five Ways to Wellbeing suggested by the New Economic Foundation (NEF 2008):

- Take notice: People — that is the whole group — have an intense sensory experience of the historic landscape; they touch, smell, taste, listen, look and hear. They care about each other's welfare, they feel for each other, they watch out for each other.
- Be active: Walking once a week, the groups get out and about in the landscapes surrounding ancient monuments. They walk further and more confidently, session by session; they climb hills, go underground, cross streams and plunge into snowdrifts. They are walking with intent.

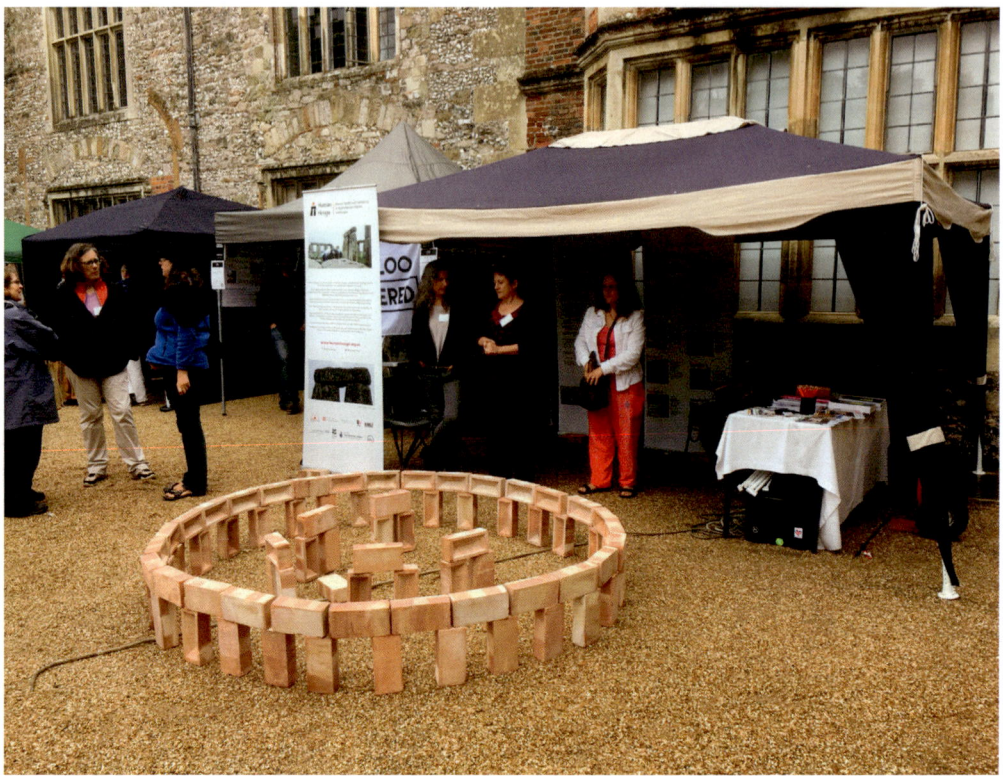

Figure 5.2 'Brickhenge' at the Festival of Archaeology in Salisbury, July 2017. (Photograph by Timothy Darvill, Human Henge project. Copyright reserved)

- Connect: People make connections across deep time; with the ancestors, with the stars, the stones and the music, with the place they live, and with each other. Connecting is a risk because it always threatens loss, and people do really feel that loss when the sessions end. Imagine the courage to take that risk, when loss has been so dangerous in the past.
- Learn: People learn about archaeology, music, nature and the history of a place that matters to them. This is a real learning experience, a real encounter with knowledge that can be trusted. We believe in English Heritage's values: 'We seek to be true to the story of the places and artefacts that we look after and present. We don't exaggerate or make things up for entertainment's sake. Instead, through careful research, we separate fact from fiction and bring fascinating truth to light' (EH 2018). People also learn how to be with a group again, meeting new people and getting to know them.
- Give: The whole group shares stories, music, poetry, experiences and songs. Individuals disclose things about their personal lives, they give their fellows time, help others get to sessions, speak in public, write on the blog and take photographs.

Jane Willis, Director of the arts and health consultancy Willis Newson and commissioned as a critical friend to Human Henge, theorizes that Human Henge worked because it established a cycle of transformative processes. These can be summarized as: safety and trust; challenge and risk; achievement and confidence; connection; structures; and good communication. Safety and trust are built by secure partnerships. Challenge and risk are mediated through expert facilitation. Achievement is gained through having met and overcome challenges that lead to increased self-confidence and self-esteem. The experience of taking part — of being seen — is shared. Positive feedback in response to this visibility enhances the sense of connectedness. Enhanced connection leads to an increased feeling of safety and trust. New risk and challenge is introduced, and the cycle continues. A deeper sense of achievement leads to increased self-esteem, continued sharing leads to deeper connections, deeper connection and bonding leads to an increased sense of safety. And so on.

It seems that many people with mental health problems would feel better if they engaged with heritage in a meaningful way. And from the other end of the telescope, many heritage assets could be used to help people with mental health problems feel better.

A psychodynamic view of Human Henge

Human Henge also meets the Restoration Trust's own self-defined criteria for success, which can be summarized as follows:

- Participants have problems with their mental health
- Participants are included in management
- Partnership with cultural and health organisations
- Groupwork is the core
- Safe framework and practice
- Proper measurement of impact and outcomes
- Sustained and regular involvement
- Privileged access to real cultural assets and expertise
- Encouragement to be creative
- Learning for staff and volunteers
- Progression for participants

Some are obvious, some less so, but here I want to look at three in more detail in relation to the experiences of Human Henge: Groupwork; Privileged access to real cultural assets and expertise; and Encouragement to be creative.

Groupwork is the core

Over ten weeks of sustained and regular involvement within a context of safe frameworks and practice, and with expert facilitation from Yvette Staelens with Daniel O'Donoghue, a group began to form. Foulkes (1946) describes what happens when a collection of individuals meets routinely together with someone he named a conductor:

> 'They will begin to live, feel, think, act and talk more in terms of "we" than in terms of "I", "you", and "he". At the same time, and I want to stress this point, the individuals do not become submerged but, on the contrary, show up their personal characteristics more and more distinctly within the dynamic interplay of an every changing and often highly dramatic scene. As soon as this little sample community shows signs of organization and structure in the way described, we will call it a group'. (Foulkes 1946, *)

This is what we were trying to achieve through Human Henge.

Privileged access to real cultural assets and expertise

How does a historic or archaeological landscape help? It is only human to be in nature, to use our bodies and minds, to connect with each other and to be creative. It is certainly better than some of the alternatives, such as loneliness, boredom, and sadness. But why 'historic'? Why 'archaeological'? Why 'ancient'? Why does it help to have the company of people who know a lot about it?

Mental illness can attack mental space, filling it with rumination or psychosis, or negating it with both restlessness and passivity in depression. It makes space malignant, so that it cannot be traversed to connect with others. Flashbacks in post-traumatic stress disorder (PTSD) collapse time, as the past overwhelms the present. Without space to think, to act, nothing creative can happen; there can be no imagination, no relating. A group experience of a historic or archaeological landscape, illuminated by people who know about it, opens up multiple vistas of temporal, topographical and psychological space. These are based on reality rather than on disabling fantasy or memory. It is not a universal prescription, for not everyone is interested in the past. But for those who are, and who can find the strength to face the daunting prospect of a project like Human Henge, historic and archaeological landscapes are one way to face down mental illness's erosion of the self.

Encouragement to be creative

Human Henge's music, photography, clay work, and creative writing activities occupy what Winnicott (1971) called 'potential space'. This is the place between subject and object that he saw as the crucible of creativity, where frustration can be tolerated and thought can thrive. Expanding into potential space from the restrictions of mental illness enables people to be playful, curious and rebellious, private and personal, spiritual and sensual. If we share these characteristics with the ancestors who made and used these irreducibly mysterious places, perhaps Human Henge echoes something of their existence in its physical embodiment of an interior landscape.

Call to action

We plan to run or to mentor more Human Henge projects, with more participants, in more ancient landscapes. The aim of this is to gather sufficient robust quantitative and qualitative data that we persuade health and social care commissioners to confidently prescribe this as a therapeutic activity. It is intended that the facilitated experiences of walking with intent in historic landscapes on the Human Henge model should be an accepted approach to improve the well-being of people living with mental health problems.

As other papers in this volume illustrate, archaeology and historic landscapes can offer distinct mental health benefits to people who have the lowest levels of well-being in our society. Such intriguing initiatives, with their common ethos of accessibility, inclusion, and well-being, are far more than mere fireworks in the night sky, blazing brightly before disappearing without trace. The Culture, Health and Wellbeing Alliance shows what can be achieved by assimilating case studies and evidence accrued over many years so that the results become politically visible. We now need a comprehensive initiative to integrate archaeology and historic landscapes into mental health and well-being provision through NHS social prescribing, local authority cultural commissioning, and through the actions of the heritage sector itself.

To draw these ideas together I will finish with three short poems by Chris Jessup, a volunteer in Human Henge.

I

Early in our first encounter,
Claire declared herself a nutter
Ten weeks have passed without a sign
Of anything like, so malign.

II

We all went on the cursus, walking
Tim guiding us, with much talking.
In the eve the stars shone bright
Giving us a gentle light.
Later on, a mist arose,
Making all mysterious.

III

Are your emotions healthy?
Have you had your MOT?
I expect that you are wondering
What on earth these letters be.
Why, it's the Mental Opportunities Tuning
From the Human Henge Degree.

Bibliography

Abdallah, S., H. Wheatley and A. Quick 2017. Drivers of wellbeing inequality. Inequality in life satisfaction across local authorities in Great Britain [Webpage]. Viewed 6 December 2018, <https://whatworkswellbeing.org/product/drivers-of-wellbeing-inequality/>.

APPGAHW 2017. The arts for health and wellbeing [Webpage]. Viewed 6 December 2018, <https://www.artshealthandwellbeing.org.uk/appg-inquiry/>.

BBC 2017. Open Country: Stonehenge and mental health [Webpage]. Viewed 6 December 2018, <https://www.bbc.co.uk/programmes/b08md98n>.

Centre for Mental Health 2018. What would a long-term funding settlement for the NHS mean for mental health? [Blog]. Viewed 23 October 2018, <https://www.centreformentalhealth.org.uk/blog/centre-mental-health-blog/what-would-long-term-funding-settlement-nhs-mean-mental-health>.

CHWA 2018. *The Culture, Health and Wellbeing Alliance Business Plan 2018–22* [Online document]. Topsham, Devon: Arts and Health South West. Viewed 6 December 2018, <https://ahsw.org.uk/userfiles/CHWA/CHWA%20Business%20Plan%20January%2031%202018.pdf>.

EH 2017. Human Henge: How can historic landscapes be good for you? [Webpage]. Viewed 6 December 2018, <http://blog.english-heritage.org.uk/human-henge-how-can-a-historic-landscape-be-good-for-you/>.

EH 2018. Our vision & values: Authenticity [Webpage]. Viewed 6 December 2018, <https://www.english-heritage.org.uk/about-us/our-values/>.

Foulkes, S.H. 1946. On group analysis. *International Journal of Psychoanalysis* 27: 46–51.

The Guardian 2017. Hundreds gather for Stonehenge sunrise after winter solstice [Webpage]. Viewed 6 December 2018, <https://www.theguardian.com/uk-news/2017/dec/22/hundreds-gather-for-stonehenge-sunrise-after-winter-solstice>.
HACT 2018. UK Social Value Bank Calculator 4.0 [Webpage]. Viewed 6 December 2018, <https://www.hact.org.uk/value-calculator>.
HLF 2018. Human Henge: Historic landscapes and mental health at Stonehenge [Webpage]. Viewed 6 December 2018, <https://www.hlf.org.uk/our-projects/human-henge-historic-landscapes-and-mental-health-stonehenge>.
Mental Health Foundation 2015. *Fundamental facts about mental health 2015* [Online document]. London: Mental Health Foundation. Viewed 6 December 2018, <https://www.mentalhealth.org.uk/sites/default/files/fundamental-facts-15.pdf>.
Mind 2017. Mental health facts and statistics [Webpage]. Viewed 6 December 2018, <https://www.mind.org.uk/information-support/types-of-mental-health-problems/statistics-and-facts-about-mental-health/how-common-are-mental-health-problems/>.
NEF 2008. Five ways to wellbeing: The evidence [Webpage]. Viewed 6 December 2018, <https://neweconomics.org/2008/10/five-ways-to-wellbeing-the-evidence>.
Winnicott, D.W. 1971. *Playing and reality*. London: Tavistock Publications.

Chapter 6

Monuments for life: Building Human Henge at Stonehenge and Avebury

Timothy Darvill

Abstract

Human Henge was built from two key ideas. First, that Stonehenge, and many other prehistoric and later sites like it, were originally places of healing. And second, that ancient sites can and should have a wide range of societally relevant uses in the modern world. Both ideas are explored here in some detail in order to highlight key themes that were woven together in the development of Human Henge's cultural heritage therapy. This used the iconic sites of Stonehenge and Avebury and their surrounding landscapes as arenas within which participants could be creative while safely exploring places in unfamiliar ways. Through programmes of participant-led activities, local people living with mental health problems came together for fun and therapeutic adventures, assisted by experts, carers, support workers, and contributors from a range of different cultures. By journeying through the World Heritage Site, spending time at a selection of the monuments, thinking, talking, singing, dancing, and making music, it became possible for them to connect with the landscape, the skyscape, the archaeology, and, most importantly, to re-connect with themselves and with other participants.

Keywords: Avebury; Healing; Mental health; Stonehenge; Well-being

Introduction

Two quite different strands of thinking, one interpretative and one creative, came together in an unexpected coalition in response to the question of how heritage could be used to enhance mental well-being. They provided the theoretical and academic underpinnings for what became Human Henge. First, was the idea that, like many ancient sites, Stonehenge was a place of healing whose importance to prehistoric people was derived in no small measure from the power of the exotic bluestones imported to the site from the Preseli Mountains of southwest Wales (Darvill 2007; Darvill and Wainwright 2014). Second, an axiom of the intersection between archaeological resource management, sustainable development, creative conservation, and the realization of public value, was the idea that heritage assets need a purpose and a role in the modern world (EH 2008; Hill 2016). Ancient monuments, and the historic landscapes in which they lie, should somehow 'pay their way' by contributing to the needs of today's society; not just as curiosities of the ancient world but also as arenas for social action, creative spaces, re-creation/recreation zones, places of memory, pathways to the past, and potentially much more beside.

In fact both these ideas connect with wider webs of study and debate; they are explored in the following sections and provide the background to the ways in which Human Henge took form and developed. Attention is then directed to the pilot programmes of cultural heritage therapy undertaken in the Stonehenge and Avebury World Heritage Site. The elements examined include the programmes' aims, how they were created, and what they comprised, from theoretical and operational perspectives. The activities themselves are described and illustrated from the view-points of the facilitators and the participants in Chapters 7 and 8 by Yvette Staelens and Danny O'Donoghue respectively; the well-being outcomes of the programmes are discussed in Chapter 9 by Vanessa Heaslip. Finally, in considering cultural heritage therapy in this way we ask what can be learnt from the pilot programmes, and whether there is a role for developing the idea further as a contribution to the societal needs of the twenty-first century.

Heritage, Health, and Healing

Health and well-being are amongst the most fundamental of human concerns, fully embracing the welfare of body, mind, and soul. They relate not only to the individual self but also to a shared emotional state that extends to fellow human beings — especially close family and loved-ones. Natural and constructed places connected with healing the body, mind, and soul have existed for millennia, although archaeological interpretations of such places have tended to favour generalizing notions of 'ritual' and 'ceremony'. This avoids the specifics of what those people who built and used such places were actually doing; what were their intentions, and their hopes and dreams. With a few notable exceptions (e.g. Gemi-Iordanou *et al.* 2014; Michaelides 2014), archaeologists have tended to circumvent the reality that many monuments were built as venues for healing. Stepping outside the twenty-first century western world, whether into the traditions of non-western contemporary societies or into the customs of earlier societies, is illuminating and emphasizes the non-medicalized nature of many approaches to health and well-being.

Enforcing modern binary oppositions between science and religious beliefs presents a fundamental stumbling block in the search for ways of improving well-being in general, and mental health well-being in particular. It obstructs the recognition and understanding of the potential power afforded by integrative approaches. Important here is the idea of building bridges between the physical and the spiritual in order to promote and enhance health and healing. Benjamin Koen vividly shows how this is done using music and prayer amongst communities living in the towering Pamir Mountains of Badakhshan straddling parts of Tajikistan, Afghanistan, and China (Koen 2009). In other cases water becomes the bridge, and it is notable that scared springs and holy wells have been widely recognized as powerful and therapeutic places for generations. Many have biographies stretching deep into ancient times, as illustrated for example by sites in Ireland (Foley 2010; Ray 2014) and Wales (Jones 1992). Interestingly, it was ancient and historic sites closely connected with springs — the birthplace of Asclepius the Healer at Epidauros in Greece, and the Marian Apparitio at the Massabielle Grotto at Lourdes in France — that provided the case studies from which Will Gesler developed the valuable and almost universal bridging concept of the *therapeutic landscape* (Gesler 1993; 1996; 2003; Kearns and Gesler 1998). Such areas, whether large or small, constructed or natural, embrace the healing powers of specific sites, the activities undertaken there, connections between place and well-being, and how the process of healing works itself out through people's subjective experiences of their surroundings.

Variously drawing on ideas from cultural ecology, structuralism, phenomenology, and humanism, the study of therapeutic landscapes has become a major interdisciplinary field. It creates intersections between geography, anthropology, health-care, nursing, architecture, landscape design, and many other disciplines beside (Gesler 2003; Williams 2007). Sadly, in keeping with rather guarded attitudes to such matters, archaeology as a discipline has contributed very little to the debate so far. But from an archaeological perspective it is interesting that, right across the world, places associated with healing and miracles often have roots running deep into the ancient past. These places have been appropriated and re-appropriated by successive cultures that valued and understood the traditions, power, and meanings in terms of human well-being that they inherited (literally, their heritage).

Re-winding the history of therapeutic places and landscapes in Britain involves a journey through some of its most famous historic environments. Only a small selection can be considered here, but they illustrate the point that so much of what we see as heritage assets relate in one way or another to well-being, health, and healing for the body and mind. As a starting point it may be noted that during the late seventeenth, eighteenth, nineteenth, and early twentieth centuries, the architectural design of many hospitals and asylums focused on ways of facilitating the healing process (Rutherford 2004; 2005; Stevenson 2000). Buildings, many of which are still with us, were constructed with such purposes to the fore, as too the associated gardens and recreational area (Hickman 2013). One of the best documented examples from the nineteenth century is Brislington House in Bristol, opened as a private asylum in 1806 (Hickman 2005: 47). Landscape features designed by Edward Long Fox included pathways, walks, leisure facilities, and a grotto, all created in the hope of improving the emotional state of the resident patients (Hickman 2005: 59). Spas also featured strongly in the therapeutic landscapes of the post-medieval period. The fashionable and widely experienced London doctor Augustus Granville published a guide to English spas in 1841, documenting hundreds of examples large and small in three volumes (Granville 1841). Bath was one of the most famous with its hot springs bubbling out mineral-rich water at a constant 46 degrees centigrade, and a history of use stretching back into prehistory (Cunliffe 1986; Gesler 1998).

In medieval times the Christian Church played a leading role in healthcare, with its many nunneries, monasteries, minsters, and abbeys providing support through the provision of hospitals and infirmaries. As Roberta Gilchrist has remarked, all hospitals were at least semi-religious due to the believed connection between spiritual and physical disease (1994: 173). The Knights Hospitallers, also known as the Order of Knights of the Hospital of St John of Jerusalem, emerged in the early twelfth century, initially to care for the sick, poor or injured on pilgrimage to the Holy Land. Its influence and patronage spread, and around 40 priories, preceptories, and commanderies of the Order are known in England (King 1967: 83–84). It has been estimated that by the time of Dissolution in the 1530s there were more 800 hospitals of all denominations in England (Gilchrist 1994: 173). Archaeologically, it has been possible to examine the form and layout of the buildings within and around the cloister, and of course the well-filled burial grounds where, sooner or later, many of the patients ended up (Gilchrist and Sloane 2005). Gardens were important as recuperative places, and as sources for herbal remedies. And from well before AD 1400, specialists such as the physicians of Meddygon Myddfai in northern Carmarthenshire built their reputation by fusing traditional knowledge with borrowings from the classical literature to create a magico-medical science (Davies and Owen 1975).

Alongside the routine treatment and care of the sick and infirm in hospitals and infirmaries were the healing centres or cult places famous for miraculous cures through associations with holy relics, and, in more recent times, the work of those deemed close to God (Duffin 2009; Scott 2010). Many healing centres great and small were associated with the act of pilgrimage:

a physical journey to a place that is significant to a person's beliefs, made in order to connect with the power of the place or imitate the actions of archetypal beings. The aim is usually spiritual renewal, emotional enrichment, renunciation of the past, guidance about the future, performing a rite of passage, or seeking physical and spiritual healing (Armstrong 2012; Darvill 2016: 155). At a local level Nicholas Orme lists more than 80 such destinations in the five counties of southwest England alone (2018). Beyond them were many nationally recognized centres, for example: Canterbury, Kent, with the tomb of Archbishop Thomas Beckett; Walsingham, Norfolk, with its shrines to the Virgin Mary and a phial of her milk; or Salisbury, Wiltshire, with the shrine of Bishop Osmund offering medical cures (Webb 2000). Further afield still there was: Santiago d'Compostella in Galicia, northern Spain, with a finger-bone of St James (Roux 2004; Shaver-Crandell and Gerson 1995); Rome, Italy, with the tombs of the apostles St Peter and St Paul (Birch 2000); and of course Jerusalem, Israel, where the Pool of Siloam and Temple Mount are sacred in Judaism, Christianity, and Islam (Chareyron 2005). Pilgrimage also features in many major religions across the world, for example: the Islamic Hajj to Mecca with its holy spring (Well of Abraham) and central Kaaba with the sacred Black Stone on its eastern corner (Peters 1994; Porter 2012); Cahuachi, Peru, as a centre for early Nasca cults (Silverman 1994); and the Buddhist temples at Kanhari in western India (Ray 1994). Journeying, being out in the open air, and exploring new places, are all core themes running through the therapeutic value of pilgrimage at all scales.

Of course the Christian Church often appropriated and reused existing holy places, sites that were already well-known as healing centres and which take us back into the pre-Christian era. An example is the convent established at Bath around AD 675 that became a Benedictine monastery in the late tenth century. It gained cathedral status in 1090, by which time its cherished possessions included chains that (allegedly) fettered St Peter in prison, that were shown or lent to pregnant women to ensure an easy delivery. But the popularity, power, wealth, and prestige of Bath Abbey in medieval times arguably derived from its proximity to, and connections with, the far earlier Roman bath complex. Parts of these earlier structures continued to be used, and Bishop Reginald (1174–1191) founded the hospital of St John nearby to care for the poor and sick (Orme 2018: 142). Excavations directed by Barry Cunliffe around the King's Bath Spring revealed substantial accumulations of votive offerings starting in the late first century BC. By the early first century AD, a polygonal stone-walled reservoir was built to contain the hot water from the spring before it was channelled off for use in the adjacent bath-block to the south (Cunliffe 1980: 190–193; Cunliffe and Davenport 1985: 39–45). Dedicated to the goddess Sulis-Minerva, the temple precinct to the north of the spring was no doubt the source of both the votive offerings and the divine power invoked to promote healing and wisdom (Cunliffe 1995: 55).

Bath was not unique in being a centre of healing during Romano-British times, and Anne Ross and Miranda Green emphasize the important link between healing cults and water and sacred springs at this time, and back into the first millennium BC (Green 1986: 150–166; Ross 1967: 20–33). Sites such as Coventina's Well beside Hadrian's Wall, Northumberland (Allason-Jones and McKay 1985) and the temple of the healer-god Nodens at Lydney beside the River Severn in Gloucestershire (Aldhouse-Green and Aldhouse-Green 2005: 162) represent prime examples. But how far back can we go?

Direct evidence for healing rituals at sites going back into prehistory is slight, although, as noted above, that may in part result from a reluctance on the part of prehistorians to explore such topics.

There may have been a belief in the healing power of supernatural forces mediated through talismanic objects such as charms or amulets, or spiritual guides such as might be referred to as shamans, magicians, sorcerers, priests, medicine-men/women, or witch-doctors. It is tempting to push the significance of Bath as a healing centre back into the Mesolithic and Neolithic as worked flints were found scattered on the natural gravel bank surrounding the spring at the King's Bath (Cunliffe and Davenport 1985: 8–9) and in greater quantities near the Cross Bath Spring (Davenport *et al.* 2007: 145–149). An early Bronze Age axe-hammer made of rock from the Lake District was found at Coventina's Well hinting at early use of the site, although again its context and associations are far from clear (Allason-Jones and McKay 1985: 19–20).

Folklore and ethnography support the idea that many prehistoric sites across northwest Europe included healing amongst their key roles as perceived by those who built and used them. Leslie Grinsell (1976: 15–16) notes that, right across Britain, standing stones, stone settings, and appropriated natural rocks are believed to have healing properties, especially those with holes in them such as: the Long Stone at Minchinhampton, Gloucestershire; the Men-an-Tol, Cornwall (Figure 6.1); and the Tolvan Stone, Cornwall. Mention has already been made of sacred springs and holy wells with Roman and later associations that are associated with healing; it is notable that a few examples are associated with cup-marks and cup-and-ring style rock art broadly datable to the fourth, third, and second millennia BC. Amongst recorded examples are two in Pembrokeshire: St Non's Well near St David's (Bennett-Samuels and Evans 2008) and Ffynnon Beswch on Carn Sian (Darvill *et al.* 2004: 106–108).

The case for thinking about Stonehenge, Wiltshire, as a place of healing partly rests on the folklore embedded in the writings of the twelfth century monk Geoffrey of Monmouth. He

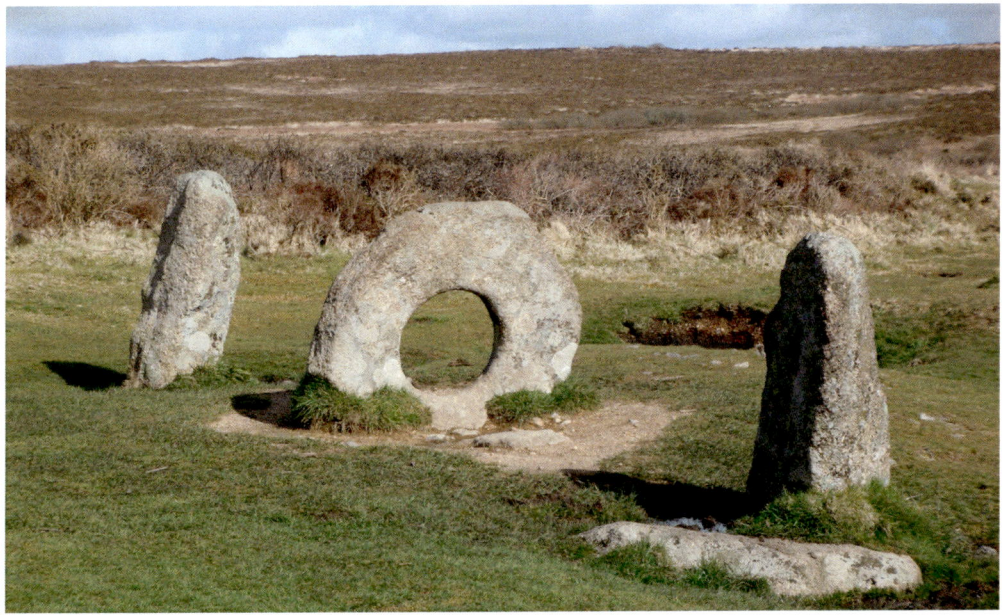

Figure 6.1. The Men-an-Tol, Ladron, Cornwall. The stones were possibly once part of a stone circle. Tradition holds that the central perforated stone has healing powers. (Photograph by Timothy Darvill. Copyright reserved)

asserted, through the voice of Merlin the Magician, that particular stones were brought to Salisbury Plain because of their healing powers (Thorpe 1966: 196). Sacred springs and holy wells are closely associated with the source outcrops of these 'Bluestones' in the Preseli Hills of west Wales, and water is associated with Stonehenge by way of the Avenue that physically connects the monument with Stonehenge Bottom and the River Avon (Darvill 2006: 158–161). The arrangement of the small Bluestone pillars forming the Outer Bluestone Circle just inside the ring of 30 massive sarsen uprights with gaps between (the Sarsen Circle), restricts access to them. It means that anyone standing on the outside can see the Bluestones, feel their presence, experience their power, but cannot quite touch them. Curiously, less than 10 km south of Stonehenge is the prehistoric and later fortified hilltop settlement of Old Sarum, where healing miracles are well attested. In the early Norman period a magnificent cathedral was built by Bishop Osmund, a holy man who was buried there in AD 1099 (RCHME 1980: 19). Accordingly to Papal records, healing miracles began to occur at his tomb about a century after his death, and Daphne Stroud (1984: 51) suggests that the tomb was already a place of resort for the sick and afflicted well before that time, and that locally at least, Osmund was considered a saint by the early thirteenth century even though he was not officially canonized until AD 1457. His remains were translated to the new cathedral at Salisbury in 1226 where they were incorporated into an elaborate shrine within the Lady Chapel. Healing miracles continued (see Scott 2010: xv–xvi for examples), but the cult of the saint was abolished at the

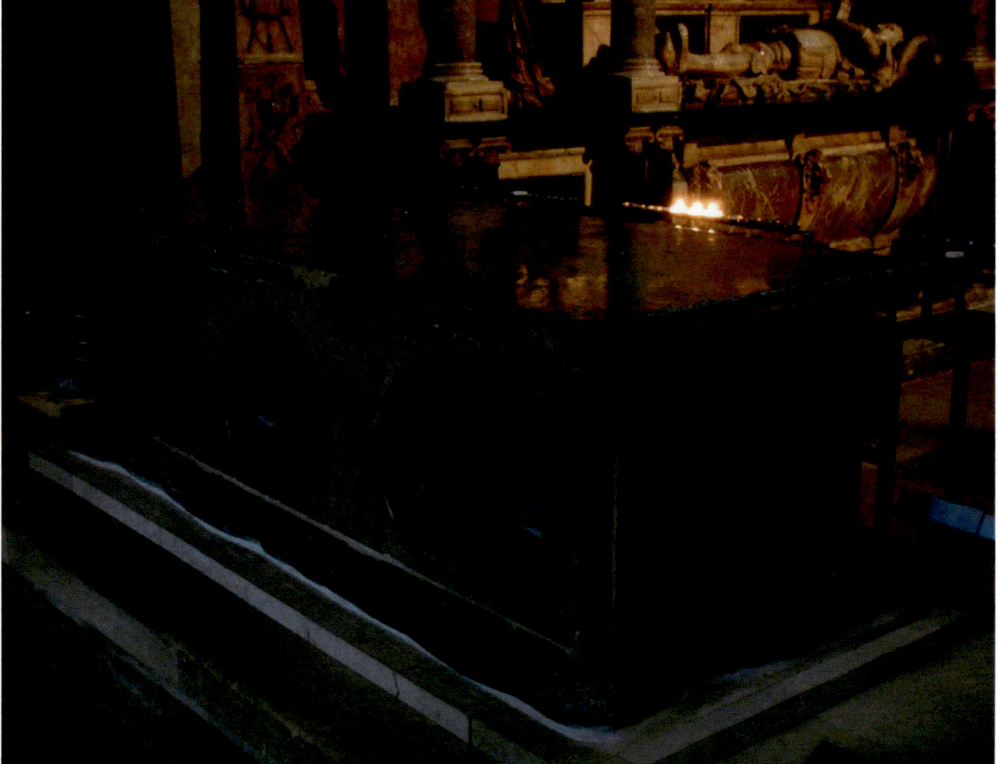

Figure 6.2. The remains of St Osmond's Shrine in the south aisle of Salisbury Cathedral, Wiltshire, showing three round kneeling-holes (foramina) allowing pilgrims to place parts of their body close to the central sarcophagus. (Photograph by Timothy Darvill. Copyright reserved)

Reformation and little of the shrine survived the Dissolution. What remained now lies in the south nave arcade: a Purbeck marble table-topped structure, probably the base of the shrine (Figure 6.2). It has three round kneeling-holes (*foramina*) on each side, common at the time but very reminiscent of the arrangement of sarsens and bluestones at Stonehenge, allowing sick or crippled pilgrims to place parts of their body against the central sarcophagus in the hope that proximity to the bones would effect a miraculous cure (Stroud 1984: 50).

Connections between the world of the living and power over life and death was held in the hands of the gods (for example Lug, Thor, and Wodan), and are central themes of North European folklore and tradition (Davidson 1988: 91). This may be reflected in the architecture, construction, and placement of shrines and sanctuaries. In the Mediterranean, the Bronze Age Cretan peak sanctuaries, for example, rich in finds of anatomical models, have long been recognized as healing centres (Morris and Peatfield 2014). Likewise, Ömür Harmanşah has argued that Hittite spring sanctuaries and rock monuments in Anatolia were powerful places where miraculous healing events took place, in the same way as those at later healing sites (2015: 9). No doubt similar events played out at Neolithic and early Bronze Age sites across Britain. Following excavations and surveys at the Thornborough Henges, North Yorkshire, for example, Jan Harding rather cautiously concluded that the 'monuments served to impress the spirit world and worshipper alike, and by so doing, enabled a meaningful religious dialogue between both parties' (Harding 2013: 217). Drawing on early Neolithic finds from within and around the main causewayed enclosure on Hambledon Hill, Dorset, Ffion Reynolds (2014) suggests that the manipulation of human remains here indicates shamanic rituals connected with healing.

All this takes us back to the need for 'bridges' within the therapeutic landscape so that things and behaviours can connect participants with the powers of the cosmos. These are in a sense the 'ritual' items so beloved of archaeology that are so much more (see Merrifield 1987: 1–21): badges and insignia were worn by pilgrims (Blick 2007); sacred stones carried to small islands (Harbison 1994: 102) or used to franchise shrines far away from their magical sources (Insoll 2006); or flasks of holy water collected at sacred springs or rivers taken home to transmit purity and holiness (Oestigaard 2017). And behind these physical traits it is also worth remembering the intangible cultural heritage of healing that bridges time and space: the food, drink, dress, song, and music, as well as ceremonies and rituals preparing the body for its journey through washing, shaving, and perfuming (Haleem 2012).

There is much more to be done in thinking about both the tangible and intangible heritage of healing in prehistoric times. However, emerging out the many and varied current understandings of the archaeological, ethnographic, and historical record, are a handful of key themes that were carried forward as contributions to building the Human Henge experience:

- Journeying with aim of moving through landscapes in space and time
- Stimulating the imagination through sensory activities
- Creating new positive and worthwhile memories to hold onto
- Bonding individuals with each other to create larger groupings
- Bridging physical and emotional states of being

All of these elements are important in their own right, but combining them involves creating something new, something for the modern world and living participants; it involves making heritage work for today.

Living Heritage

Through the 1980s and 1990s traditional (largely positivist) attitudes to the management of archaeological sites, aimed at simply protecting and preserving physical remains, were challenged and superseded by more dynamic and democratic (largely relativist) approaches. These were grounded in what might be called 'constructive conservation' and the recognition that heritage management is much more than looking after the fossilized remains of the past (Darvill 1987; Ucko 1994). Implicit in much of this new thinking was an acceptance that the Western Gaze gave a distorted view of the past by perpetuating an essentially imperialist perspective of heritage in which there was just one authorized take on how it should be looked after and what it all meant (Richardson and Almansa-Sánchez 2015: 194–195). David Lowenthal memorably referred to the 'past as a foreign country' in his book of the same name, arguing forcefully that the past had ceased to be a sanction for inherited power or privilege, but rather had become a focus for personal and national identity and a bulwark against distressing change (Lowenthal 1985). Flowing from these new approaches is a focus on two intersecting themes: sustainability, and public value.

Sustainability means reconciling the desire to achieve economic development in order to secure higher standards of living now and for future generations, with the need to protect and enhance the environment both now and in the longer term (Brundtland Commission 1987). Working out the application of sustainability within the heritage sector involved forging close links to the so-called Green Debate (MacInnes and Wickham-Jones 1992). In the specifically archaeological context sustainability is taken to mean making good and appropriate use of heritage resources for the needs of today, without compromising the ability of future generations to enjoy the same benefits.

Public value refers to understanding the relative importance that people place on the changes they experience in their lives and the overall contribution to the common good made by particular actions or activities (Barber 2017; Moore 1995). Usefully, this takes us away from the idea that everything should be measured in monetary or economic terms using reductionist metrics. Instead, it moves towards greater awareness of value in areas such as, well-being, a sense of place, and contributions to the wider concept of sustainable development, many of which have become central to public policy and appear in a wide range of strategies and policy documents at many organizational scales (see Chapter 1).

Axiomatic to both sustainability and public value is the idea of using sites, monuments, and landscapes for ethically sound and societally relevant purposes, increasing inclusivity, accessibility, personal and communal identity, and public benefit; what Nick Merriman (2004) refers to as the 'multiple perspectives' model of public archaeology. The set of *Conservation Principles* negotiated with the heritage profession by English Heritage in the mid-2000s, emphasize that the historic environment is a shared resource, that everyone should be able to participate in sustaining it, and that significant places should be managed to sustain their values (EH 2008: 7, Principles 1, 2, and 4). Particularly important here is the area of communal value that derives from the meanings of a place for the people who relate to it or for whom it figures in their collective experience or memory, commemorative and symbolic values, social values, and spiritual values (EH 2008: 31–32). It is a perspective that connects very well with what Siân Jones (2006) was talking about when she argued that we should think about sites and monuments, and archaeological materials generally, as 'living things'; their very existence forms part of a process in which social values and contemporary cultural significance drive our approaches to them, and serves to integrate the remains of the past, both tangible and intangible, with contemporary social life. As Susana Alves has discussed (2018) intangible experiences and values can be linked to physical aspects of heritage through active imagination, a relationship that promotes different ways of knowing, being, and doing. This encourages diversity and opens up the potential to connect or re-connect with ideas and situations both within and beyond the self.

Initially, the focus of much constructive conservation was the built environment as represented by historic buildings and associated townscapes. Work by conservation architects such as James Strike (1994) and John Ashurst (2006) focused on how to produce new developments at historic sites that took account of the character of places and related to shared perceptions of history. On a wider scale work on what has become known as 'place-making' allows the broad sweep of history and culture to influence the ways in which public and private spaces are created or re-purposed, by revealing, reflecting, embedding, or reinforcing meanings, understandings, and values (Darvill 2014; Schneekloth and Shibley 1995). Through place-making, aspects of the past and present are fused together in a way that echoes some of the ideas set out in Noha Nasser's book *Bridging cultures* (2015). Here she explores creative social innovation in cosmopolitan cities where public spaces provide a critical setting for inter-cultural encounters. She encourages the use of light-touch choreography to make public spaces arenas of inter-cultural mixing, re-activating them with the creative pulse of inter-culturalism.

Such approaches need not be confined to urban areas, the built environment, or indeed historic times. Place-making need not involve permanent creations as places and spaces can hold temporary or transient meanings and values. And when we think of inter-culturalism we are potentially looking at a very broad spectrum of people and communities, some of whom have previously been marginalized through the hegemony of traditional styles of heritage management. Using elements of the historic environment in sustainable ways to provide worthwhile public value does not necessarily involve physical changes to their form or structure; using them as arenas for real-time immersive engagements and as platforms upon which to build new ways of thinking, does no harm. Rather it creatively expands how people experience the historic environment, draw inspiration from it, and use understandings of it to help negotiate contemporary social and personal issues. This kind of place-making accords well with Johann Hari's unexpected solutions to the treatment of depression and mental health issues through social prescribing in which people are encouraged to re-connect with others, with their work, and with meaningful places around about, thereby finding a kind of sympathetic joy (Hari 2018).

Emerging out of these reflections on current and innovative approaches archaeological resource management are a handful of key themes that were carried forward as contributions to building the Human Henge experience:

- Combining the use of tangible and intangible cultural heritage
- Re-connecting people with landscapes and monuments through active imagination
- Treading lightly on sites and landscape in ways that are sustainable and non-destructive
- Place-making, albeit temporarily, through performance and association
- Creating public value through adaptive uses of sites and monuments to stimulate well-being

Combining these themes with those noted above around understanding something of the archaeological dimensions of healing places provides the conceptual building blocks from which Human Henge was constructed.

Building Human Henge

Human Henge combines archaeology and creativity, in order to take local people living with mental health problems on journeys of discovery through ancient landscapes as a way of improving mental health well-being. The work to date is essentially a series of pilot programmes; feasibility studies. The organizational context and wide network of collaborators is discussed by the project manager Laura Drysdale in Chapter 5. Here we focus on the cultural heritage therapy programme that ran three times over the course of the project, twice in the Stonehenge landscape and once in the Avebury landscape. The participants in all three programmes were referred to the project by outside organizations.

As a starting point it is important to emphasize that Human Henge is not based on archaeological investigation; participants did not engage in excavation, survey, or any form of direct intervention with the archaeological resource. Such work is something participants might consider engaging with later, and it is recognized that volunteering within the heritage sector is something that appears to offer positive well-being effects (Bennett 2018; Darvill *et al.* 2018: 117–119). Nor was the project based on talking heads explaining the development of the landscape or the sites within it. Certainly the archaeology of the target venues was explored by those knowledgeable about them, but we wanted to avoid the traditional route-march around the landscape, describing what could be seen and speculating about what could not. Instead, sites and monuments and their surrounding landscapes provided spaces for encounters and experiences, arenas for performative reflective engagement, and props through which to explore emotions, feelings, and understandings. Using prehistoric sites and ancient landscapes provided something that was at once familiar and yet distant; known and yet unknown. Areas rich in Neolithic and early Bronze Age sites and monuments provide the perfect environment as the places and their associations are quite different from anything more recent. Thus they open up cognitive vistas that stimulate active imagination.

Journeying was important to Human Henge, and a critical starting point. Physically, travelling to sites in a minibus and then on foot took participants out of the daily home/work/domestic world that they normally inhabited and brought them into another space, a different world. Twisting slightly the much-quoted words opening L.P. Hartley's 1953 novel *The Go-Between*, travelling to the venues for each session meant that the past became a foreign country and participants did things differently there. Intellectually, the sites selected as venues allowed parallel narratives and multi-voiced perspectives to emerge into the open, and be discussed and debated by all those present: participants, facilitators, and helpers. No one else was listening beyond the group. Every contribution counted. Every contribution took its author on a mental journey into new realms of thought, potentially opening doors and windows in the dark corridors of the mind to let the wind blow through and the sun shine in.

Re-connection was also recognized as important. Understanding the past is a high-order mental challenge; one that underpins the phenomenal interest in the what the popular media often dub 'enigmas', 'puzzles', and 'riddles'. They are not terms that academic archaeologists might apply to their studies, but Stonehenge and Avebury in particular are no strangers to journalistic inquiries under such headlines, and even popular accounts of scholarly studies sometimes stray in this direction to ensure interest. And why not? The point is that the intellectual processes underlying such inquiry are powerful, deep, challenging, and universal. Stimulating the mind, creating synaptic links, and energizing neural networks, is a recognized non-medicated approach to enhancing mental health and promoting well-being through processes of re-connection (Hari 2018). Grasping the past means simultaneously building up pictures at different scales, often from the minutiae of single actions. This might involve, say, decorating a pot with a familiar motif, then considering the broad sweep of cosmological references that give meaning to that pot motif as referencing the rising sun – the beginning of the day :: the beginning of life. And importantly, the dataset that prehistoric archaeology draws upon to build these pictures is constantly changing because of new discoveries, new analyses, and new ways of thinking about the human condition. Re-connection to the past is an ongoing dynamic process involving cyclical iterations, analysis, and synthesis, just as with re-connecting to a landscape, a site, a community, or one's self.

Human Henge began from the idea of using some well-known prehistoric landscapes, and foremost in our mind was the World Heritage Site of Stonehenge, Avebury, and associated monuments in Wiltshire. Inscribed on the World Heritage List in 1986, the two parcels of land that it comprises contain one of the most dense concentrations of upstanding Neolithic and Bronze Age monuments in northwest Europe. The outstanding universal value (OUV) of the site includes the idea that 'the monuments and landscape have had an unwavering influence on architects, artists, historians and archaeologists, and still retain a huge potential for future research' (UNESCO 2019: Criterion II). Moreover, the central sites themselves, and large tracts of their surrounding landscapes, are variously in the care of English Heritage and the National Trust, and thus potentially accessible for zero-impact activities such as the Human Henge programmes. Walking the landscape, seeing the monuments, touching the earth, hearing nature, smelling the air, and tasting the weather is part of experiencing the environment; these are central to the re-creational role that such places play and the mandate of the organizations that care for them (see Chapters 10 and 11 for discussion of the commitment and benefits accruing to these organizations).

The first iteration of Human Henge focused on the Stonehenge landscape. The education room in the Visitor Centre at Airman's Corner became base-camp: an orientation centre with comfort facilities, opportunities to mingle and chat over refreshments, and the starting point for all the journeys in the landscape. The programme comprised ten half-day sessions, one per week, run by a facilitator with support from helpers and volunteers, all of whom had mental health first aid training. Guest experts, artists, and musicians would contribute to specific sessions. Most sessions were during day-time, but one took place after dark in order to explore skyscapes as well as landscapes. It is easy to forget that prehistoric people's access to their monuments was not confined to the day-time or to formal opening-hours (although other taboos and restrictions might have applied!). The culmination of the programme was a performance within Stonehenge itself, near to the winter solstice, and designed by the participants based on their experiences of the landscape and re-connections to the prehistoric past over preceding sessions.

In such archaeologically rich landscapes, selecting which sites to visit was itself quite a challenge, with numerous contenders. But the process of selection turned out to be quite intuitive. There were no fixed criteria beyond the question of easy access, diversity and variety of opportunity, and a recognition of their potential for exploring ideas rather than simply their prehistory. There was no attempt to tell the 'big' story of culture-history or landscape development; these were narratives that the participants could beneficially piece together for themselves through whatever means suited them. Our task in selecting sites was to provide cognitive headroom; space to think and tools with which to think.

After brain-storming a list of possible sites to use, and the journeys these would involve, the exact order and the themes to be explored at each developed organically through discussions within the wider project team, the facilitators, and the professionals engaged along the way. What emerged was part planned and part extemporary, focused around taking the participants on meaningful journeys and activating their imaginations. So, for example, visiting the Cuckoo Stone we introduced Chartwell Dutiro, a Zimbabwean musician and mbira master, knowing that he had stories to tell about colour, stone, music, and song from Shona culture. Mbira music plays an important role in Shona ceremonies connected with rain-making and funerals, is used to call-up animal spirits or wandering spirits, and is widely used in *bira* ceremonies where a common ancestor is summoned to discern the cause of illness or misfortune and help remedy it (Berliner 1978: 187–188). As the participants walked towards the stone the sound of the mbira came to their ears, and as they drew near they saw that Chartwell was wearing his traditional dress (Figure 6.3). The cross-cultural references and music became the bridge. It

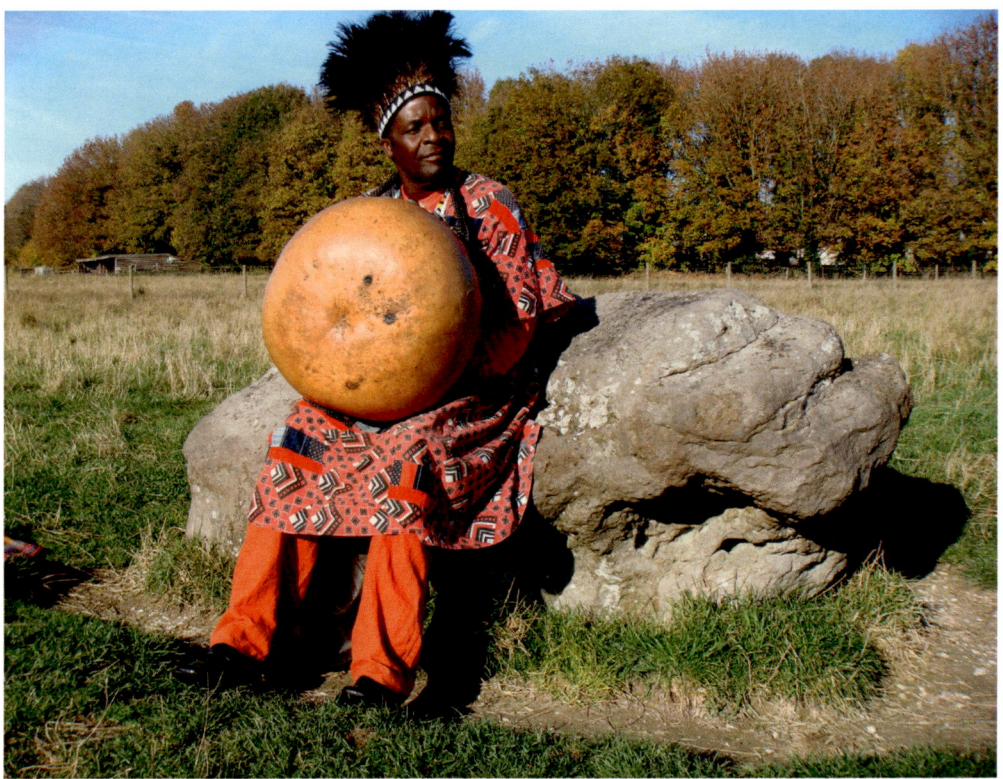

Figure 6.3 Chartwell Dutiro playing his mbira on the Cuckoo Stone, near Stonehenge, Wiltshire. (Photograph by Timothy Darvill, Human Henge project. Copyright reserved)

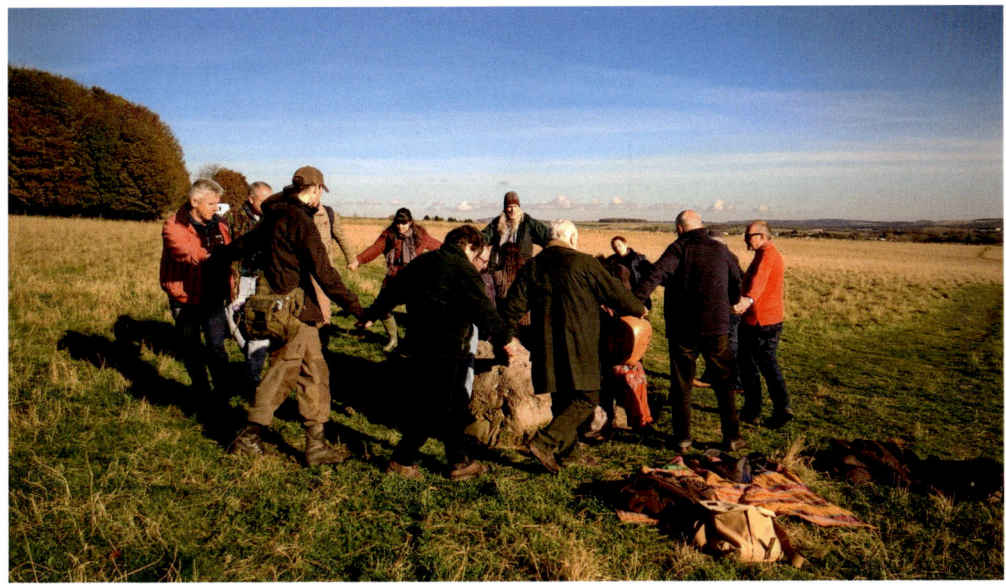

Figure 6.4 Human Henge in motion: Dancing at the Cuckoo Stone, near Stonehenge, Wiltshire. (Photograph by Yvette Staelens, Human Henge project. Copyright reserved)

was possible to explore what in archaeological theory would be called 'materiality'; in practical terms this means thinking about the many varied meanings attaching to the stuff we call stone, the idea of 'stoniness', its colour, texture, feel, and the past and present place of stone in the landscape. From this part-choreographed start emerged the possibility of exploring feelings and emotions prompted by thinking about stone and, importantly, using these thoughts to draw out passion and excitement from the minds of the participants. In this way, the ancient Cuckoo Stone in the modern landscape became a conduit through which they could explore their own thoughts, express themselves verbally and through motion and dance (Figure 6.4), and make new connections and re-connections.

Table 6.A summarizes the venues used for the first iteration of the Stonehenge programme in October, November, and December 2016, and the themes associated with each. The night-walk allowed the opportunity to journey along the Stonehenge Cursus thereby providing a chance to experience the largest monument in the landscape under a star-lit sky. Constellations were identified, and prehistoric astronomy and the extraordinary Nebra Disk provided a starting point for discussing wider issues of cosmology, being, and time. The ceremony at the end of the programme involved an early-morning event inside Stonehenge a few days before the winter solstice. Designed and executed by the participants themselves, there was music, singing, dancing, and chanting.

The second iteration of the programme took place in the Stonehenge landscape in January, February, and March 2017. It followed much the same pattern as the first, although the order of site visits changed slightly and different guests were brought in. The closing ceremony was linked to the spring equinox. The third iteration used venues within the Avebury landscape in January, February, and March 2018, again ending with a ceremony at the spring equinox that on this occasion took place inside a wintery Avebury Henge (Figure 6.5). Table 6.B summarizes the venues used.

Table 6. A Summary of the venues used for Human Henge events in the first iteration of the Programme in the Stonehenge landscape, October to December 2016.

Session	Activity
Orientation	Stonehenge Visitor Centre. Meet the project team. Introduction to the programme and the research, and complete the baseline questionnaire. Practising trip to Stonehenge and familiarization with the Visitor Centre facilities
1	Woodhenge and Durrington Walls. Introduction to Human Henge, making noise in the landscape and boasting
2	Cursus Barrow Cemetery. Walk in the historic landscape, guided meditation, sitting between the barrows
3	Fargo Wood. Walk to Fargo Wood, explore the woodland, practice woodcraft.
4	Cuckoo Stone. Drive to Woodhenge and then walk to the Cuckoo Stone, meet Chartwell Dutiro and hear the music of the mbira. Discuss stone and it meanings
5	Stonehenge Cursus. An evening walk along the cursus from east to west, exploring skyscapes and the movements of the celestial bodies
6	Reconstructed Neolithic houses and displays at the Visitor Centre. Meet staff and volunteers. Mid-point questionnaire
7	Pottery and reflection on the experience so far. Make pots with Mark Vyvyan-Penney and fire them outside
8	Stonehenge Avenue and King Barrow Ridge. Drive to the National Trust Cottage, and then walk in the landscape thinking about barrows and processions
9	Stonehenge Visitor Centre. Creative workshop with Chartwell Dutiro preparing for the celebration to be held within the stones of Stonehenge
10	Stonehenge. Final celebration near the winter solstice. Walk to the stones, music and performance. End of programme questionnaire
Monitoring	Focus groups and surveys with Dr Vanessa Heaslip

From an archaeological perspective, the programmes were successful in introducing people who had previously had little access to these rich historic landscapes and to the wonders and understandings of prehistory. The archaeological sites provided bridges between past and present, people and place, time and space, body and mind. In this way, through journeying and connection/re-connection, people's lives were changed. In Chapters 7 and 8 Yvette Staelens and Daniel O'Donoghue reflect in different ways on the organization and running of the programmes, their strengths and weaknesses. They use the words of the participants themselves to convey something of the variety, excitement and depth of the experiences they had. In Chapter 9 Vanessa Heaslip describes and contextualizes the results of carefully and systematically monitoring the participants' mental health well-being before, during, and after the programmes. And in Chapters 10 and 11 Martin Allfrey and Briony Clifford look outwards from the project in the work of English Heritage and the National Trust respectively.

Table 6.B Summary of the venues used for Human Henge events in the third iteration of the Programme in the Avebury landscape, January to March 2018.

Session	Activity
Orientation	Avebury Education Room. Meet the project team. Introduction to the programme and the research, and complete the baseline questionnaire. Practising trip to the Avebury area and familiarization with the facilities
1	Windmill Hill. Introduction to Human Henge, guided meditation at the Neolithic enclosure and sitting on the Bronze Age barrows
2	Silbury Hill and the Swallowhead Springs. Walk in the historic landscape and along the river south of Avebury, sacred water, hidden Roman town, sarsen stepping stones and the rag-tree beside the spring
3	West Kennet Long Barrow, tomb of the ancestors, monuments in the landscape, soundscapes, marking time, ancient sounds and songs with Max des Oiseaux
4	Lockeridge Down. Stone and its meanings, sarsen working, making axes
5	The Sanctuary and the Ridgeway Round Barrows. Circular structures, linear routes. Midpoint questionnaire
6	Night walk through the stones of Avebury Henge and then down the West Kennet Avenue. Skyscapes and constellations
7	Fired earth. Making pots and clay tree-figures in the landscape. Led by Briony Clifton
8	Collections in the museum. Pottery, flints, stone. Handling and exploring ancient artefacts. Led by Ros Cleal
9	Planning the ceremony
10	Avebury Henge. Final celebration at the spring equinox. Walk to the stones, music and performance. End of programme questionnaire
Monitoring	Focus groups and surveys with Dr Vanessa Heaslip

Discussion

The three iterations of the Human Henge programme, which can loosely be termed a kind of cultural heritage therapy, clearly show how Neolithic and early Bronze Age sites with well-known historic environments can be used to enhance mental health well-being. In this it is not the sites themselves *per se* but the opportunities given by those places to explore ways of being. The aim was to open up new ways of looking at the landscape, and at ourselves. Thinking about how people might have used ancient places, coming together for communal endeavours, interacting and creating social networks, and finding opportunities to break down some of the emotional barriers that underpin many mental health issues. Building on the idea that Stonehenge and many other ancient sites were designed and constructed as places for healing opens up new ways of exploring the relationships between people and place in the past and in the present. Using dynamic ideas from constructive conservation, place-making, sustainability, and public value both underpins the ethics of using archaeological sites in these ways and shows how monuments can and should have a wide range of uses in the modern world. They can be important for communities that were either poorly represented or marginalized because of the prevailing, but now outdated, concepts of management and access. By spending time at a selection of sites, singing, dancing, making music, and looking both inwards and outwards, it becomes possible to connect with the landscape, the skyscape, the monuments, and, most importantly, with other participants, and with one's self. In that sense, Human Henge allowed participants to do things and explore places in safe but unfamiliar ways, rejuvenating and revitalizing identities and bolstering self-esteem.

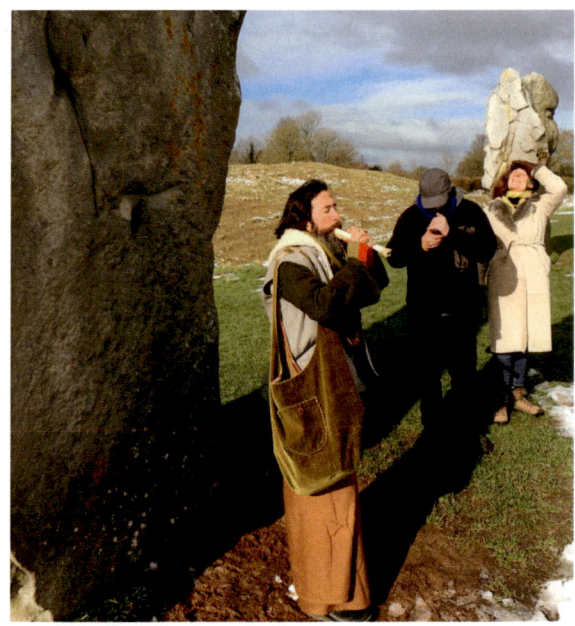

Figure 6.5. Maxence des Oiseaux playing a bone flute beside Stone 9 in the southwest sector at Avebury, Wiltshire. (Photograph by Timothy Darvill, Human Henge project. Copyright reserved)

Conclusions

So what have we learnt? Prehistoric sites and landscapes certainly make good venues for this kind of work, their detachment and difference from today's world being a significant factor. Practical and fairly fixed routines for the delivery of the programme seem to be important in terms of timetable, duration, and arrangements. This stability builds confidence on the part of the participants as well as a special kind of trust in the delivery team who can then take participants on the journeys described here. Treating everyone present at programme events as equal strengthens self-esteem. A sense of shared discovery illustrates the process that individuals can later use on their own. On the basis of the three iterations undertaken to date the Human Henge programme worked for many of those that took part, although how representative that sample is remains to be seen.

And what about the future? In terms of the programme itself, lessons have been leant about the nature and range of sites that can be used, the processes of delivery, and the needs of the participants. It is also clear that we underestimated the need for support after each ten-week programme ended. This has partly been addressed through self-help initiatives, but there needs to be a more structured approach involving follow-up events at intervals over the course of a year or two beyond the structured intensive programmes. Such events would be stepping stones from the Human Henge programme into the wider world; a continuation of the participants' journeys. They would undoubtedly be beneficial and enhance the power and reach of the programmes. Such activities could involve a wide range of heritage organizations including museums, heritage centres, and heritage properties of various kinds, widening the network of partnerships and expanding both sustainability and public value. The next step is to try similar programmes in less well-known landscapes, and to increase the sample of participants to allow a more meaningful assessment of the power and impact of using the historic environment in this innovative way.

Acknowledgements

Human Henge could not have happened without the unstinting support of so many individuals and organizations, all of whom deserve thanks for their contributions and insights: Martin Allfrey; Kerry Barrass; Briony Clifton; Laura Drysdale; Vanessa Heaslip; Danny O'Donoghue; Yvette Stalens; and Toby Sutcliffe; members of the various advisory boards and panels; staff at English Heritage, HLF, and the National Trust; and the many participants, facilitators, performers, and helpers that made the events such an extraordinary experience.

Bibliography

Aldhouse-Green, M. and S. Aldhouse-Green 2005. *The quest for the shaman*. London: Thames and Hudson.
Allason-Jones, L. and B. McKay 1985. *Coventina's Well: A shrine on Hadrian's Wall*. Oxford: Oxbow Books.
Alves, S. 2018. Understanding intangible aspects of cultural heritage: The role of active imagination. *The Historic Environment: Policy and Practice* 9(3–4): 207–228.
Armstrong, K. 2012. Pilgrimage: Why do they do it?, in V. Porter (ed.) *Hajj. Journey to the heart of Islam*: 18–25. London: The British Museum Press.
Ashurst, J. 2006. *Conservation of ruins*. London: Butterworth-Heinemann.
Barber, M. 2017. *Delivering better outcomes for citizens: Practice steps for unlocking public value* [Online document]. Viewed 11 March 2019, <https://www.gov.uk/government/publications/delivering-better-outcomes-for-citizens-practical-steps-for-unlocking-public-value>.
Bennett, R. 2018. Saving lives: Breaking ground heritage. *British Archaeology* 161 (July–August 2018): 50–55.
Bennett-Samuels, M. and D.M. Evans 2008. Is this the fingerprint of St Non? *Current Archaeology* 19 (Issue 233): 5.
Berliner, P.F. 1978. *The soul of mbira. Music and traditions of the Shona people of Zimbabwe*. Berkeley, CA: University of California Press.
Birch, D.J. 2000. *Pilgrimage to Rome in the Middle Ages: Continuity and change*. London: Boydell and Brewer.
Blick, S. (ed.) 2007. *Beyond pilgrim souvenirs and secular badges. Essays in honour of Brian Spencer*. Oxford: Oxbow Books.
Brundtland Commission 1987. *Our Common Future: The Report of the World Commission on Environment and Development*. Oxford: Oxford University Press.
Chareyron, N. 2005. *Pilgrims to Jerusalem in the Middle Ages*. New York: Columbia University Press.
Cunliffe, B. 1980. The excavation of the Roman spring at Bath 1979. A preliminary discussion. *Antiquaries Journal* 40: 187–206.
Cunliffe, B. 1986. *The city of Bath*. Gloucester: Alan Sutton.
Cunliffe, B. 1995. *Roman Bath*. London: Batsford and English Heritage.
Cunliffe, B. and P. Davenport 1985. *The Temple of Sulis Minerva at Bath. Volume 1: The site*. Oxford: Oxford University Committee for Archaeology (2 volumes).

Darvill, T. 1987. *Ancient monuments in the countryside: An archaeological management review* (HBMCE Archaeological Report 9). London: English Heritage.
Darvill, T. 2006. *Stonehenge: The biography of a landscape*. Stroud: Tempus / History Press.
Darvill, T. 2007. Towards the within: Stonehenge and its purpose, in D.A. Barrowclough and C. Malone (eds.) *Cult in context. Reconsidering ritual in archaeology*: 148–157. Oxford: Oxbow Books.
Darvill, T. 2014. Rock and soul: Humanizing heritage, memorializing music, and producing places. *World Archaeology* 46(3): 462–476.
Darvill, T. 2016. Roads to Stonehenge: A prehistoric healing centre and pilgrimage site in southern Britain, in A. Ranft and W. Schenkluhn (eds.) *Kulturstraßen als Konzept. 20 Jahre Straße der Romani* (More Romano. Schriften des Europäischen Romanik Zentrums 5): 155–166. Regensburg: Schell and Steiner.
Darvill, T. and G. Wainwright 2014. Beyond Stonehenge: Carn Menyn Quarry and the origin and date of bluestone extraction in the Preseli Hills of southwest Wales. *Antiquity* 88: 1099–1114.
Darvill, T., D.M. Evans and G. Wainwright 2004. Strumble-Preseli Ancient Communities and Environment Study (SPACES): Third Report 2004. *Archaeology in Wales* 44: 104–109.
Darvill, T., V. Heaslip and K. Barrass 2018. Heritage and well-being: Therapeutic places, past and present, in K.T. Galvin (ed.) *Routledge Handbook of Well-being*: 112–23. Abingdon: Routledge.
Davenport, P., C. Poole and D. Jordon 2007. *Archaeology in Bath. Excavations at the New Royal Baths (the Spa), and Bellott's Hospital 1998-1999* (Oxford Archaeology Monograph 3). Oxford: Oxford Archaeology.
Davidson, H.R.E. 1988. *Myths and symbols in Pagan Europe: Early Scandinavian and Celtic religions*. Manchester: Manchester University Press.
Davies, H.E.F. and M.E. Owen 1975. Meddygon Myddfai, in J. Cule (ed.) *Wales and medicine*: 156–168. London: British Society for the History of Medicine.
Duffin, J. 2009. *Medical miracles. Doctors, saints, and healing in the modern world*. Oxford: Oxford University Press.
EH 2008. *Conservation principles. Policy and Guidance* [Online document]. London: English Heritage. Viewed 11 March 2019, <https://historicengland.org.uk/images-books/publications/conservation-principles-sustainable-management-historic-environment/>.
Foley, R. 2010. *Healing waters. Therapeutic landscapes in historic and contemporary Ireland*. Abingdon: Routledge.
Gesler, W.M. 1993. Therapeutic landscapes: Theory and a case study of Epidauros, Greece. *Environment and Planning* D11: 171–189.
Gesler, W.M. 1996. Lourdes: Healing in a place of pilgrimage. *Health and Place* 2: 95–105.
Gesler, W.M. 1998. Bath's reputation as a healing place, in R.A. Kearns and W.M. Gesler (eds.) *Putting Health into Place*: 17–35. Syracuse: Syracuse University Press.
Gesler, W.M. 2003. *Healing places*. Lanham, MD: Rowman and Littlefield.
Gemi-Iordanou, E., S. Gordon, R. Matthew, E. McInnes and R. Pettitt (eds.), 2014. *Medicine, healing and performance*. Oxford: Oxbow Books.
Gilchrist, R. 1994. *Gender and material culture. The Archaeology of religious women*. London: Routledge.
Gilchrist, R. and B. Sloane 2005. *Requiem: The medieval monastic cemetery in Britain*. London: Museum of London Archaeology Service.
Granville, A.B. 1841. *The Spas of England and principal sea-bathing places*. London: Henry Colburn. Three volumes. (Reprinted 1971 with an introduction by G. Martin, by Adams and Dart).
Green, M. 1986. *The Gods of the Celts*. Gloucester: Alan Sutton.

Grinsell, L.V. 1976. *The folklore of prehistoric sites in Britain*. Newton Abbot: David and Charles.

Haleem, M.A.S.A. 2012. The importance of Hajj: Spirit and rituals, in V. Porter (ed.) *Hajj. Journey to the heart of Islam*: 26–67. London: The British Museum Press.

Harbison, P. 1994. Early Irish pilgrim archaeology in the Dingle Peninsula. *World Archaeology* 26(1): 90–103.

Harding, J. 2013. *Cult, religion, and pilgrimage. Archaeological investigations at the Neolithic and Bronze Age monument complex of Thornborough, North Yorkshire* (CBA Research Report 174). York: Council for British Archaeology.

Hari, J. 2018. *Lost connections. Uncovering the real Causes of depression – and the unexpected solutions*. London: Bloomsbury Circus.

Harmanşah, O. 2015. *Place, memory, and healing. An archaeology of Anatolian rock monuments*. London: Routledge.

Hickman, C. 2005. The picturesque at Brislington House, Bristol: The role of landscape in relation to the treatment of mental illness in the early nineteenth-century asylum. *Garden History* 33: 47–60.

Hickman, C. 2013. *Therapeutic landscapes: A history of English hospital gardens since 1800*. Manchester: Manchester University Press.

Hill, S. 2016. Constructive conservation – a model for developing heritage assets. *Journal of Cultural Heritage Management and Sustainable Development* 6(1): 34–46.

Insoll, T. 2006. Shrine franchising and the Neolithic in the British Isles: Some observations based upon the Tallensi, northern Ghana. *Cambridge Archaeological Journal* 16(2): 223–238.

Jones, F. 1992. *The holy wells of Wales*. Cardiff: University of Wales Press.

Jones, S. 2006. 'They made it a living thing didn't they...': The growth of things and the fossilization of heritage, in R. Layton, S. Shennan and P. Stone (eds.) *A future for archaeology. The past in the present*: 107–126. London: UCL Press.

Kearns, R.A. and W.M. Gesler (eds.) 1998. *Putting health into place. Landscape, identity, and well-being*. Syracuse: Syracuse University Press.

King, E.J. 1967. *The Knights of St John in the British realm* (Third edition). London: St John's Gate.

Koen, B.D. 2009. *Beyond the roof of the world. Music, prayer and healing in the Pamir Mountains*. Oxford: Oxford University Press.

Lowenthal, D. 1985. *The past is a foreign country*. Cambridge: Cambridge University Press.

MacInnes, L. and C.R. Wickham-Jones (eds.) 1992. *All natural things. Archaeology and the Green Debate*. Oxford: Oxbow Books.

Merrifield, R. 1987. *The archaeology of ritual and magic*. London: Batsford.

Merriman, N. 2004. Introduction: Diversity and dissonance in public archaeology, in N. Merriman (ed.) *Public archaeology*: 1–17. London: Routledge.

Michaelides, D. (ed.) 2014. *Medicine and healing in the ancient Mediterranean*. Oxford: Oxbow.

Moore, M. 1995. *Creating public value — Strategic management in government*. Cambridge, MA: Harvard University Press.

Morris, C. and A. Peatfield 2014. Health and healing on Cretan Bronze Age peak sanctuaries, in D. Michaelides (ed.) *Medicine and healing in the ancient Mediterranean*: 54–63. Oxford: Oxbow.

Nasser, N. 2015. *Bridging cultures. The guide to social innovation in cosmopolitan cities*. Markham (ON): 10-10-10 Publishing.

Oestigaard, T. 2017. Holy water: The works of water in defining and understanding holiness. *WIREswater* 4(3): e1205 [Online publication]. Viewed 11 March 2019, <doi: 10.1002/wat2.1205>.

Orme, N. 2018. *Medieval pilgrimage*. Exeter: Impress Books.

Peters, F.E. 1994. *The Hajj: The Muslim pilgrimage to Mecca and the holy places*. Princeton University Press.
Porter, V. (ed.) 2012. *Hajj. Journey to the heart of Islam*. London: The British Museum Press.
Ray, C. 2014. *The origins of Ireland's holy wells*. Oxford: Archaeopress Archaeology.
Ray, H.P. 1994. Kanheri: The archaeology of an early Buddhist pilgrimage centre in western India. *World Archaeology* 26(1): 35-46.
RCHME 1980. *Ancient and Historical Monuments in the City of Salisbury. Volume 1*. London: Royal Commission on Historical Monuments (England).
Reynolds, F. 2014. Early Neolithic shamans? Performance, healing and the power of skulls at Hambledon Hill, Dorset, in E. Gemi-Iordanou, S. Gordon, R. Matthew, E. McInnes and R. Pettitt (eds.) *Medicine, healing and performance*: 6-24. Oxford: Oxbow Books.
Richardson, L-J. and J. Almansa-Sánchez 2015. Do you even know what public archaeology is? Trends, theory, practice, ethics. *World Archaeology* 47(2): 194-211.
Roux, J. 2004. *The roads to Santiago de Compostela*. Vic-en-Bigorre: MSM.
Ross, A. 1967. *Pagan Celtic Britain. Studies in iconography and tradition*. London: Routledge.
Rutherford, S. 2004. Victorian and Edwardian institutional landscapes in England. *Landscapes* 5(2): 25-41.
Rutherford, S. 2005. Landscapers for the mind: English asylum designers, 1845-1914. *Garden History* 33(1): 61-86.
Schneekloth, L.H. and R.G. Shibley 1995. *Placemaking. The art and practice of building communities*. New York: John Wiley and Sons.
Scott, R.A. 2010. *Miracle cures. Saints, pilgrimage and the healing power of belief*. Berkeley (CA): University of California Press.
Shaver-Crandell, A. and P. Gerson 1995. *The pilgrim's guide to Santiago de Compostela*. London: Harvey Miller.
Silverman, H. 1994. The archaeological identification of an ancient Peruvian pilgrimage center. *World Archaeology* 26(1): 1-18.
Stevenson, C. 2000. *Medicine and magnificence. British hospital and asylum architecture 1660-1815*. New Haven and London: Yale University Press.
Strike, J. 1994. *Architecture in conservation*. London: Routledge.
Stroud, D. 1984. The cult and tombs of St Osmund at Salisbury. *Wiltshire Archaeological and Natural History Magazine* 78: 50-54.
Thorpe, L. (trans.) 1966. *Geoffrey of Monmouth: The history of the kings of Britain*. Harmondsworth: Penguin Books.
Ucko, P.J. 1994. Museums and sites: Cultures of the past within education - Zimbabwe, some ten years on, in P.G. Stone and B.L. Molyneaux (eds.) *The presented past: Heritage, museums, and education*: 237-282. London: Routledge.
UNESCO 2019, Stonehenge, Avebury and associated sites. World Heritage List [Webpage]. Viewed 11 March 2019, <https://whc.unesco.org/en/list/373>.
Webb, D. 2000. *Pilgrimage in medieval England*. London: Hambledon and London.
Williams, A.M. 2007. Introduction: The continuing maturation of the therapeutic landscape concept, in A.M. Williams (ed.) *Therapeutic landscapes*: 1-12. London: Ashgate (Geographies of Health).

Chapter 7

'What did you do today mummy?': Human Henge and mental well-being

Yvette Staelens

Abstract

As the co-ordinator of Human Henge, the author describes the ethos behind the project and the many ways in which this was put into practice around the landscapes and monuments of Stonehenge and Avebury in Wiltshire. Comments from participants are included to illuminate memories of this unique project. This chapter aims to gives a flavour of the project's sights, sounds, sensations, joys, challenges, and achievements. There are adventures in the rain and on night walks, surprise meetings with music from other cultures, a close encounter with a hare, copious quantities of tea, and a person who finally gains a satisfying answer to the question 'What did you do today mummy?' Personal reflections on the activities and rich experiences afforded to 'Human Hengers' give powerful insights into the potential for enhancing mental well-being furnished by this project's innovative approach.

Keywords: Adventure; Healing; Human Henge; Landscape; Prehistory

Introduction

In this chapter I will attempt to unfold the events and journeying that took place during three iterations of Human Henge: two centred at Stonehenge, and one at Avebury. Much has been said about the context, partnerships, and aims of Human Henge in Chapters 5 and 6, and there is an on-going research programme tracking participants discussed in Chapter 9. Here I will try to develop an understanding of what made these three programmes unlike any other undertaken on prehistoric sites, and will try to answer the question: 'What did we do at the monuments to enhance participant's mental well-being?'

First though it is important to acknowledge that this was an experiment, a feasibility study, with all the inherent risks that experimentation entails. We were exploring uncharted territory, a journey into the unknown, and due acknowledgment must be give right at the outset to all the brave participants who took part. Throughout this narrative I will draw on the actual words of some of those who participated; they are indented and separate from the flow of the text but for safeguarding reasons individual contributors will not be identified here (they will know who they are: thank you).

Why Stonehenge?

The Stonehenge landscape was chosen for the following reasons: its world renown; its visitor resources; and the willingness of English Heritage (EH) and the National Trust (NT) to partner and participate. From an archaeological perspective we were following up a theory propounded by Tim Darvill that Stonehenge was, and perhaps still is, 'a healing landscape' (Darvill 2007; 2016; and see Chapter 6). Stonehenge and other henges like it were special places acknowledged and

Historic Landscapes and Mental Well-being

in part created by prehistoric people who for generations travelled to them for a whole range of reasons: seasonal gathering for exchange, social interaction and cohesion, ceremony and celebration, feasting, and rituals connected with healing the body, mind, and spirit.

Pitching and rolling

Human Henge had specified aims, objectives, outcomes, a budget, and all the usual requisites of a 'project'— and then there was a void, a space for debate about the group activities, discussions, and ideas pitching and rolling around. The focus shifting. Shimmering suggestions. What about an epic poem written by participants? A procession along the Avenue to the Stones? Walking by night? Burying made things? Singing and music? Everything was on the table. There was a creative, stimulating, buzz and all the time the discourse was underpinned by understandings of prehistoric archaeology. As both an archaeologist and a creative practitioner it was easy for me to navigate these waters. Others probably felt less comfortable, but crucial to our success was the trust in what we doing that permeated the team. There was mutual respect from all partners, and a deep-felt commitment to seeing Human Henge succeed. New and experimental ideas can sometimes be unsettling to agencies delivering public access to heritage, and in this respect enormous credit must be given to those involved in bringing our project to the attention of their management teams and governing bodies, and championing it at every twist and turn.

Tea

Initially, each of the three Human Henge groups met mostly as strangers to each other. There were a few existing connections because participants had sometimes worked together on projects run by the Richmond Fellowship and therefore knew Danny and his team. No-one knew me or the volunteers recruited from EH, NT and BU. My first and ongoing practical role was to welcome them, to create safe spaces within which to work, and to oversee and weave together the explorations ahead.

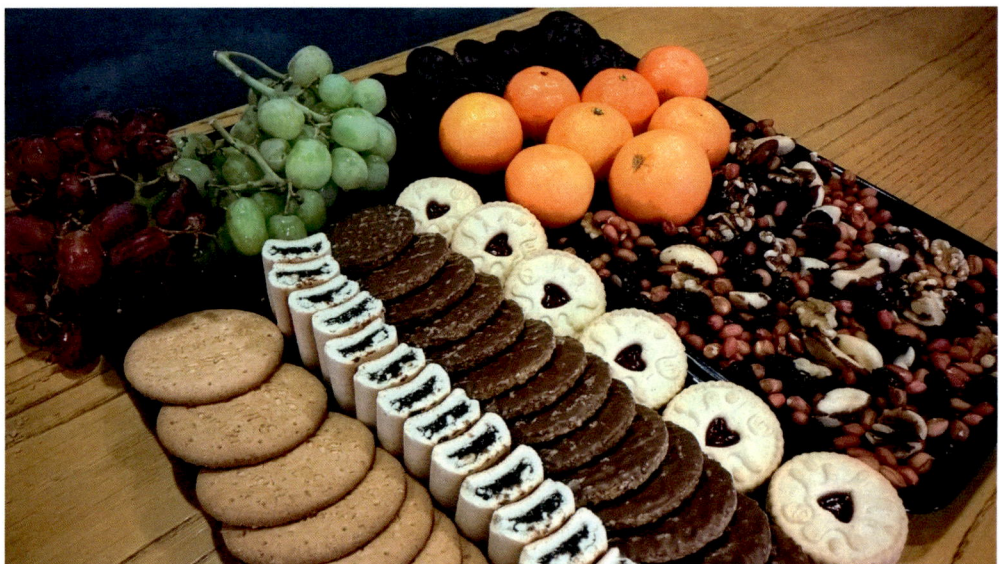

Figure 7.1. Human Henge fruit and biscuits served with love. (Photograph by Yvette Staelens. Copyright reserved)

'Tea was an important part of Human Henge.'

We needed a starting point, a place of arrival, in order to be 'here', to meet, to chat, and then to return to in order to relax and recoup after each session. For some getting up and out of bed was itself a challenge, others were looming; the journey from home, the prospect of meeting strangers, participation in group activity, and being active in a strange space. A welcome drink and beautifully arranged fresh and dried fruit, biscuits, and healthy treats (including specific dietary options) told them they were special and that their well-being was our primary concern (Figure 7.1). Importantly, neither I nor the volunteer team had any prior knowledge of the participants; they were simply people like everyone else in the project.

Another critical factor was that the participants were fully-supported by care workers and volunteers. In addition, there was the Human Henge (unspoken) ground rule that there was no 'us and them'. If you were present, then you participated. There was no opting out; we were a 'tribe' and we did things together.

'If you are here, you are doing it.'

Group One

The real pioneers were those in the first Human Henge group: HH1. These were people who challenged themselves to do something completely new and who placed their trust in those who told them that it would be a good experience and that it would be of help to their well-being. How did we plan the sessions? Following discussions between myself as co-ordinator and creative director and Tim Darvill as prehistorian and quixotic leader, we selected ten destinations for the HH1 sessions in the Stonehenge landscape:

1. Woodhenge and Durrington Walls henge
2. Cursus barrow cemetery
3. Fargo Plantation
4. Cuckoo Stone
5. Cursus night walk
6. Reconstructed huts and visitor centre collections
7. Epic poetry and pottery
8. The Avenue and King Barrow Ridge
9. Creative workshop
10. Solstice celebration ceremony inside the stones of Stonehenge

They were repeated although not in quite the same order for the HH2 sessions. HH3 met at Avebury and their journey will be described below. For HH1 and HH2 at Stonehenge, the ten sessions were preceded by an orientation visit to the Stonehenge Visitor Centre in order to familiarize participants and care workers with the site and facilities.

Less than a speck

At this point in my narrative I ask you to place yourself in the position of an HH1 participant. Over the next three months you will be guided by archaeologists, curators, creatives, and your fellow travellers. You will have session destinations, but no route. You will be asked to use your imagination, to open your heart, to sing, to join hands, to play a musical instrument, and to work clay, wood, or plant fibre. You may shelter, run, incant, grumble, say a blessing, dance, or whatever you feel like. You have a mental health issue; this may be the scariest thing you have ever done. You will make friends, you will have the support of your fellow travellers, and in turn you will support them. Because you understand. The inexplicable will happen, you will witness beauty, you will craft and create, you may write or capture an image, or perhaps tie a ribbon on a rag tree. You will discover that you are braver than you think. You will share your knowledge, you will make string, a beaker, share laughter. Pigs and dogs will have new significance. You will 'be in the green' come all weathers. Your inner world will be usurped by the power of place, the landscape, and the humans, your ancestors, who trod it first. You will ponder the details of their daily life and their beliefs, and you will find yourself less than a speck in the cosmos on a starlit night.

The essence of Human Henge is that it engages participants in a journey to a known destination, with a leader and guides. Leadership and guidance ensure that safety and support are ever present. However, the route will be partly self-determined by the participants' needs, wants, abilities, and desires. In addition, challenges will be introduced along the way. The journeying is reflective and reactive, always didactic and creative but never prescriptive. The constant is the prehistoric archaeology all around. Referenced continuously to provide evidence and understandings of past lives and different worlds. We were people seeking people as well as 'pots'. We sought to connect with the ancestors and with each other.

Elemental beings and the soundscape

Striding out on wet days was important. We went out into the landscape whatever the weather. Being outside was recognized as being beneficial on many levels health-wise. The soundscape was also important. As well as our own noise we were mindful of 'silence' and the stillness found in some activities, of the sound of flowing water and rain dripping through trees, and sometimes, when the wind decreed, the traffic on the A303.

From the outset my intention was to introduce music, beliefs, and traditions from cultures beyond these shores to expand our thinking about the prehistoric past. For this I invited three international musician friends and collaborators to participate. Chartwell Dutiro from Zimbabwe (HH1), Alphonse Tourna from Cameroon (HH2), and Maxence des Oiseaux from France (HH3). Their role was to surprise, delight and excite participants, through sharing their unique talents and cultural gifts. They were sited in specific locations in the prehistoric landscape. Each musician was deliberately concealed from the participants as they approached, and introduced in a surprise manner.

Chartwell, dressed in his ceremonial Shona robes, was seated on the Cuckoo Stone, a recumbent menhir near Woodhenge (Figure 7.2). He played his mbira and sang. We saw him from afar and our ears led us to him. This was a fabulous interaction. It led eventually to movement, joining of hands and circling him as he performed. You can hear his music if you access Sound File 1 on the website linked to this publication.

Equally powerful was meeting Alphonse at the King Barrow Ridge. Again, the participants had no inkling about what was about to happen. As we approached the barrow cemetery they just heard music and song from an unknown source. The music was of a kind they had never

Sound File 1. Chartwell Dutiro playing his mbira and singing - https://tinyurl.com/Dutiro

heard before, and a gentle voice singing in an unknown language, soft on the air. Alphonse was playing balafon (Figure 7.3). He subsequently told us stories and shared his ancestral beliefs and traditions about sacred stones delighting both the prehistorians present and the Human Hengers alike.

Maxence brought his mouth-blown instruments, crafted from bones and horns as they would have been in the prehistoric period, including flutes made from swan bones like those discovered in Upper Palaeolithic and later contexts (Figure 7.4). He was experienced in playing in prehistoric caves and we secretly located him in the West Kennet Long Barrow. You can hear a sample of his music if you access Sound File 2 on the website linked to this publication.

Again, participants heard him from afar and simply followed their ears; a magical journey. Once inside the long barrow's burial chamber, we all enjoyed hearing the unique music from each instrument reverberating around the stones, the space

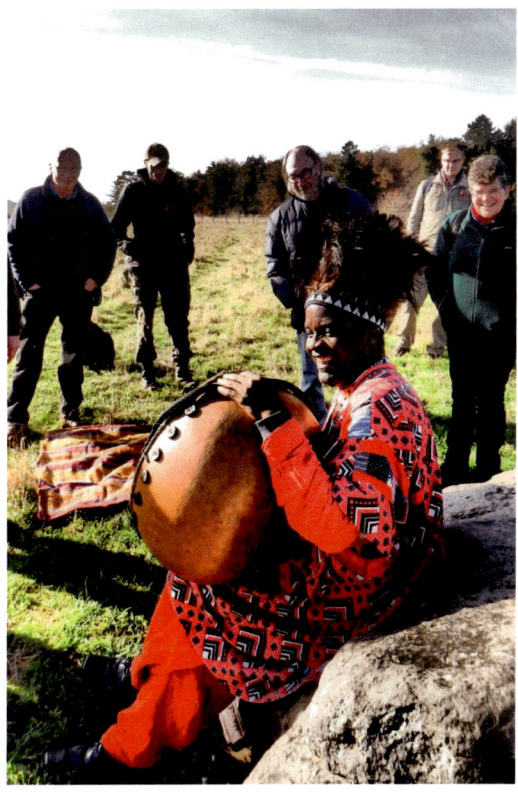

Figure 7.2 Chartwell Dutiro playing mbira on the Cuckoo Stone. (Photograph by Yvette Staelens. Copyright reserved)

and us. One Human Henger disclosed that she had lived in France, spoke fluent French, and thus offered to help translate. This is a typical example of the 'reveals' that occurred during Human Henge as one participant after another brought forward a set of skills that no-one guessed they had. As they have become more relaxed with their Human Henge companions, participants shared their skills, knowledge, experiences, and stories. Within this sharing lies deep connection powered by trust.

Avebury

Sessions in the Avebury landscape followed the established ten week pattern, ending with a celebration amongst the circles within the henge at the spring equinox. The venues were:

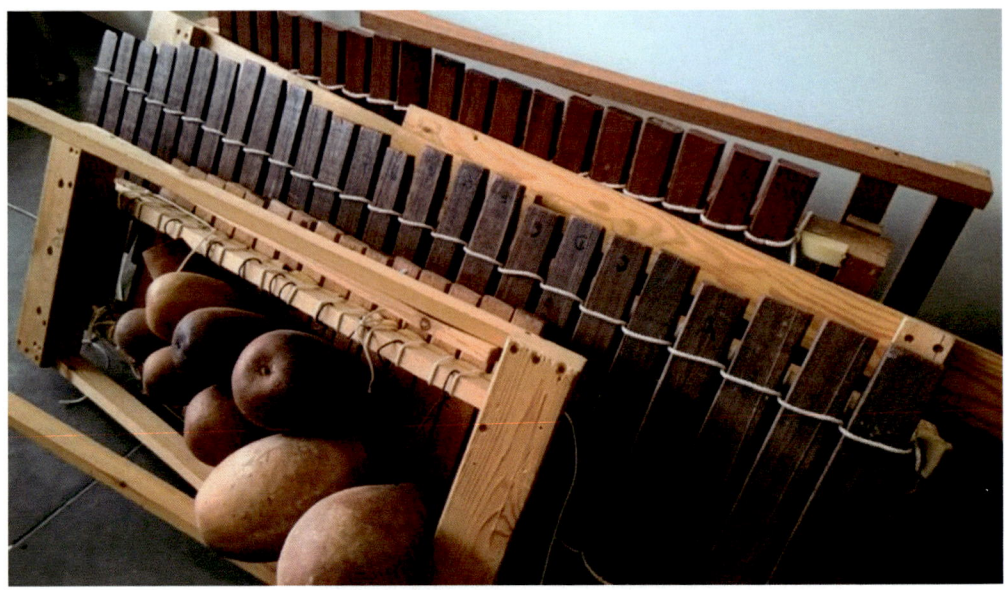

Figure 7.3. Balafons made by Alphonse Tourna and played by Human Hengers. (Photograph by Yvette Staelens. Copyright reserved)

Sound File 2. Maxence des Oiseaux playing his bone flute for the Human Henge project - https://tinyurl.com/desOiseaux

1. Windmill Hill
2. Swallowhead Springs
3. West Kennet Long Barrow
4. Lockeridge sarsen stone field
5. Sanctuary and Ridgeway Barrows
6. Night walk along the Avenue
7. Fired earth at Avebury Manor
8. Alexander Keiller Museum, Avebury
9. Ceremony planning
10. Equinox ceremony at Avebury Henge

Again, we rambled whatever the weather. We also had access to the stored collections at the Alexander Keiller Museum. Every session brought challenges, connections, and adventure. The route to Windmill Hill was a muddy

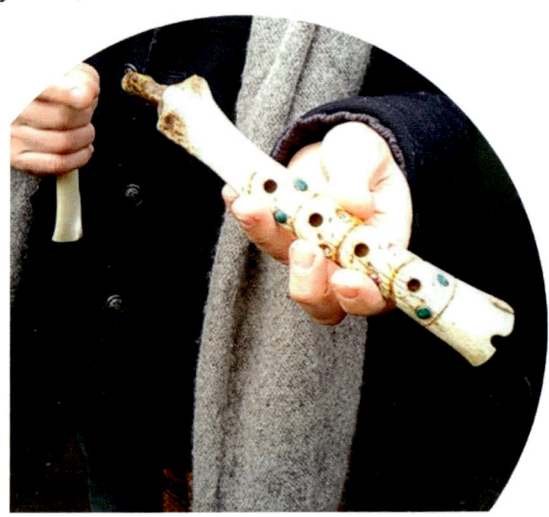

Figure 7.4. Bone flute played by Maxence des Oiseaux for the Human Henge project. (Photograph by Yvette Staelens. Copyright reserved)

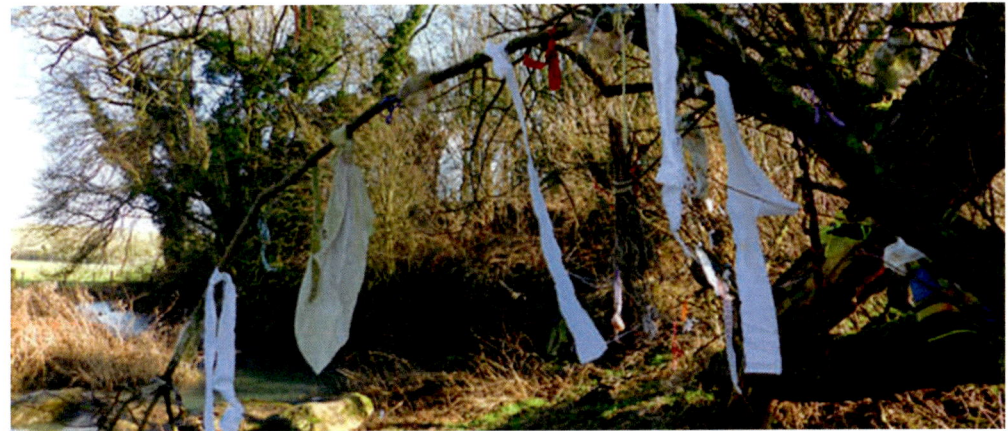

*Figure 7.5. Rag-tree at Swallowhead Springs, near Avebury, Wiltshire.
(Photograph by Yvette Staelens. Copyright reserved)*

trek for all, and no-one expected a song-share at the end. We found a crystal and a smashed mobile phone on top of one of the barrows — offerings ancient and modern. Wishes, intents and promises were tied with (biodegradable) 'ribbons' onto the rag-tree at Swallowhead Springs (Figure 7.5). And help was on hand to guide people safely across the slippery sarsen stepping stones and over the fast-flowing River Kennet. Discreet support of all kinds was always available, and our team of volunteers were invaluable in this respect.

The field of sarsen stones at Lockeridge inspired wanderings and discussions and we learned that for one Human Henger this was fairyland since his daughter saw the stones as fairy castles.

Walking the landscape at night has been a powerful manifestation of the Human Henge ethos 'to be connected' — to the cosmos, each other, the ancestors, and prehistoric landscapes. Darkness provided the mind with new ways of being with the stones of Avebury. We grouped a little more tightly together perhaps. A mist of rain provided a welcoming veil across the entrance to the Avenue; it disappeared during our walk but was there again on our return. Stones were touched, telescopes mounted on stands, voices asked 'is that a male or a female stone?' The Nebra Sky Disc from 1600 BC was discussed alongside a modern planisphere. Mid-way down the avenue the cloud cover present at the start of the walk scudded off to reveal the starscape, as we knew it would (Figure 7.6). This was Human Henge: we carry our magic with us!

Handling collections at the Museum felt very special (Figure 7.7). Here was access to the tangible prehistoric past, in our hands, and with curatorial expertise to introduce it. Everyone seemed totally engaged. For one person this activity was a highlight:

'I thought Human Henge peaked with the night walk — it didn't.'

Then things got mucky. Briony Clifton (NT) led a creative session with clay. We made masks and mounted them on an avenue of trees near Avebury Manor. Everyone created their own — sometimes more than one — and the process was totally engaging and somewhat addictive. Here they are (Figure 7.8).

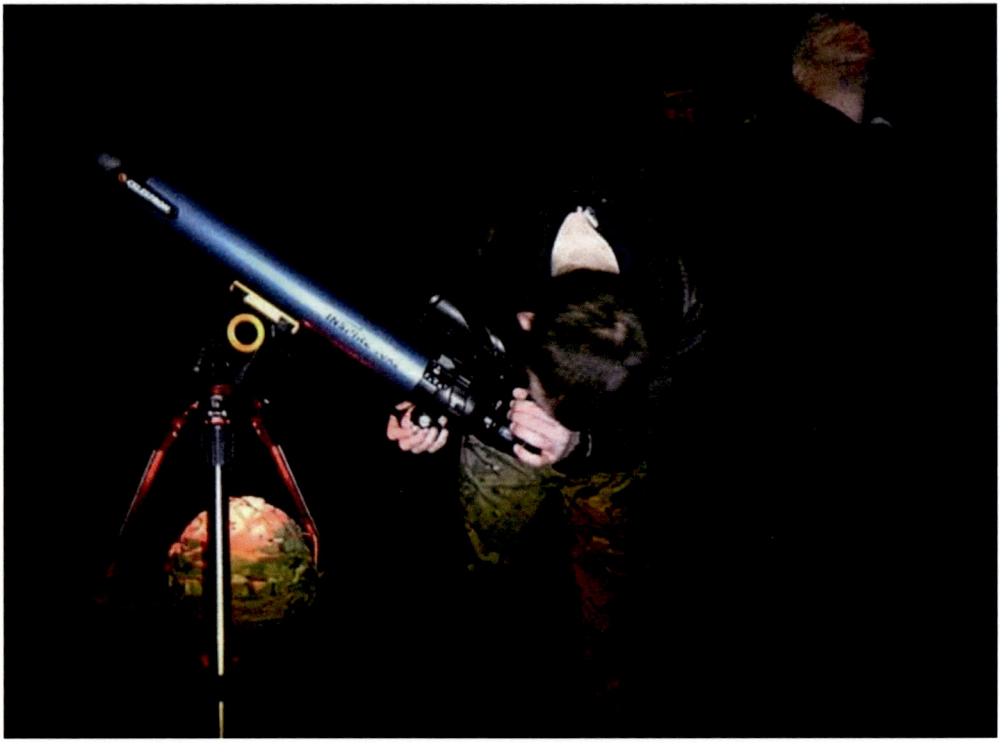

Figure 7.6. 'Skyscape inner problems recede as sense of self feels part of the endless universe'. (Photograph by Yvette Staelens. Copyright reserved)

'With my focus on the tree trunk and the clay and with birds singing in the distance, I experienced rare moments of internal peace. The creative therapy was engrossing, making me lose myself in the process, thus leaving worries and stresses at the gate.'

The Mum's tale

Reflecting upon other highlights from the three 'journeys', various happenings spring to mind. Telling stories in the reconstructed Neolithic houses at Stonehenge, whilst we made fire and string was one (Figure 7.9).

Another was the hare that fled from the ditch and up over the barrow

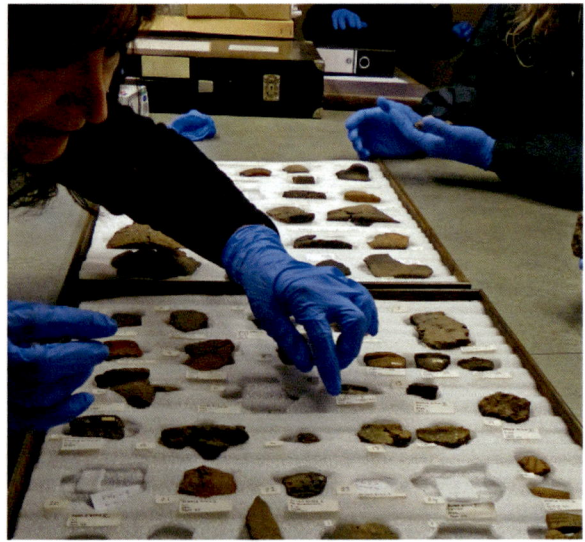

Figure 7.7. Handling prehistoric collections at the Alexander Keiller Museum, Avebury. (Photograph by Yvette Staelens. Copyright reserved)

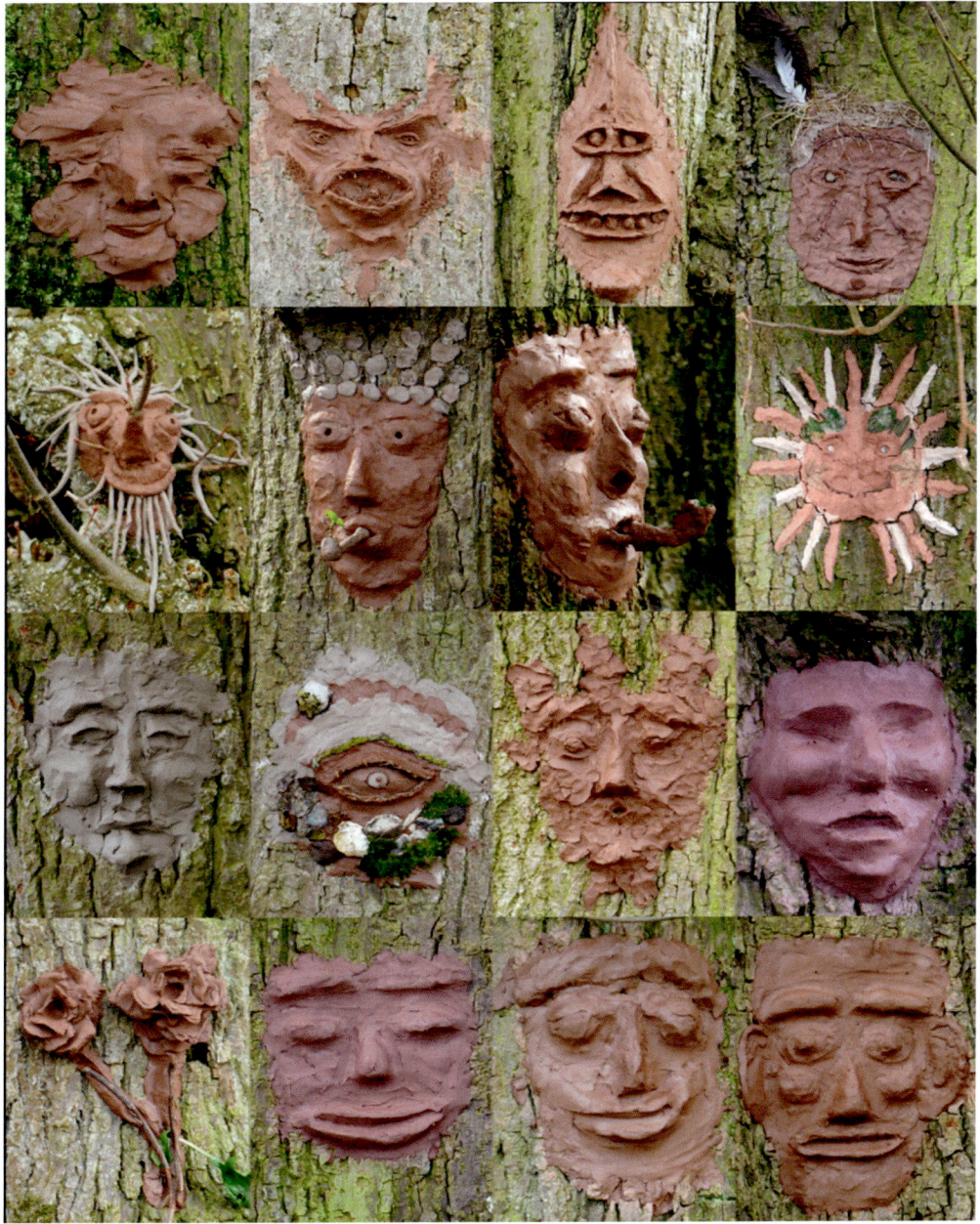

Figure 7.8. Clay masks made by Human Hengers at Avebury. (Photograph by Yvette Staelens. Copyright reserved)

that we had chosen for our guided meditation (Figure 7.10). A mythical creature of folktales, folklore, and pagan belief.

Sheltering and singing under Poundland umbrellas in Roman testudo formation in Fargo Plantation was yet another highlight (Figure 7.11).

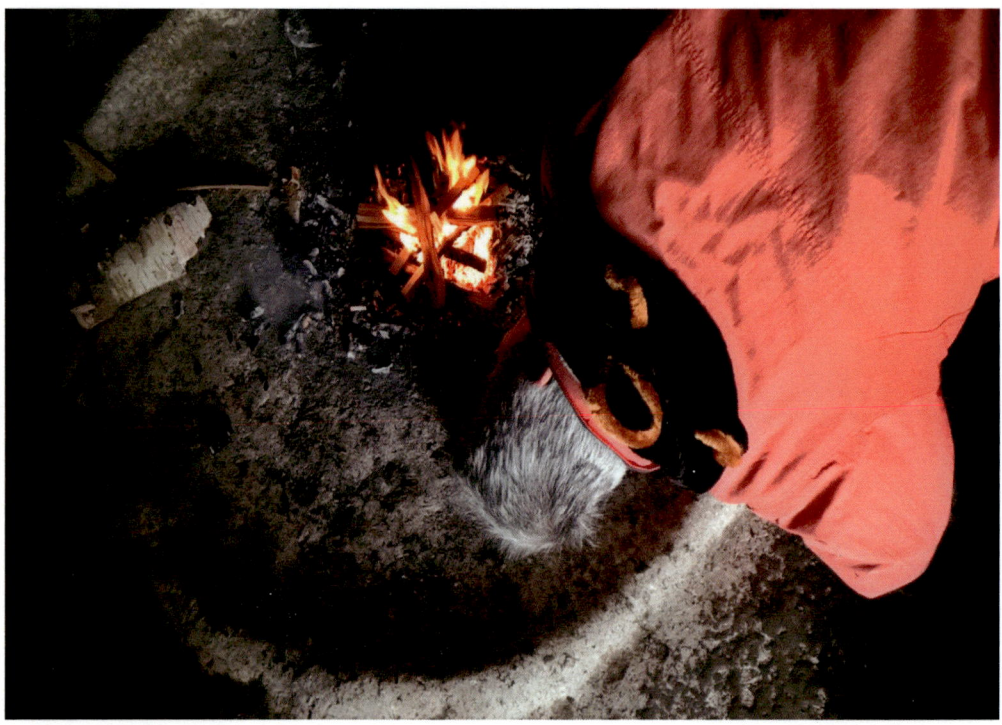

Figure 7.9. Firemaking in a Neolithic home. (Photograph by Yvette Staelens. Copyright reserved)

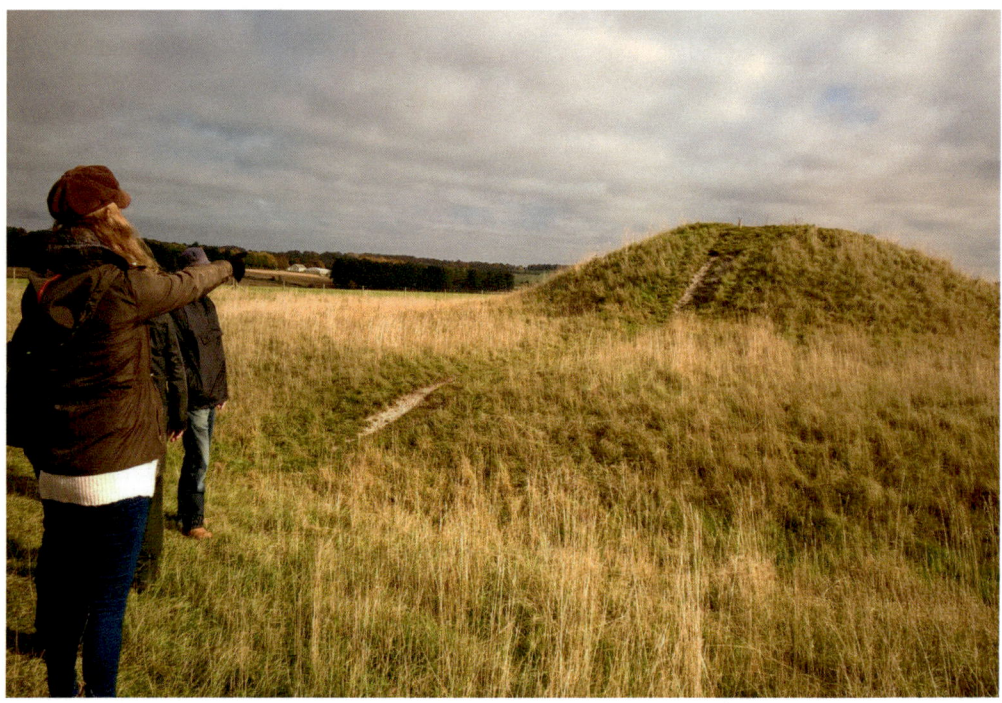

Figure 7.10. The hare on the barrow. (Photograph by Yvette Staelens. Copyright reserved)

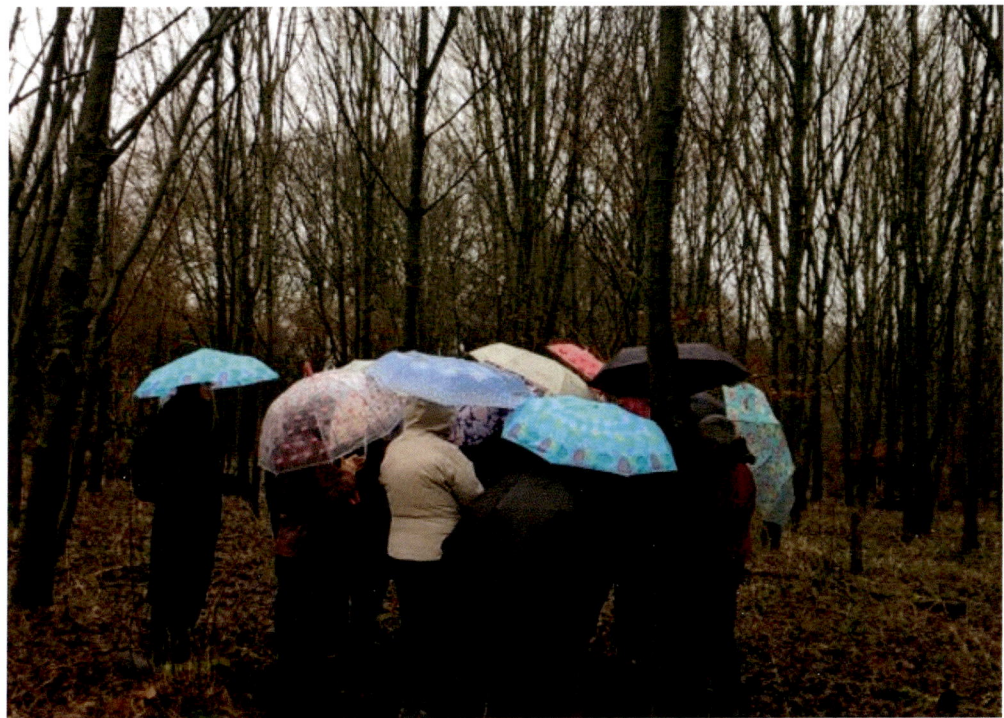

Figure 7.11. 'Getting soaked and chilled — loving it.' (Photograph by Yvette Staelens. Copyright reserved)

But one story stands out. A participant, a single parent, told me that she loved coming every week, and an important reason was because she now had something to share with her young daughter who would come home from school and ask 'What did you do today mummy?' Normally the answer was 'not much'. Now there was lots to tell, and soon mum and daughter were making visits to Human Henge sites together.

Conclusion

In some senses Human Henge felt like an oasis; a little place of safety, with fun and adventure and new knowledge. I certainly learned a great deal from the participants. It was a shared journey and I, too, felt the excitement of anticipation each Friday when I left home at dawn to drive to Human Henge. Where would our explorations lead today? The best sound of all, for me, was the chat. The merry babble that ensued each time we met and had our hot drink upon arrival. People catching up, the kindling of friendships, and an overwhelming sensation that what was really in the room was love. Even folks disinclined to articulate were engaged, and sometimes smiling. Intuitively, I felt that they were also participating in their own way, and comfortable. Here were people for whom life from time to time was truly intolerable, finding themselves in a place with others who cared. Journeying and exploring together, immersed in prehistoric archaeology and a healing landscape, was a very special privilege (Figure 7.12). We were all changed by the experience.

'Human Henge has saved lives'.

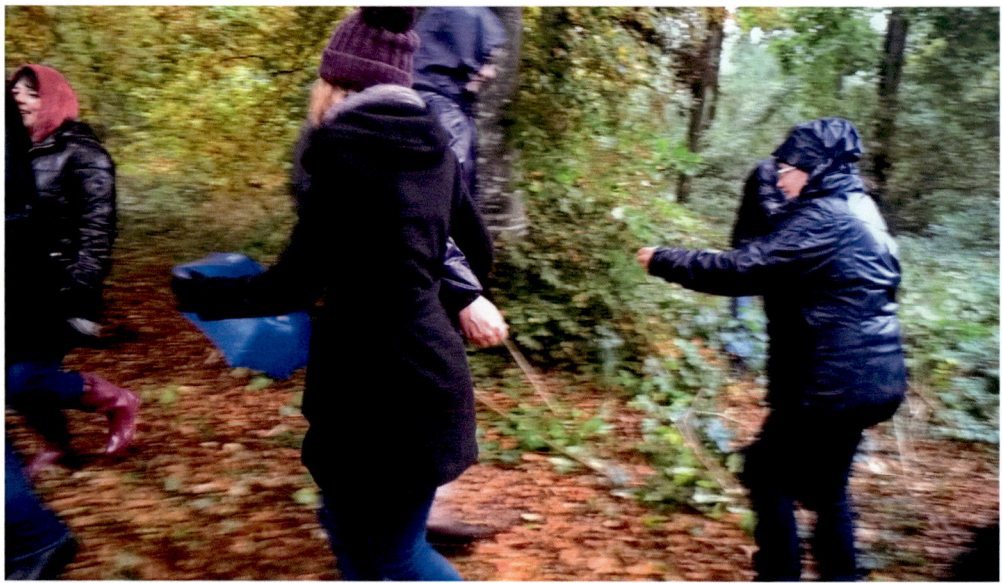

Figure 7.12 'Rain in the woods. Sweet chaos. Stripping hazel.' (Photograph by Jessica Swinburne. Copyright reserved)

Acknowledgements

Human Henge was devised and developed by the Restoration Trust (RT) in collaboration with Bournemouth University (BU). It was managed by Laura Drysdale (RT) with a Board chaired by Sarah Lunt (RT). Board membership included Toby Sutcliffe (Avon and Wiltshire Mental Health Partnership), Daniel O'Donoghue, (Richmond Fellowship; RF), Tim Darvill (BU) Vanessa Heaslip (BU), Briony Clifton (NT), Martin Allfrey (EH), Jane Willis (Willis Newson), and Katherine Snell (EH).

Bibliography

Darvill, T. 2007. Towards the within: Stonehenge and its purpose, in D.A. Barraclough and C. Malone (eds.) *Cult in Context: Reconsidering Ritual in Archaeology:* 148–157. Oxford: Oxbow.

Darvill, T. 2016. Roads to Stonehenge: A prehistoric healing centre and pilgrimage site in southern Britain, in A. Ranft and W. Schenkluhn (eds.) *Kulturstraßen als Konzept. 20 Jahre Straße der Romani* (More Romano. Schriften des Europäischen Romanik Zentrums 5): 155–166. Regensburg: Schell and Steiner.

Chapter 8

High value, short intervention historic landscape projects: Practical considerations for voluntary mental-health providers

Daniel O'Donoghue

Abstract

This paper presents a reflection on the Human Henge project and offers broad practical advice for similar projects. It is a profoundly personal commentary on the project, by a mental health and social inclusion practitioner working for Richmond Fellowship Wiltshire — part of the Richmond Fellowship, founded in 1959, one of the largest voluntary sector providers of mental health support in England, that champions recovery and social inclusion and engages with 9000 people each year. The concepts of possibility, privilege, expectation, and space are discussed as significant aspects of the Human Henge project. Particular attention is directed towards the practical considerations involved with such work. It gives an insight into the requirements of both participants and organizations, suggesting ways in which these might be successfully met during future projects that involve working in and around archaeological and historic landscapes. Extracts of poetry written by Human Henge participants illustrate the paper and it concludes with two full-length pieces.

Keywords: Delivery; Engagement; Expectations; Future developments; Privilege

The proposal

> 'Unhatched in the field's palm
> a stone calling —
> *Cuckoo! Cuckoo!*'

In my own fanciful recollection I pick up the phone to a woman I haven't met before. I listen while she enthuses over the potential therapeutic value of privileged access to Stonehenge, and a shared experience of historic landscapes for promoting mental and emotional well-being for people living with and recovering from mental health issues. There will be ten or twelve fortnightly sessions. There will be an element of academic research to which participants will hopefully agree. A high profile archaeological site such as Stonehenge is certainly the ideal — but at this stage I'm still a little unclear as to whether full agreement has been reached for this. And, of course, it all still needs funding, for which we would need prospective participants.

> 'Would you be interested?'

It feels a little bit speculative. But a good rule of thumb for Richmond Fellowship Wiltshire over the last few years has been: 'Say Yes, unless you have a very good reason to say No.' So I say 'Yes' to the nice lady on the phone, comfortable in the knowledge that this project is essentially someone else's responsibility and, if it proves to have legs, well, we can cross that bridge when we come to it.

That conversation was in July 2015 with Laura Drysdale from the Restoration Trust. In collaboration with Bournemouth University, English Heritage, and the National Trust we successfully completed the third and, for Richmond Fellowship Wiltshire, the final Human Henge sequence in March 2018.

In this book of academic papers I have the privilege — or licence — of providing a more informal account from the point of view of the voluntary sector. I was involved in each of the three Human Henge sequences as a member of staff with Richmond Fellowship and also, inevitably as it turns out, as an active participant. It would have been nigh on impossible to stand apart from what proved to be such a thoroughly engaging, immersive and inclusive experience.

I should also add, in fairness, that the proposal was already much more detailed and developed than my preamble might lead you to believe. The partnership between the Restoration Trust and Bournemouth University — which aimed to provide high quality academic and creative archaeological input — was already established, as was the research support from Bournemouth University's School of Health and Social Care. Despite my initial uncertainty, agreements were already in place with English Heritage for both privileged access to Stonehenge and also our use of the educational facilities there. Moreover, Laura Drysdale had already engaged with the Avon and Wiltshire Mental Health Partnership NHS Trust (AWP) for ways to engage participants. It was AWP who had suggested she approach Richmond Fellowship for active participation as Richmond Fellowship Wiltshire already had a reasonable track record of delivering land-based conservation projects with partner organizations.The sessions ran weekly in two sequences of 10 weeks each, at Stonehenge in late 2016 and early 2017 and for a third time in early 2018 at Avebury. Each of these culminated in either a solstice or equinox celebration. For the Richmond Fellowship then, this is the view from the bridge.

The feeling of it

> 'What shiver down her spine —
> feeling the first drops of rain
> on her newly discovered bones.'

Trying to capture the overall feeling of a project like Human Henge is necessarily subjective. With that in mind I've alighted upon feelings of possibility and privilege and of expectation and of space to try and focus my own impressions of what was, with the benefit of hindsight, significant to me about the Human Henge experience as a whole.

Possibility

There was a wonderful sense of possibility in the range of ideas and responses we allowed ourselves — and that we were encouraged to have — over a period of three months on each Human Henge sequence. We returned afresh each week, testing and exploring and testing again, our own ideas of what it was to be human — in both the past and the present. We listened to others; we sought to find expression for thoughts and feelings, and for a way of sharing and storing them away again for future recollection.

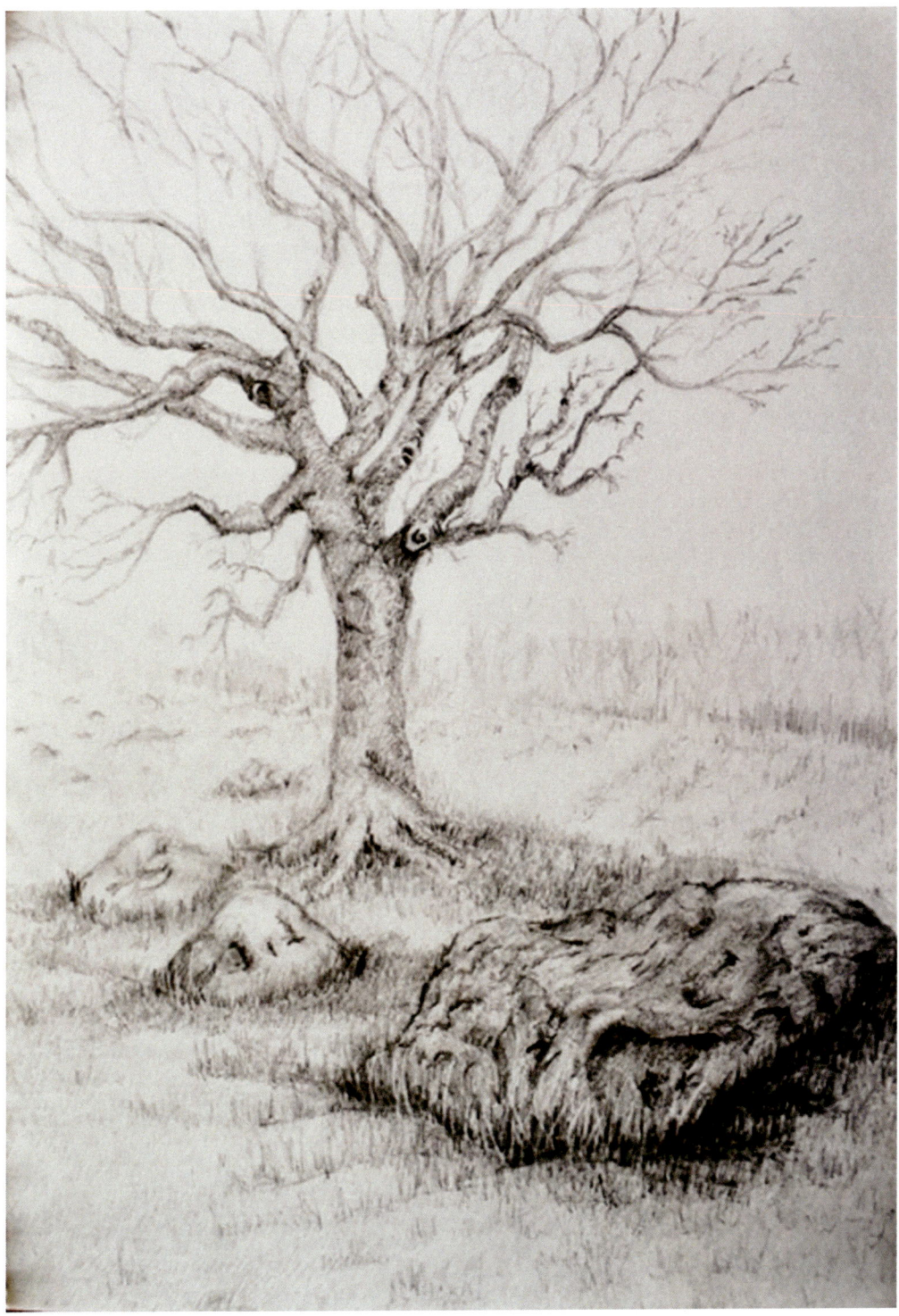

Figure 8.1. Sarsen strewn landscape at Lockeridge, Wiltshire. (Drawing by Donna Songhurst. Copyright reserved)

Privilege

There was privilege in terms of access to academic and creative expertise — professors, curators, experienced facilitators — and access to artefacts. At Stonehenge this culminated in access to the stone circle itself. At Avebury privilege was experienced in being guided through archaeological fragments curated above the public museum galleries in areas normally reserved for experts, or in sifting through material recently removed from beneath floorboards at the Manor and not yet sieved and catalogued. Recent history, brimming with questions and answers and more questions making the past feel contemporary

We were invited by experts into a kind of 'middle distance'. A landscape to be explored somewhere between tangible 'hard facts' — 'Look, a big stone!' — and the cumulative product of years of academic research that helped to set the outer bounds for what might constitute reasonable conjectures — 'Yes, but not just any stone. Let me tell you something about what we think we know about it.'

We had the anchor of those megalithic structures, silently dominating the landscapes of Stonehenge and Avebury, surrounded by voices that flitted around them gently outlining the limits of our current collective understanding. The voices of 'The Tame Professor' Tim Darvill, and others — Yvette, Steve, Nick, Briony, Ben — who helped to frame our experience of landscape and history.

Alongside these we had music from Chartwell, Alphonse, and Max on each of the respective Human Henge sequences, each of whom helped simultaneously to evoke and to articulate something of our emotional response to these places.

Expectation

There was expectation in terms of the language — and in the attitude and disposition of the facilitators on the project — that all discussions would be assumed to be perfectly understandable by each of us. It did not need to be translated or toned down, according to perceptions or misconceptions about us as participants. It was egalitarian to be addressed by specialists as being perfectly capable of understanding and assimilating what was being said, regardless of our own previous academic experience. It was empowering to realize that our own views, coming to the subject fresh or with experience, had their own natural validity.

Space

There was so much room in all of this for personal projections - from lived experience and for our own feeling of what was credible and what was incredible — different for each individual. Room for exploring what it means to be a human being, then and now. Room for exploring ideas of society, of groups and social structures.

There was room to speculate and reflect on what it means to be privileged, both for our ancestors and for ourselves, a small group of people given unprecedented access to publicly held but typically restricted cultural icons, as part of a well-being initiative. There was something of 'the wisdom of crowds' in appreciating how, collectively, we know much more than we do individually. An experience that reminds us of our own abilities; abilities we may have lost, or lost confidence in, like a gentle gauntlet thrown down for us to pick up so that we might cultivate new ones.

Hopefully, these are the charms of any good archaeology or history-based mental health project — the intrigue of exploring the space between the known and the unknown — and the open invitation to step into it, with Everyman as your guide.

And realizing that, in some sense, you knew this all along.

But what was it *really* like? The practical considerations

What follows are some basic practical considerations for people who have their feet more firmly rooted on *terra firma*, and who might be wondering how they could use the Human Henge approach, or aspects of it, as a basis for their own historical or cultural initiatives. These points are by no means exhaustive or systematic, but hopefully they will provide some useful bearings and help ensure that some of the more obvious aspects of the project are taken into account by prospective organizers.

Engagement

> 'A flock of stones.
> And herding them —
> a meadow pipit.'

Zero exclusion and self selection

We pitched the project as close to a 'zero exclusion' policy as we could make it (see also *Physical access*, below). Participants themselves made the decision as to whether they would join or not. We were fortunate in that we did not have to make that decision on behalf of any applicant. Everyone effectively self selected once they understood both the character of the project and our modest expectations. Baseline criteria were: applicants must be a minimum of 18 years of age; have recognized, though not necessarily formally diagnosed, mental health support needs; be resident in Wiltshire. Referral could be made on behalf of an applicant by a referring agency or by self referral, as is usual with the services of Richmond Fellowship Wiltshire overall. Applications were made using a form specific to the Human Henge initiative.

Once enrolled, participants were, for the duration of each Human Henge sequence, clients of Richmond Fellowship Wiltshire. This ensured accountability, appropriate risk management and support. Some participants were already clients with Richmond Fellowship prior to Human Henge involvement, and some engaged with Richmond Fellowship services subsequent to their involvement with Human Henge. For approximately half of all participants, their engagement with Human Henge would have marked their first engagement with any Richmond Fellowship staff member. For others their Human Henge participation was unique and sufficient and did not extend beyond the final sessions.

Sign up

A lot of useful work was done ahead of the first meeting with participants — with Richmond Fellowship staff calling to speak with participants in person, more than once, ahead of the first session. This was in addition to any regular contact they might have with key workers from the same service. A courtesy call a couple of weeks before the start date helped to allay anxieties as the start date approached.

Interest in the project was driven more by intellectual or emotional engagement with the subject matter rather than, for example, existing personal or social connections. A significant number of participants — between two thirds and three quarters — had not met each other prior to their involvement with Human Henge. It is testimony to the quality and value of the experience that participants gelled quickly, and it was entertaining putting faces to names when we only met in person for the first time on the orientation session.

Primary and secondary needs

We were aware of the multitude of 'secondary' needs that people might present with — and remembered that it is the person, not the diagnosis or condition, that we were engaging with. We aimed to be pragmatic, flexible, open and honest about the best way to navigate and work around secondary health, primarily physical, or social issues to ensure inclusion. Most people are pretty good at making decisions regarding participation for themselves, assuming that they have been given enough information in the first place. Not many people enjoy putting themselves in compromising or difficult situations on a weekly basis. Once participants had signed up, it was a case of working together as a group to support one another and to allow each other space when some of the issues — mental, emotional or physical — presented themselves.

Risk management

Basic risk information was collected for individuals; we felt comfortable that we could manage all significant risks that might present themselves. From a person-centred perspective it was useful to understand this in terms of the potential support required, rather than as a set of risks to be managed. We were working alongside very ordinary people with their own unique challenges, which they have a great deal of experience managing. 'What do you want us to do — if anything — to help?' was the best approach.

Practical on-site risk assessments were carried out by host organizations English Heritage and the National Trust at their respective sites. In addition, Richmond Fellowship Wiltshire had a number of assessments appropriate to travel, and Human Henge facilitators were responsible for assessing the range of activities that they were experienced in delivering.

Mental health training

Introductory mental health 'First Aid' training was provided to volunteers on the project, which included Bournemouth University and English Heritage volunteers and staff, as well as project facilitators. In addition, Richmond Fellowship was able to provide two or more staff members per session; people experienced in working in a mental health context.

'Uniquity'

What a great word, couldn't resist it. When a project has a unique character and some 'scarcity value' participants are likely to demonstrate a higher level of commitment than if there is the chance to catch up next week, or in a couple of weeks time. The fact that these were occasional or intensive projects only added to their allure against a background of more conventional projects or support.

If the offer doesn't feel special to you then ask yourself: Why do I think this offer will be appealing to someone else? Then: What's missing? What must you add in order to create the sense of opportunity and appeal essential to successful engagement? Your staff ought to be as excited about being involved as any other participants.

Horizons

Often the remoteness of the location is part of their attraction. How many of us have lived close to a tourist destination we've never or rarely visited ourselves? We'll often travel long distances for something special whilst we overlook what is unique locally. Sometimes a spurious sense of familiarity, quietly breeds contempt. Having to make an effort can help make the objective itself seem more worthwhile — being supported to make the effort, then makes achieving the objective feasible.

Delivering Human Henge

> 'Barrow builders —
> following the same gradient a leaf takes
> when it falls.'

Transport

We were fortunate to already have the use of a small minibus at Richmond Fellowship as well as project workers familiar with picking up and dropping off clients to ensure access to a project. We also had a lot of lifts being offered between participants once a sequence was underway — a natural gesture that made it easier to rationalize travel once the project started. Easy access is a basic provision to ensure success and a pre-arranged pick-up has the further advantage of increasing the likelihood of continued and consistent attendance. Public transport in Wiltshire, especially given the comparatively remote locations of Stonehenge and Avebury, was not a viable option for any of the participants. This may be a different proposition in urban areas, for example for museum or cathedral access in city landscapes, but this was an everyday tale of country folk.

An additional benefit of being able to provide our own transport was that, from a participant's perspective, the day began at the point at which they were picked up through to when they were dropped off again or we parted company. This allows for all manner of easy and informal conversations about anything and everything. Clinical colleagues in the Early Intervention in Psychosis (EIP) teams used to joke 'We do our best work in the car'. You can easily believe it.

Orientation session

We had a separate orientation session before each of the Human Henge sequences began. During these, we trialled pick ups and met together for the first time as a group. It gave us a chance to stress test our arrangements, to begin to get to know each other, to talk together about what we could expect from the project and what it might expect from us. We could more easily provide clarity about facilities, appropriate clothing, refreshments and lunchtime arrangements etc. and by now we were doing this in real time.

Having no previous immediate experience to draw on for the first Human Henge it was obvious to participants that we weren't entirely sure of some of the details ourselves. We were open about this. Whilst this gave us a reputation for having little or no idea of what was going on, we were, by way of compensation, credited with a degree of honesty and the sense that whatever happened 'it'll be fine'. In subsequent Human Henge sequences we were much better able to tell our coccyx from our cuckoo, but I can't help feeling that we lost a little in the way of charm as a result.

Physical access

Not everyone could participate to the same extent physically. This wasn't due to unreasonable distances or unnecessarily difficult terrain but, if you have mobility issues, it can be sobering to realize that even a short walk with gentle gradients can leave you breathless if you're not used to being active out of doors. Some prospective participants withdrew before the start of the sessions due to physical health issues, after reflecting on the integral character of a landscape based project. One lady persevered, and whilst she struggled with some of the outdoor sessions, she continued to involve herself by attending the building-based sessions that she felt more comfortable navigating. This was another aspect of self-management for project participants — allowing them to exercise flexibility. Accommodating different levels of physical ability was important, where possible.

Social anxiety

Social anxiety was a challenge for a significant proportion of participants — exceeding half — as this typically fuelled their social exclusion in the first instance. However, the desire to directly address this provided a motivating factor for their engagement in Human Henge.

Challenging their anxiety by becoming involved in group activity didn't work for everyone. One participant attended and then withdrew after three sessions on the grounds that the negative impact — feelings of inadequacy and self-reproach after a session — was greater than the achievement experienced in having faced their demons by attending. Whilst this could not be overcome within the project, which was inherently rooted in group activity, the decision to withdraw could still be acknowledged and respected.

Punctuality

Sessions normally ran from 10am to 1pm and then we finished with lunch. We would typically be on the move again by 2pm, with drop-offs finishing around 3–3:30pm. We tried to make sure we were clear about pick ups and end times and to keep to these after an early complaint from one participant. However we still needed to allow for a degree of flexibility — socially as well in practical terms. At the beginning of the day, pick ups could easily be delayed by one person oversleeping. A phone call ahead of time the following week might guard against this happening again, but participants may continue to struggle with the new set of expectations or with the effects of medication in early mornings. If a session ran over, we needed to be proactive in ensuring that all participants were comfortable with this and that there was not someone worrying in silence about a missed transport link or child pick up.

Timings

If you can vary the times of your sessions, why not? Mix it up a little bit. We had one night time session walking out in the landscape in each sequence, looking at constellations where breaks in the cloud cover allowed and pondering on how things like night time, the darkness and the night sky might have affected people in the past. We also had an early morning start to accommodate privileged access at 8am for the two culminating dates at Stonehenge. Similar arrangements were made for the Avebury-based group. You'd be surprised how few people go out walking after dark — and not just from a sense of anxiety over personal security. Opportunity knocks, especially in a group setting, for creating new and stimulating experiences that are out of the ordinary in simple but evocative ways.

Food and drink

Tea and coffee were always provided with the natural variations — de-caff and non-dairy — to ensure a sense of hospitality and welcome. Biscuits were there right beside them. Sometimes basic provisions like this gave an opportunity for demonstrations of kindness and consideration. After one participant expressed a preference for fig rolls, these were provided the following week and were greatly appreciated. Small gestures like this can contribute to the positive atmosphere of a group and lets participants know that they are being heard. Little things count.

After that the provision of food was down to the budget — we were able to provide extras like fruit and nuts, which were appreciated. A focus on a particular day, or a culminating event, when people can bring and share food or have some food provided lends itself to the feeling of communion; that basic social bond of sharing food together.

Facilities

Loos are great! People really like to know that they will have access to toilet facilities and can be disconcerted when they unexpectedly find that none are available. Some might have health issues which make toilets vital to their participation. Others react with surprising fortitude and a willingness to make do and mend, given the easy availability of decent shrub cover. Considering the potential anxiety around the availability of these facilities it was obviously important to be clear about when they would and would not be easily available and to give this information ahead of time. People have all sorts of techniques and approaches to managing their own functions but only if they have a reasonable idea of what to expect and when. For example, if you know in advance that you won't see a toilet until lunchtime you might just decide to have a smaller than usual tea or coffee with breakfast. If you give people the opportunity to plan ahead they can prove more resilient than you might expect when it becomes necessary.

Security

Being able to leave your belongings in a safe place — especially when setting out across the landscape — was liberating. Locked rooms, cupboards, and at a pinch car boots for excess baggage are a real boon to participants.

Weather

We took the rough with the smooth. If you are expecting to spend a significant amount of time outdoors, especially in winter, you should ensure that everyone has been well briefed on what to wear. Where possible, you should try to bring additional waterproofs for the occasional but inevitable oversight. Again, advance notice is key. People who don't habitually spend much time outdoors might need a few days' warning to find things like waterproofs and boots. A stock of cheap umbrellas provided by the project made a handy *testudo* against sudden downpours - as well as providing opportunities for silly behaviour and photo opportunities.

Our third Human Henge sequence at Avebury culminated with a snowy Spring Equinox. Knock yourself out when the weather is like this — there's still a child inside most of us.

Creative projects

Human Henge encouraged open thinking and creativity with practical projects using methods contemporary with the period we were exploring — cooking, pottery, cordage, fire lighting. People were happy to get their hands dirty for the most part. The idea was to encourage participants to open up, so it really didn't matter if your Beaker pot had all the characteristics of an ashtray or your cordage looked more like something the cat just coughed up.

> 'From the edge of my seat I watch
> my pot
> consigned to flames.'

We had an extra dimension in that our co-ordinator and facilitator Yvette Staelens, an archaeologist by training, was also a natural voice practitioner. I think it is fair to say that whilst not everyone can sing, regardless of what they tell you, everyone has a voice. In open fields you can sound like a crow and nobody really minds (although to be fair, Yvette has a great voice!). The rest of us stopped caring what we sounded like after the first couple of weeks.

> 'Bone flutes
> still long for the smell of honey
> on warm breath.'

We started our first Human Henge sequence with a notion of generating our own epic poem — which became an epic worry until we realized that we simply had the wrong approach. We relaxed and ended up with a range of creative results which had every bit as much merit — and probably greater meaning to participants. Group One wrote a charming saga composed on Post-it notes which is reproduced below. Group Two produced an individually-authored epic, also reproduced, and a short story. I've added a handful of haiku in this article. By the time we got to Group Three there was no written record to refer back to at all and we reverted to oral history instead. We all have fond memories of Flo's marvellous and unexpected singing on the final day.

'If I sing
let it be like fire
in dry brush.'

Improvise

One of our best sessions was when another facilitator failed to arrive due to unforeseen circumstances. A brief question and answer session was scheduled before taking advantage of hastily arranged access to an exhibition. However, we never left the Education Room. With maps spread out across the tables, one question led to another as participants explored all manner of ideas with Professor Tim Darvill, in what was an especially lively tutorial which we couldn't have arranged to such great effect if we'd tried. Sometimes situations which start as problems, transform into ideal opportunities.

Facebook

There are angels and devils in Facebook and other social media as everyone knows but, handled sensitively, Facebook can be a really useful tool for closed or short lived groups and projects. It worked especially effectively for Group Two who cohered around the possibilities created by a closed group and shared experience. Its development was very much participant led and is something which might actively be encouraged. For some, Facebook offered a useful way of staying in contact once the formal sessions had ended.

www.humanhenge.org

Human Henge also had a public face — www.humanhenge.org — which allowed for input from participants in terms of blogs, photographs, creative writing, pictures and commentary. It allowed people outside the project a window into its activities, and provided a way for participants to share their thoughts if they chose to do so.

When managing a website it is an obvious point to make to remember to be clear about consent from those appearing in pictures and video footage and get permission to reproduce material. The Restoration Trust working with participants, staff and volunteers, managed this aspect without incident and the pages generated remain as a testimony to the experience.

Step down

After a comparatively intense experience, it was obvious that we needed to provide opportunities to meet and reflect at a later date, in order to mitigate the impact of 'The End'. Anxiety about the withdrawal of interaction and support provided by Human Henge was clear amongst participants and we learned to address this. Scheduling dates and events subsequent to the core group experience did meant that closure of each sequence was delayed. However this allowed people to revive, reflect and assimilate the lessons and experiences of a quality experience.

Remember to begin talking about the end soon after the mid-point — if not before. Advance notice helps people to assimilate the coming change of circumstances, and to prepare themselves for it. This is especially true if there are genuine opportunities for continued participation in other contexts, such as volunteering with a partner organization, a local affordable membership to the facilities or sites which had been used, or perhaps informal group visits to other places of interest under participants' own steam (see the use of Facebook above).

Where to from here?

> "uman 'enge.
> The uprights and lintels lost
> Only the apostrophes remain, like crows.'

Individuals

In terms of individual successes these are necessarily anonymized and muted in publications. However, for those present, there were clearly some tremendous positive and sustained outcomes notwithstanding the fact that, at the time of writing, analysis of the most recent Human Henge sequence is still ongoing. See Vanessa Heaslip's Chapter 9 in this volume for the quantitative data. The Human Henge website gives a qualitative flavour.

Not everyone enjoys a feeling of personal achievement and recovery, and you can usually sense when others seem to receive much more from an experience than you do. However projects like Human Henge create a sense of possibility; highlighting the potential for a positive impact is an important prerequisite for any prospect of success for the individual.

It is important to recognize that whatever you offer won't be for everyone; there is no 'one size fits all' approach. Anticipate and respect this. Be mindful that participants may need support after not being able to access a project and that it is not just a matter of giving support to enable people to access your project. Reflecting now, I do wonder whether we might have done more for those individuals who did not progress with Human Henge. Having said that, Human Henge had a good attendance rate and a number of those who did not maintain attendance were able to access, or were already in receipt of support from Richmond Fellowship or other agencies.

Partners

Look around. There are numerous publicly-funded cultural providers — museums, galleries, libraries, trusts — all of whom are genuinely looking to broaden and improve access to their resources. They don't necessarily know how best to do this, or how to reach particular groups. If you are a voluntary sector provider looking to improve social inclusion for any given client group then there could be a winning partnership just waiting to happen.

We have recently been exploring and developing a partnership with Salisbury Cathedral around privileged access for clients through a sequence of workshops. These workshops, modelled broadly on a Human Henge approach, aim to share something of the life and history of the cathedral from the Middle Ages to the present, from the sacred to the secular, recognizing the enormous cultural capital of the cathedral for everyone in the community. The Salisbury Cathedral Outreach team, motivated by their own desire for social inclusion, initiated this proposal and we are only too happy to encourage people to participate to attend.

Short term interventions and commissioning strategies

We are using some of the approaches and outcomes from Human Henge to inform the development of a range of higher value/shorter term interventions on behalf of clients. We are doing this in order to meet commissioning demands for services that clearly demonstrate improved outcomes and increased throughput. The Human Henge experience has been useful in formulating ideas and also increasing confidence in providing shorter term interventions in services that have previously provided more open ended support over longer periods.

It will be interesting to explore how we can incorporate the unique with the ordinary as part of our everyday delivery of support. We aim to offer more structured, sequenced and time limited interventions that are open and responsive to different individuals' needs alongside the offer of more conventional one to one support in pursuit of greater social inclusion.

Final thoughts

> 'Mind like a lizard
> on the sunny side
> of these old stones.'

Time and transport remained the biggest challenges for Richmond Fellowship Wiltshire, as they often are for any organization. But where there's a will there's a way. Be prepared to put in more than you expect and be prepared to get more out of it than you expect and all the sums will add up!

I realize I have said nothing about our current partners in Human Henge — except to add here that they have all, without exception, been marvellous. Each of them worked with a willingness, intelligence and understanding of our requirements in terms of the people we support that was at all times natural and commendable. If we were able to reciprocate in any way it was always the least that we could do.

I might add: Beware the woman from The Restoration Trust bearing gifts! But that would be unfair given the fabulous return we have had from this partnership. So much so that we have recently agreed to participate in a new provisional project focussed around exploring the old Wiltshire asylum archives — as part of a broader national initiative — sharing and developing the archivist's skills and techniques with participants over a period of 15 weeks, with a view to reviving and developing personal, professional and creative skills and experience. No umbrella needed.

And finally... The only joke I remember from Human Henge came from walking back from the circle at Stonehenge after winter solstice and three of us imagining Stone Age teenagers complaining about their parents and talking about their new mobile technology.

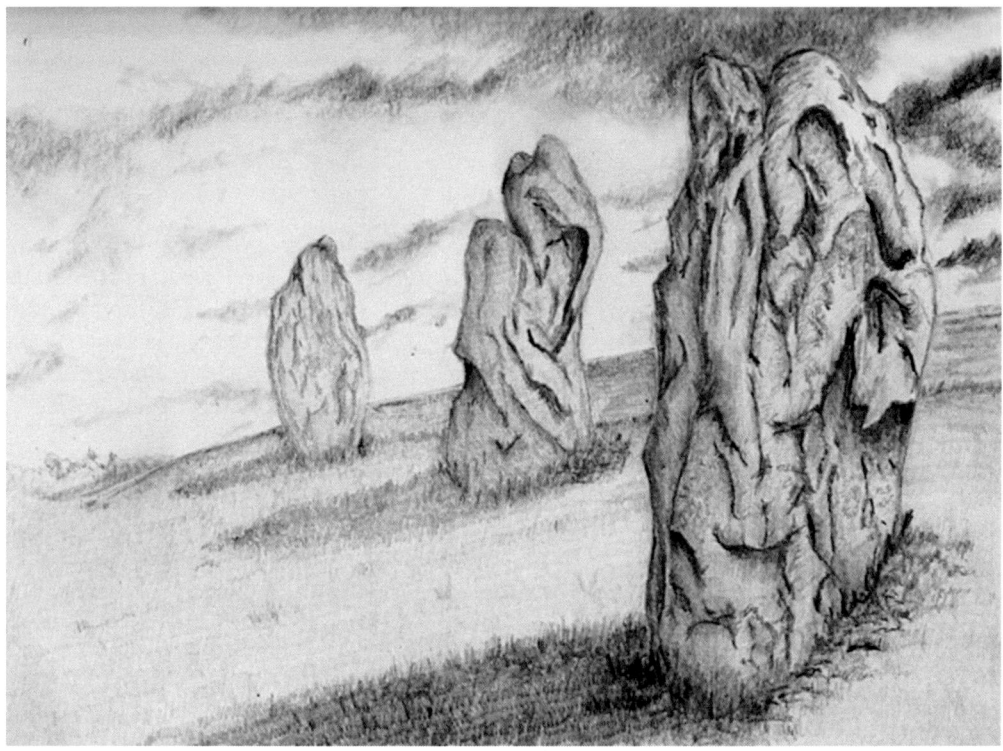

Figure 8.2. Avebury Henge, Wiltshire. (Drawing by Donna Songhurst. Copyright reserved)

'Ooh, is that a brick'?
'Nah, its a smart stone'.
'Is it on contract'?
'No. Pay as you throw'.

Hey, it was still early in the morning and it made us laugh...

'The builders gone —
the sun setting
between these standing stones'

Human Henge – The Post-it Note Saga
or
'Song of Ourselves'
Group 1, Stonehenge

Woodhenge

WENT TO WOODHENGE.
Durrington bowl.
Open Space
Views
Wind
Natural landscape
Cold Clear Sunny.

INVERTED MOAT,
walking the henge feeling history — the ancient contact with our ancestors

No wood at Woodhenge

A SPACE FULL OF STATUES
Posts, timber posts, plunged into the earth.
Standing on posts.
concrete posts
Standing on woodhenge

Photos taken.getting to know each other.
Whats it all about this human henge
Nice feelings of getting together.

Horrid Histories film.
Funny boasting
Boast battle video — nuts!
What could be my boast?

The Cuckoo Stone

Sneaking a peek at the cuckoo stone!

WE CAME & SUNG AND WENT AWAY
Piggy Pig Dog Dog 🎵

Barrow burial

WENT TO MOUNDS & WOODS
Standing on the Plain
Barrow walk Barrow burial

One barrow looks much like any other

Monarchs & meditation.
bronze warriors/kings
This Monarch of the Plain what strange rites were conducted near you, who were you for and why were you made.
What about the little people — where buried?

I saw a male adult stood on top of the round barrow. He was just looking south. He had a feather in his hair.

White hare
wet dog
feeling cold
Trees dripping water
Silence
Peace
Burials

SANG A SONG IN THE RAIN
Autumn leaves song
Singing 'leaves are falling'

COMMUNING WITH OUR ANCESTORS ON THE GRAVES OF THE WHITE HARE!

Woodland walk

Wet
Cold
Fargo Woods
All these trees, so different, grow as one matt beneath the sounding sky.
RAIN
Rain in the woods.
Sweet chaos.

Fargo wood like a broken umbrella in the autumn letting the rain in

Stripping hazel.
Strip willow
Stripped the Willow dance —
Sapping the willow.
Waving Wands of hazel.
What did wood get used for — hazel rings
Alfred Cake.
ancient knowledge passed down.
— our heritage

Rain, Rain, glorious rain.
Getting soaked & cold chilled — loving it.

Wet wet wet — singing in the rain!

A WOVEN DANCE
TO FORGET ABOUT THE RAIN
PEACE.
THE LEAVES ARE FALLING falling

Pissing rain.
Can't do singing in a group.

Walking & talking along the road.
Walking back to a cup of tea.
We talked of how the Neolithic people might not have hot tea.

Chartwell singing at Cuckoo Stone

Chartwell and his gourd making sweet sounds
CUCKOO STONE,
like an unhatched egg in the palm of the fiddler hand.
Sun — hot!
I watched a hawk fly and hover behind him.
We sang his ancestral 'welcome' song.

CLEAR DAY,
BEAUTIFUL WEATHER,
SUN
Tim: The cuckoo song and bluestone.
Fallen stones and tailbones.

Chartwell's robe.
Black — grandfather's line
White — grandmothers' line
red — other.
honour the ancestors

Singing and now dancing together
Holding hands — beautiful.
We circled the stone in a ring together.
SINGING/CHANTING AROUND THE STONE.
I turned round & around feeling the bright sun.
People moving in an eddy, a whirl, a circle on orbit....

Ancient music
Joy of Singing, joy of dancing spontaneous.
Ancestors
were
with
Us.

SINGING FOR THE ANCESTORS, IN HUMBLE RECOGNITION.

RESPECTING OUR PAST.

Night walk at the Cursus

Night walk on Cursus
Painfully cold
CLOUDY NIGHT,
SOME STARS,

Nebra disc — so cold & beautiful glimpses of the cosmos as the clouds cleared.

Frosty night

STARS WERE BRIGHT

WALK OF THE DEAD

DEAD OF THE NIGHT

Nebra Sky Disk held safe in the earth for centuries, uncovered showing up the Seven sisters and the Sun barge carrying that glowing mass under the world to rise again.

The Seven Sisters
Little children lost in the woods....
Skyscape.
Seeing further in darkness than you can in broad daylight.
inner problems recede as sense of self feels part of the endless universe

I missed the night cursus.
I had a raging toothache.
An abscess in my jaw.
How the people of stonehenge must have endured physical pain.

Ancient Sky — a sense of being so small and fleeting — but in a good way
Walking.

Cold cold but happy

ate doughnuts.

The red/white ribbons of cars on 303.

Round houses, collections, and making mats

HUTS AND COLLECTIONS

Museum day.
Today I realised how the ancients never put any figurative work on their pots.
Always the same. Were they slaves?
Were they lacking expression.
Were they avoiding animal plant & people marks.
Nick digeridoo pot.

smelting, bronze, malachite
what extraordinary ability is this — running metal from stone!! Veins in the rock.....
Monuments of mankind.
Turn back the night sky but not see the sweat running which raised them up.

HOUSES AND ROUND HUTS
Really glad to be inside a Neolithic house.
Handling a shirt of nettle fibres.
ECHOES FROM THE PAST

ESCAPE FROM THE POTS.
HAD FIRE & DID REED WEAVING
MAKING MATS
making things from reeds.
I'm really useless at weaving
LAYING ON A VERY FIRM YET COMFORTABLE BED, GETTING A TASTE OF STONEAGE LIFE.
WEAVING IN THE CONSCIOUS THOUGHTS ABOUT THE UNCONSCIOUS.

Smoke, fire, heat, huts, needles
Fire in the hut buyo!
told stories around the fire
Albert's ghost story in the other hut.
Why is it always in the other place?
sense of community round the fire, weaving, talking —
sense of peace and simplicity
a sense of living/working/being all at the same time — a natural life.
Broken key in minibus

Making pots

We all made pots for firing
Made thumb pot & decorated it.
WRITING MY MEMOIRES.

What dreams are these on beaker pots inside and out…..?
Recreate the way of ancestors. See through their eyes and shape the clay.
ancient artisans
THUMBING OUR WAY AROUND TO MAKE A VESSEL THAT CAN TAKE US BACK IN TIME!

Lovely to sit together & create, range of skills just what a treat to get mucky & make with Mark.
Lovely chap who costumed up for us.

Why can everyone else make a better pot than me
How difficult to make a beaker — I made a bucket.
> My pot was OK. I am not good at handy crafts. It felt good. And making the patterns was easy.
>> this is real life real living — making pots in order to eat and drink.

I helped weave the willow enclosure for his test — loved that.
Something new I can do.

WATCHING AN ANCIENT FORGE.
fire pit kiln.
Watched fire maker
Nick making fire with a stick and bow.
Fire in the hold buyo!
this is living/working at the same time
bellows demo with open bags & bone hole.
Smoking pots.
SMOKING THE POTS

King Barrows and walk up The Avenue

VERY ENJOYABLE WALK ALONG THE KING BARROWS
CONNECTING WITH ANCESTORS
singing — climbing the hill song —
Manytimes……
Open your heart. Lift up your voice!!!!
 let us sing together for a while…

Kings barrow to bury pots — but didn't.
Pot in a tree stump

Walking up & down the line of barrows
Kicking over mole hills.
I am enjoying my time at Stonehenge.
The singing is OK
also the walking
The fields are pitted with these ancient men,
how they came to their ends puzzles us
as does why they were lodged for eternity at such places.

I sat on a fallen tree and started to drum my djembe.
We danced as others joined in.
DRUMMING, MAGICAL, TRANCE — WITH THE STONES IN THE DISTANCE
bells with drums & Danny up in the tree.
American hikers
Then trying to get Dan out of the tree

THE FALLEN BUT STILL GROWING YEW TREE

Find the avenue.
Liz leading us to the Avenue
the walk up the Avenue
to Stonehenge.

BURYING THE POTS.
—hiding the pots!
Nic's smiley pot — fool the archaeologists?
CREATIVE REBELS BURY THEIR CREATIVE MINDS.
PERSPECTIVES OF THE FUTURE!

Looking at the stones so close.
But we have to wait.
Leave .....
Shadow on the stones.....

Discussion

Very relaxed get together.
Reflections on the henge experience,
easy to recollect as such days seep into one's being.

Chit chat
laughing with Chartwell

DISCUSSING RELIGION
PAGAN, WICCA, DRUIDIC,
DRESS CODE PAST PRESENT AND FUTURE
NUDITY IN RELIGION AND CULTURE.

MOST BORING 2 HOURS OF MY LIFE

Silence is golden

Ceremony at the Stones

Dawn at the Stones!

The big day.

I didn't sleep much.

Waited for lift in the dark.
Very early start.
A quiet sense of anticipation
as we met in the dark.
Early Start!

On to the minibus.
and before we know it we are in the henge!
Within the centre of antiquity.

What those people saw we see part of.
Opacity veils our comprehension,
the chain is forever broken, though some try to forge it once more
only guessing with profundity at what it may all mean.

Took photos
ACHIEVED MY AIM OF PHOTOGRAPHING EVERY STONE.
I brought a picture in a frame of my friend Adrian who died in the summer.
He loved Stonehenge

Running round the Stones
weaving amongst the stones
WALKING IN AND AROUND THE STONE CIRCLE.
walk round clockwise.
Running running running rings around the circle

Open your heart song at stones 'leaving shadow on stones'
What a wonderful time.
So open and relaxed and sweet sweet music from Chartwell
ma wee ah! Chartwell's welcome song

SONGS SONGS SONG
DRUMS DRUMS DRUMS many songs & drums.
THE BEATS ECHO ROUND THE STONES
THE SUNRISE OVER THE STONES
THE SPIRITS CHEERS AS WE CELEBRATE
MEMORIES OF PAST TIMES

Dancing
Singing
Laughing
hugging

SUCH CLOSENESS QUITE FRIGHTENS ME

WONDERFUL CELEBRATION

Dreamlike.
Special moment of my life.
Whacky.
Bravery.
Openheart ♥

We leave our shadow on the Stones.

CHANTING AND SINGING THE LAST SUN OF THE WINTER SOLSTICE.
HUMBLED AND SACRED
A VORTEX OF ENERGY
RELIEF....RELIEF!!
AWARENESS, JOY, AND SILENCE,
AS WE LEAVE OUR SHADOWS UPON THE STONES.
TIME...TIME...

A Stonehenge Saga
(Group 2, Stonehenge)

In darkness the creature stalks and fear takes many forms,
From winter's kiss to spring reborn,
A fellowship will form.
The seven sisters dance in glory of the midnight,
One by one, a call is sent,
Only hope replies.

The wisdom council assembled to guide and advise
Men and women of bone and stone,
The enchantress of time,
Along with the rich men of the universe of henge.
Gathered combined — a mind to mend
Across land and time spent.

A fellowship so newly formed, must find its true start,
At wall of Durham and wood henge —
Old and new piggy songs
Walking, talking — old robin follows the mystery
And good friendships start to form,
So into the past we see.

Fifteen true souls were called to quest the deep hidden land,
From pre-history to the modern day,
Walking in comradeship —
Walking! So much walking to bare, in the wet and wind,
Each session a united task,
So soon those ten weeks past.

With barrows and bones the monarch of the plain is proud,
The Cursus calls once more —
A minute in the brain.
In the distance the future they will see — the Stonehenge,
And time and space reveals so much,
But still so far to go.

From Cursus to Fargo, in woods they sang and they played.
Ringing the living bell in voice,
With barrows and bodies.
The far past resurrected in a moment of time,
Poundland umbrellas keep them dry,
And the wind and rain stayed.

The people of bone and stone send a teacher so wise
Darvill had danced in dirt —

And unearth a real truth,
His words carried true wisdom and knowledge in their wake,
While questions quickly filled the air,
Fact a deep discussion.

As day becomes night to the star and Cursus set flight,
Pleiades stars, and laser light,
Revealing nights secrets.
Calm with the darkness and sky full of stars as mists roll,
The Nebra disc... a story told,
The clues of our past form.

The task is half done, what more learning and fun to come,
United in knowledge and mirth
The group now all as one,
In house of round with roof of thatch the fellowship rest,
Fur and fire and stone-baked bread —
Weaving like ancient dead

As Time moved back for all to see how life then would be.
They built up and tore down fences
Smoothed with wattle white clay.
Time moves fast but this fellowship cant stay — spring awaits,
To earth secrets they must return
Lessons in mastery,

With lumps of clay a bowl is sort, fingers as tools craft,
Decorated the oldest ways,
To fire... they put their pots.
In tent of the boar, the man of fire and wind baked clay
Future artefacts we did make,
And they all came closer.

Unity disrupted by digital eyes and ears,
The dark beast hunts our fellowship,
Some fear from camera
The Balafon played lightness over the king barrow,
And the man from Cameroon played.
Piggy certificates!

The fellowship stood on the burial mounds of kings
And claimed their true place and full strength
And walked the Avenue
Over hill, across fields of sheep, in honour they marched,
Off towards the heal stone setting,
The stone circle at hand .

A plan to break the cordon and access stones was hatched,
The fellowship played loud music,
Driving back the darkness.
In joyous anticipation they await the dawn,
Some dream of old gods and blue stones
Some in sleepless slumber.

The sun rises as the fellowship takes the circle.
Four elements called to protect
A circle newly formed,
Gifts of friendship bestowed from new appointed keepers,
A given blessing not forgot.
A dream frozen in time,

All together the fellowship held back the darkness,
Found strength and knowledge and true will,
True hope and real friendships.
Through history and the earth you can find a healing rebirth
And even a little magick
And a fellowship of kind

Author: Mr BPD
Website http://www.my-dark-lyrics.uk
About the author: I have Borderline Personality Disorder and as a writer and poet I explore my madness through the creative arts. I have a personal belief that even in darkness light exists and it is a personal responsibility to always seek the light and I find the light in creating something.

Chapter 9

Human Henge: The impact of Neolithic healing landscapes on mental health and well-being

Vanessa Heaslip

Abstract

Throughout history there have been links between the environment and cultural landscapes in aiding mental health recovery. However, as clinically-based approaches to mental health gained popularity, the focus on these declined. Recently, there has been a re-emergence of interest in the benefits of cultural landscapes and historical artefacts on mental health and well-being, although as yet, empirical examination as to the health benefits of these interventions have been limited. This paper reports upon the Human Henge programme, in which 36 people living with mental illness were involved in an innovative, creative programme over ten weeks, at the Neolithic sites of Stonehenge and Avebury in Wiltshire. The impact of the project on participants' mental health and well-being was evaluated over a one year period, using mixed method research. Quantitative data was collated using the shortened version of the Warwick Edinburgh Mental Well-being Scale over four occasions, whilst qualitative data was collated through focus groups interviews and creative methodologies based upon photo elicitation. This paper presents the findings of the qualitative and quantitative analysis, highlighting how the creative exploration of a historic landscape can achieve measurable mental health and well-being outcomes for people with mental health conditions.

Keywords: Marginalization; Mental health; Mixed methods; Stigma; Well-being

Background

General estimates suggest that around one in four people will be affected by mental or neurological disorders at some point during their lives (WHO 2001). It is thought that around 450 million people are currently living with from a mental illness, placing it as one of the leading causes of ill-health and disability (WHO 2001). Poor mental health is also a risk factor for other diseases (Lombardo *et al.* 2018); a study by Zolezzi *et al.* (2017) of 336 patients with a severe mental illness attending a psychiatric outpatient clinic, identified that almost a third of the participants (29.2%) had at least one other medical comorbidity alongside their mental illness. This co-morbidity contributes to the lower life expectancy of people living with mental illness (Taylor and Shiers 2017). Not only do those living with mental illness have shorter life span, but they also have lower levels of life satisfaction (Lombardo *et al.* 2018). Stigma and discrimination against people with mental illness affects everyday aspects of their life (Ye *et al.* 2016), impacting on their own self-worth, their ability to socialize with others, and their capacity to integrate into their local communities.

Due to the health inequities associated with mental illness, there has been a shift in thinking at an international level towards a focus on mental health. Indeed, mental health is an integral part of well-being; it is defined as 'a state of well-being in which every individual realizes his or her own potential, can cope with the normal stresses of life, can work productively and fruitfully, and is able to make a contribution to her or his community' (WHO 2014). The WHO developed an international Mental Health Action plan 2013–2020 with a goal of promoting mental well-being, preventing mental disorders, reducing morbidity and mortality, and caring for and supporting recovery for those who are ill, whilst simultaneously promoting the human rights of individuals experiencing mental illness (WHO 2013: 9).

This shift to a focus on well-being has enabled more interdisciplinary approaches to the promotion of mental health well-being. Recent approaches have involved landscape (Abraham *et al.* 2010), heritage (Ander *et al.* 2013), museums (Camic and Chatterjee 2013; Kindleysides and Biglands 2015), and archaeology ('Operation Nightingale' from the Defence Archaeology Group (DAG) 2018; Ministry of Defence & Defence Infrastructure Organization 2019; Waterloo Uncovered 2016). This shift in emphasis led to the development of a White Paper on Culture from the Department for Culture, Media and Sport (DCMS 2016), which highlighted commitment by the cultural sector to the improvement of health and well-being. However, this paper also acknowledged the lack of robust evidence regarding the impact of these approaches (DCMS 2016).

With funding from the Heritage Lottery Fund, the Restoration Trust in partnership with Bournemouth University, the Richmond Fellowship, English Heritage, National Trust, and the Avon and Wiltshire Mental Health Partnership NHS Trust, developed the Human Henge programme as explained in Chapters 5 to 8 in this volume. Overall, the Human Henge programme aimed to improve mental health through creative explorations of historic landscapes. However, unlike other projects which use interdisciplinary approaches to promote well-being, Human Henge incorporates a systematic empirical evaluation of the health impact of the programme, which shall be presented here.

Methods

The research question framing the evaluation was: 'Does a creative exploration of historic landscape achieve sustained, measurable mental health and well-being outcomes for people with mental health conditions?' In order to address this, the study employed a mixed method approach including quantitative and qualitative data collection.

Participants

Participants were recruited to the Human Henge project via the Richmond Fellowship, with all of the participants self-identified as having an ongoing mental health issue. In total, 35 participants were involved in the research evaluation across three groups; Groups 1 and 2 were based at Stonehenge, whilst Group 3 was based at Avebury. The age and gender composition of the participant groups can be seen in Table 9.A. The age range of participants was between

Table 9.A Participants' age and gender composition.

	Group 1 (n=13) Stonehenge	Group 2 (n=10) Stonehenge	Group 3 (n=12) Avebury	Total (n=35)
Age range	26–77	35–54	21–56	21–77
Mean age	51.23	43.30	39.83	45.06
Male	9 (69.0%)	3 (30.0%)	4 (33.3%)	16 (45.7%)
Female	4 (31.0%)	7 (70.0%)	8 (66.7%)	19 (54.3%)

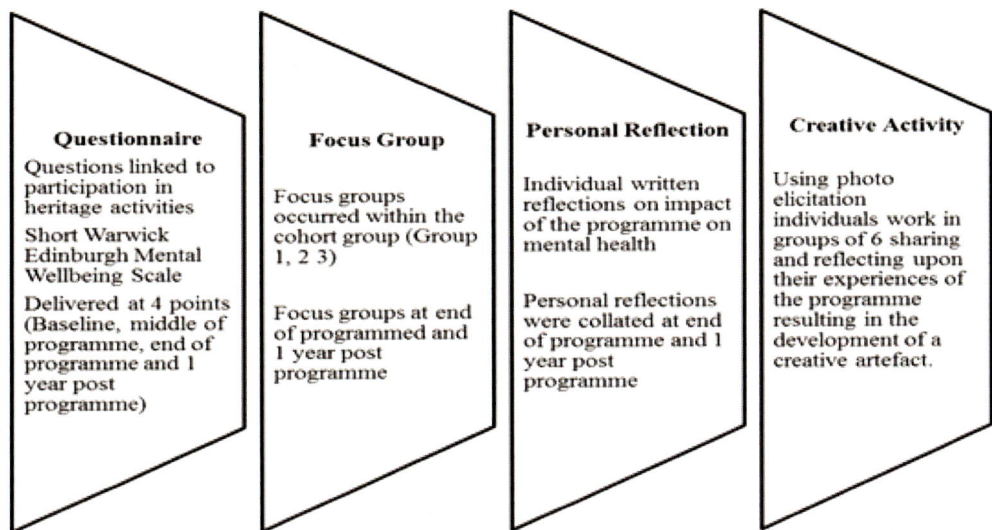

Figure 9.1 Data collection methods. (Illustration by Vanessa Heaslip. Copyright reserved)

21 and 77 years, with Group 1 on average the oldest cohort, whilst Group 3 was the youngest. In total, 16 male and 19 females were involved; Group 1 consisted of predominately more male participants whilst Groups 2 and 3 consisted of predominately more female participants.

Data collection

Multiple data collection methods were used including questionnaires, interviews, and creative activities in order to fully capture the participants' experiences of the Human Henge programme, as well as the impact of this on their mental health (Figure 9.1).

Quantitative data was obtained through a printed questionnaire using the Short Warwick Edinburgh Mental Well-being Scale (Tennant *et al.* 2007) to measure mental well-being (Table 9.B). This was supplemented with questions regarding participants' interests in history,

Table 9.B Short Warwick-Edinburgh Mental Well-being Scale. (Based on Tennant et al. 2007)

Statements	None of the time ☹	Rarely	Some of the time 🙂	Often	All of the time ☺
I've been feeling optimistic about the future					
I've been feeling useful					
I've been feeling relaxed					
I've been dealing with problems well					
I've been thinking clearly					
I've been feeling close to other people					
I've been able to make up my own mind about things					

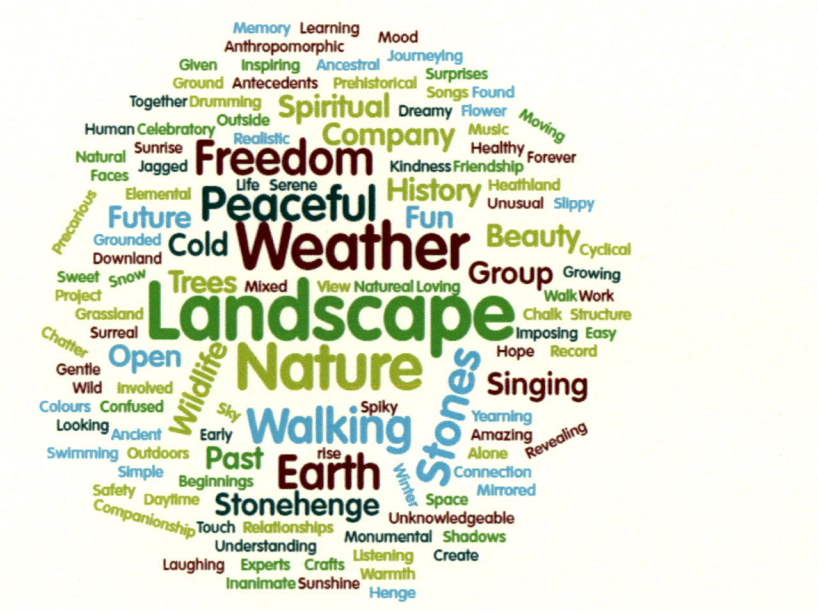

Figure 9.2 Group activity condensed into a word-cloud: Groups 1–3. (Illustration by Vanessa Heaslip. Copyright reserved)

heritage, and archaeology. The questionnaire was deployed at four intervals: a baseline assessment before the programme commenced; half way through the ten week programme; at the end of the ten week programme; and one year after completion of the programme.

Qualitative data was obtained using a variety of methods in order to facilitate engagement. The assessment consisted of a creative activity based upon the principles of photo-elicitation, in which participants chose a photograph that resonated with their Human Henge journey. After they had picked the photograph, they identified six words that reflected their Human Henge experience. The collated words resulted in a word cloud (Figure 9.2).

As can be seen, the participants used a wide variety of words during this activity, some of which were associated with geographical dimensions of the landscape (such as 'stones' and 'landscape'), activities of the programme (such as 'walking', 'outside' and 'weather'), whilst others related to states of mind (such as 'freedom', 'peaceful', 'hope' and 'fun') or the past (such as 'history', 'ancient' and 'ancestral'). All triangulate well with data obtained through scrutiny of the free-text responses from the questionnaire. Each participant shared their six words with others in a sub-group of six participants, and turned these words into sentences which then formed the basis of the next stage of the activity. In this, participants read the six sentences that the sub-group had constructed, and then used these to develop a creative output such as a picture, written prose, or a poem summing up their experiences of Human Henge. In addition to the creative activity, there was an opportunity for participants to share their personal reflections; things they may not wish to share openly in a focus group setting. This was captured twice; firstly at the end of the ten week programme and then one year post-engagement with Human Henge. The final method of eliciting qualitative data was through a focus group at the end of the ten week programme. Each of the three groups was asked the question: 'I'm interested in hearing about your experiences and your thoughts about your participation in the Human Henge, can you please tell me about it?'. One year post engagement in Human Henge, participants were asked: 'It's one year since you finished the Human Henge project, I'm interested in hearing about your reflections of your involvement one year on, and your thoughts and your experiences of participating in the project'.

Data analysis

Quantitative data was analysed using SPSS descriptive statistics. For this paper, the five point rating scale has been condensed into three points: 'none of the time/rarely', 'some of the time', and 'often/all of the time'. Qualitative data collated through personal reflections and focus groups were analysed thematically using Braun and Clarke's (2006) process of thematic analysis.

Ethics

Research Ethics committee approval was granted for the study by Bournemouth University's research committee.

Results

Quantitative data

At the time of writing, Groups 1 and 2 have completed all aspects of the data collection, whilst Group 3 have yet to complete data collection at one year post involvement in Human Henge. Data analysis using inferential statistics has begun; however, only descriptive statistics will be presented here. Table 9.C presents the descriptive statistics on the seven points of the Short Warwick Edinburgh Mental Well-being Scale (Tennant *et al.* 2007).

Considering the rating points for each dimension of the mental well-being scale from baseline to end of programme, it is evident that there is a reduction in the rating of 'none of the time/rarely' and a subsequent increase in the rating 'often/all of the' time across all seven dimensions of the Short Warwick Edinburgh Mental Well-being Scale (Tennant *et al.* 2007). This highlights that the participants felt more positive at the end of the programme in comparison to their scoring at baseline. However when the data for one year post involvement in the programme is examined, the picture is more mixed. Exploring the rating 'often/all of the time', it is evident that there has been an increase from baseline to one year post involvement in three of the seven dimensions (Feeling optimistic of the future 9.1–25.0; Feeling relaxed 9.1–25.0; Feeling close to people 12.1–25.0). Yet when examining the rating 'none of the time/rarely' from baseline to one year post the Human Henge project, there has been a decrease in five of the seven dimensions (Feeling optimistic about the future 48.5–41.7; Feeling useful 36.4–33.3; Dealing with problems well 36.4–33.3; Thinking clearly 30.3–16.7; Feeling close to people 51.5–33.3) indicating a shift in perceptions from 'none of the rime/rarely' to 'some of the time'. However caution is required at this stage as it has to be remembered that data from baseline to one year post involvement was only available for Groups 1 and 2 at the time of writing, as data had not yet been collected from Group 3.

Qualitative data: Creative activity

Whilst participants were initially nervous about the creative activity, many of them really enjoyed undertaking this, as it enabled them to draw upon other thoughts and feelings. The key factor in the approach to this activity, was reassuring participants that there was no set

Table 9.C Quantitative results

	Baseline %	Middle %	End %	1-Year F-U*
Feeling optimistic about the future				
None of the time/rarely	48.5	33.3	30.0	41.7
Some of the time	42.4	40.0	46.7	33.3
Often/all of the time	9.1	26.7	23.3	25.0
Feeling relaxed				
None of the time/rarely	39.4	40.0	20.0	41.7
Some of the time	51.5	43.3	50.0	33.3
Often/all of the time	9.1	16.7	30.0	25.0
Feeling useful				
None of the time/rarely	36.4	16.7	20.0	33.3
Some of the time	51.5	60.0	50.0	58.3
Often/all of the time	12.1	23.3	30.0	8.3
Dealing with problems well				
None of the time/rarely	36.4	13.3	23.3	33.3
Some of the time	36.4	73.3	36.7	50.0
Often/all of the time	27.3	13.3	40.0	16.7
Thinking clearly				
None of the time/rarely	30.3	10.0	26.7	16.7
Some of the time	54.5	60.0	36.7	75.0
Often/all of the time	15.2	30.0	36.7	8.3
Feeling close to people				
None of the time/rarely	51.5	23.3	30.0	33.3
Some of the time	36.4	40.0	23.3	41.7
Often/all of the time	12.1	36.7	46.7	25.0
Able to make up my own mind about things				
None of the time/rarely	24.2	16.7	20.0	25.0
Some of the time	39.4	43.3	26.7	50.0
Often/all of the time	36.4	40.0	53.3	25.0

expectation or parameter regarding what they produced; it just needed to reflect the essence of what was written in the six sentences they had collated as part of the activity. With reflection, this was an important part of the data collection; it enabled the capture of participant voices, for those who found it difficult to verbalize their thoughts and feelings in a group setting. A selection of the creative outputs is presented below (Figure 9.3).

These show the importance of the group within the Human Henge project, and how the participants felt they could be themselves within this group without judgement or shame, which was a really important to them. However, it must be acknowledged that for a very few participants, being in a group setting was challenging for them due to their mental health. This is really highlighted in the drawing at the bottom right, where there is one sad face surrounded

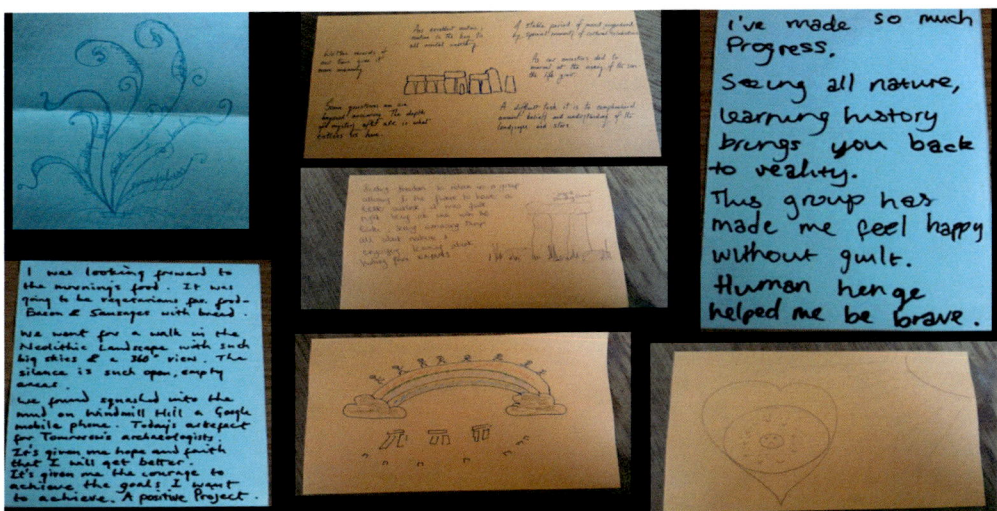

Figure 9.3 Creative activity outputs Groups 1–3. (Compiled by Vanessa Heaslip. Copyright reserved)

by happy faces located within a heart. As the participants gave their date of birth on the back of their outputs, I was able to explore this with the individual alongside their personal reflection, as well as their focus group contribution. For this participant, their involvement in the project enabled them to have a much better understanding of their personal mental health and the challenges they face when interacting socially with others.

Qualitative data: Personal reflection

Exploring data from the personal reflections, highlighted themes around 'knowing oneself' and 'connections'. In 'knowing oneself', participants expressed their improved understanding of challenges associated with their mental illness, and also their potential for recovery. They also acknowledged the inner strength they had found through engagement with the programme. This strength enabled them to reconnect both with other individuals and also with their local communities in which they lived.

> 'Helped me connect with local people socially and local places with happy memories. Feeling more connected with Wiltshire and feeling like I have a place to be/belong in Wiltshire.' (Participant 21, Group 2, one year post Human Henge)

> 'The increased motivation, creativeness and determination that I have achieved by attending Human Henge enabled me to give a successful presentation to 29 people this week. I could not have considered doing anything like this prior to my involvement with Richmond Fellowship and in particular Human Henge. In the past I would have been a shaking wreck!' (Participant 30, Group 3, End of Human Henge)

For one of the participants (Participant 3, Group 1), being part of the qualitative data collection at the end of the programme was too difficult; they had to leave and not participate in this. However, when they were contacted again one year post involvement in the Human Henge programme, their personal reflection noted:

'I learnt I was iller than I thought. I have gone on to socialize more, not much more but more. The environment made being around others easier, I became less self –conscious'

Focus group

As previously highlighted, focus groups were undertaken twice for each group; at the end of the Human Henge programme and one year post involvement in Human Henge. The data presented here focuses upon the analysis of the three groups' end of programme data, as data collation for Group 3 one year post involvement has not been collated at the time of writing.

Feeling special

The participants in Groups 1 and 2 spoke about feeling privileged and feeling special about being part of the project. This was not only reflected in the culmination of their programme (access to the interior of the Stonehenge stone circle) but also in their opportunity to use all of the facilities on offer at the Stonehenge Visitor Centre (e.g. the museum and replica Neolithic huts) on an almost daily basis. They also spoke of the access they had to experts in archaeology, and how the project made them feel special:

'...I was really impressed by what we had each week. Like, we had...obviously the climax the access to the stones, but like the museum, the exhibition, and then doing the pottery. I thought the quality, we had like VIP treatment.'(Male participant Focus Group 1)

'...being able to learn from experts and things like that' (Male participant Focus Group 2)

However, this theme of 'feeling special' was not evident when analysing Group 3 data, and this may reflect the change of location of the Human Henge project. As previously noted, the programme for Groups 1 and 2 took place at Stonehenge, where access to the stones themselves is restricted. For those groups, the programme culminated in the participants being allowed access to the stones themselves. In comparison, Group 3 was located at the Neolithic site of Avebury Henge, which is an open site where members of the public can interact with the stones. This difference in the perception of privileged access may have been reflected in the Group 3 data.

Building confidence

Participation in Human Henge gave some of the participants the confidence to step outside of their self-imposed boundaries and try something new; something they would not have contemplated before. For some, it was within the group setting itself, leading and facilitating a Human Henge session. For others, it was challenging themselves outside the group, creating new opportunities and possibilities for themselves, linked to employment or new hobbies:

'I found it difficult...really difficult to stand there in front of a group of people talking to them an' all that, but afterwards I thought... phew! I did really well there!' (Male Participant Focus group 1)

'This is the first time I've done them (taken photographs) and you've really influenced me to go into a shop and say "Look this is what I've got, do you wanna buy it off of me?"

And I think that's awesome that is. And then a couple'a weeks ago I did actually take my cards into a shop in ***** and they bought almost a hundred of my cards and it was really exciting for me' (Female Participant Focus Group 2)

The participants gained inspiration and strength from the group, which was instrumental in giving them the confidence to try new things. A female participant (Group 3) sums this up:

'... you see people grow and they overcome their personal struggles, some physical, some mental and that gives you some strength and some determination to overcome your own, you know, push yourself a little bit'.

Connections

Across all three groups, there was a strong theme regarding connection that was facilitated through their Human Henge experience. This centred on a re-connection with people. This was achieved through both connecting with others in the group and also through a connection to ancestors who had walked and lived in the landscape they were exploring. In addition to connecting with people, there was also a re-connection to their local area and landscape. These connections had previously become fractured as a result of their mental illness. Reasons for this included unhappy memories associated with time and place, as well as negative experiences of feeling discriminated against and stigmatized due to their mental illness. Both of these factors had culminated in the affected participants isolating themselves from others. In addition, the participants in Group 2 expressed how clinical mental health services focussed on their mental illness, and not them as individual people. This was in contrast to the Human Henge programme, which focused on them as individuals and not on the fact that they were living with a mental illness. Through associating with others with similar experiences, participants developed the strength and confidence to revisit local places, as well as engaging more readily with their local communities. These were positive experiences for them:

[on handling ancient pottery]'... some of that is like thousands of years old, and it has been handled exactly as we were handling it, you know they had their hands on it and now I've got my hands on it and so that was like a connection and they would have had their same worries, perhaps not in exactly the same way, but shelter, food, family, those things would have been just the same for them, so I think there's a connection.' (Male participant Focus Group 3)

'Only speaking for myself, you can get trapped up in making the world so small and protecting yourself from the world. Sometimes you don't need protecting from that. Sometimes I think it's just slowly breaking down them barriers and this is a start, you know, within these groups. (Female participant Focus Group 3)

'I mean, I feel more sort of connected to the landscape and I didn't realize how many ancient artefacts there are in Wiltshire.' (Male participant Focus Group 1)

Mental health

It was evident from qualitative data, that the majority of participants felt that their mental health and well-being had improved as a result of participating in the project. For some participants, it gave them something positive to look forward to, in that the days on which they were going to be involved with Human Henge activity, were keenly anticipated rather than dreaded:

> 'I've had quite a bad time this year…and most mornings I've woken up with my stomach churning, panic feelings… But on those Fridays when we met, you know, I woke up thinking (excited) "Right – I've got to get ready! Down to Stonehenge!" Have a little drive in my car. And then… when I drove back after we had our sessions, I felt so much better. I actually had a normal, fairly happy day on those Fridays. (Female participant Focus Group 1)

> 'This has been… more positive than anything I've done in the last two years.' (Female participant Focus Group 2)

One female participant in Group 2, had become increasingly housebound and isolated due to her mental illness. However, she found that being involved in Human Henge had not only given her a focus for the first time in years, but it had also reduced her self-harming; for her, this was very significant. She shared:

> 'No for me there was two there were two things, one I hadn't committed to anything for… over… three years, so for me to actually… commit to something was quite a big thing anyway. But then also to commit to this I also had to be disciplined because unfortunately at times I self-harm really badly so to commit to this I had to agree with my husband that on the day I come here I would not self-harm, and the first week I did but since then I haven't.'

It is important to note that participating in Human Henge does not eradicate the ongoing mental health challenges that participants faced. Instead, it provided them with more confidence and improved belief in their ability to manage these challenges. One of the female participants in Group 3 noted:

> 'I think I've learned that I can cope with like my symptoms a lot better, like before I would just run away, but now I'm like learning to deal with it.'

However, it is important to note that for some participants, being part of the project was very challenging for them and this linked to their ongoing mental health issues. One of the male participants (Group 1) expressed challenges he experienced regarding the singing in the group activities; he responded to this by walking away from the activity:

> 'all the singing and all that sort of… I found that really terribly frightening. I mean I love the history, I've always been interested in history that's why I wanted to come here but… having to take part in all the dancing an' singing an' all that… I just found that so difficult… I just had to turn round walk away.'

Individual mental health diagnoses were not explored as part of the Human Henge project. It is therefore not possible to speculate as to whether some individuals with specific types of mental health issues may find this style of programme challenging. Future research needs to explore this further.

Fear for the Future

It was evident that the impact of the ten week programme for some participants had been so profound, that they expressed anxiety and fear regarding the potential repercussions on their mental health and well-being when the project came to an end. For some participants (particularly Groups 2 and 3) this was very difficult, and some of them became distressed during the focus group session just thinking about it. They were particularly worried about two aspects. Firstly, the loss of focus and structure that the programme had given them; something to look forward to each week. Secondly and perhaps more important, was the possible loss of the sense of belonging that had developed; the social acceptance that they felt within the group sessions, and the friendships they had made:

'It's a shame to hit a dead end and then nothing.' (Female participant Focus Group 1)

'I'm devastated it's over. [Tearful] I don't want this to finish. (Female participant Focus Group 2)

'I feel like this experience as well has given us something to get ready for, something to look forward to. And I just think it's a bit hard that they're just robbing it from us and taking it all away, because after this, like **** [participant name] said, at that week where you didn't have it, it was hard. It was a hard week. You, know, because you had nothing else. But now it's going to be gone and I feel like some of you I'll probably never see again, and I don't want that.' (Female participant Focus Group 3)

The project team became aware at the end of Group 1, that a sudden withdrawal of the programme would have a negative impact on participants. As a result of this, the project implemented a variety of additional meetings, both as small groups but also as a wider Human Henge group consisting of participants from Groups 1-3. However, organically, participants also developed strategies to stay connected using social media (notably Groups 2 and 3) and they have continued to meet socially. In contrast, participants in Group 1 have not established such mechanisms to keep in contact, and this may reflect different group dynamics. Group 1 was an older cohort; as such they may use social media less than Groups 2 and 3. However, Group 1 also had a stronger group identity with the Richmond Fellowship (many of the participants were already part of Richmond Fellowship groups) and during the focus group they did discuss speaking to the Richmond Fellowship to keep the activity going; they were more reliant on the Richmond Fellowship to organize and maintain the group. By contrast, Groups 2 and 3 did not have this identity; many of the participants did not know each other prior to the Human Henge programme they joined, and as such looked within themselves to maintain contact.

Conclusion

The original research question — 'Does a creative exploration of historic landscape achieve sustained, measurable mental health and well-being outcomes for people with mental health conditions?' — is difficult to answer conclusively at the time of writing, as data collection and analysis is ongoing. Nevertheless, interim findings highlight that involvement in Human Henge had a positive impact upon participants' mental health and well-being, which was still apparent to some degree, one year post involvement in the programme. However, caution is advised due to the small sample size, and further data collection is required before any claims regarding generalizability of the findings can be made.

Bibliography

Abraham, A., K. Sommerhalder and T. Abel 2010. Landscape and well-being: A scoping study on the health-promoting impact of outdoor environments. *International Journal of Public Health* 55: 59–69.

Ander, E., L. Thomson, G. Noble, A. Lanceley, U. Menon and H. Chatterjee, H. 2013. Heritage, health and well-being: Assessing the impact of a heritage focused intervention on health and well-being. *International Journal of Heritage Studies* 19(3): 229–242.

Braun, V. and V. Clarke 2006. Using thematic analysis in psychology. *Qualitative Research in Psychology* 3: 77–101.

Camic, P. and H. Chatterjee 2013. Museums and art galleries as partners for public health interventions. *Perspectives in Public Health* 133(66): 66–71.

DAG, 2018. Defence Archaeology Group: Home [Webpage]. Viewed 22 November 2018, <http://www.dag.org.uk/index.html>.

DCMS, 2016. *The Culture White Paper* [Online document]. London: HM Government. Viewed 22 November 2018, <https://www.gov.uk/government/uploads/system/uploads/attachment_data/file/510798/DCMS_The_Culture_White_Paper__3_.pdf>.

Kindleysides, M. and E. Biglands 2015. 'Thinking outside the box, and making it too': Piloting an occupational therapy group at an open-air museum. *Arts and Health* 7(3): 271–278.

Lombardo, P., W. Jones, L. Wang, X. Shen and E. Goldner 2018. The fundamental association between mental health and life satisfaction: results from successive waves of a Canadian national survey. *BMC Public Health* 18(1): 342.

MOD and DIO, 2019. Operation Nightingale [Webpage]. Viewed 4 February 2019, <https://www.gov.uk/guidance/operation-nightingale>.

Taylor, J. and D. Shiers 2017. 'Don't Just Screen – Intervene': Protecting the cardiometabolic health of people with severe mental illness. *Diabetes & Primary Care* 19: 217–223.

Tennant, R., L. Hiller, R. Fishwick, P. Platt, S. Joseph, S. Weich, J. Parkinson, J. Secker and S. Stewart-Brown 2007. The Warwick-Edinburgh Mental Well-being Scale (WEMWBS): Development and UK validation. *Health and Quality of Life Outcomes* 5: 63. Viewed 28 February 2019, <https://doi.org/10.1186/1477-7525-5-63>.

Waterloo Uncovered, 2018. Waterloo Uncovered: Home [Webpage]. Viewed 22 November 2018, <http://www.waterloouncovered.com/>.

WHO, 2001. Mental disorders affect one in four people [Webpage]. Viewed 22 November 2018, <http://www.who.int/whr/2001/media_centre/press_release/en/>.

WHO, 2013. *Mental health action plan 2013-2020* [Online document]. Geneva: WHO. Viewed 22 November 2018, <https://www.who.int/iris/bitstream/10665/89966/1/9789241506021_eng.pdf>.

WHO, 2014. Mental health: A state of well-being [Webpage]. Viewed 22 November 2018, <http://www.who.int/features/factfiles/mental_health/en/>.

Ye, J., T. Chen, D. Paul, R. McCahon, S. Shankar, A. Rosen and C. O'Reilly 2016. Stigma and discrimination experienced by people living with severe and persistent mental illness in assertive community treatment settings. *International Journal of Social Psychiatry* 62(6): 532–541.

Zolezzi, M., S. Abdulrhim, N. Isleem, F. Zahrah and Y. Eltorki 2017. Medical comorbidities in patients with serious mental illness: A retrospective study of mental health patients attending an outpatient clinic in Qatar. *Neuropsychiatric Disease and Treatment* 13: 2411–2418.

Chapter 10

A place to heal: Past perceptions and new opportunities for using historic sites to change lives

Martin Allfrey

Abstract

English Heritage has supported Human Henge since the idea for the project, exploring how archaeological landscapes and ancient sites can be used to help people with mental health issues, was first proposed by the Restoration Trust. This paper is written from the English Heritage perspective. It initially looks back over the last century at the ways in which historic places in state care in England have contributed to mental health and well-being initiatives. It focuses on the impact of the First World War on the country, how it shaped people's views of the past and influenced the unprecedented rise in the number of sites taken into state care in the post-war years. Historic places played an important role in the country's recovery in the aftermath of the war. They were places of work and rehabilitation for ex-servicemen and they became places of order and peace in a shattered world. In 2017, Human Henge was initiated at Stonehenge. As well as the positive implications for English Heritage, this pilot study has enabled us to plan the delivery of similar well-being programmes across the English Heritage estate.

Keywords: English Heritage; First World War; Human Henge; Stonehenge; Well-being

Introduction

When Sara Lunt and Laura Drysdale from the Restoration Trust first approached English Heritage with the idea of using Stonehenge to test how historic landscapes can be used to promote well-being, it immediately felt like something that we should wholeheartedly support, for a variety of reasons. From our perspective, it was the rigorous research framework underpinning the project that drew us to it. We wanted to know whether a programme of activities in a historic landscape, with a focus on making connections with ancient places, could lead to a meaningful, measurable and sustained improvement in mental health. Although the project initially only had funding to run one pilot at Stonehenge, we were very keen not to see it as a one-off but as a starting point for something that was replicable and deliverable across other sites and areas of the country.

Stonehenge is the best known prehistoric monument in England — perhaps in the world. Today, it is cared for by the English Heritage Trust, a registered charity that manages over 400 of England's historic buildings, monuments and sites. Stonehenge is undoubtedly a special and unique place and it never fails to evoke an emotional response in anyone who visits it. Since it was first conceived and constructed, every generation has wondered at the imagination and skill of its builders, and they have attached their own meanings to those enigmatic stones. As well as posing many questions about the people who built it and those who continued to modify and use it, Stonehenge still resonates with us today and its raw power and presence make us all think about our own place in the world and our links to the past. As Jacquetta Hawkes said in 1967 'Every age gets the Stonehenge it deserves — and desires'. In welcoming

Human Henge to Stonehenge I hoped in some small way to create something positive and new; a prism through which we might gain a greater understanding of how the site can help people today and how it can continue to be relevant. Our desire was that this innovative project, using the stone circle and its surrounding landscape, would have a big impact on people's lives.

We hoped that the Human Henge model would work in any historic landscape or site but, by choosing Stonehenge, we could also capitalize on the fact that the site is so well-known. By doing something at Stonehenge, we knew that people would take notice and be interested in the results. I think this made a difference for the participants too, knowing that they would be made welcome and given special access to such an iconic landmark and that they would be exploring it with expert and passionate guides. By offering Stonehenge we also sent a strong signal to our partners the National Trust, and the external funders such as the Heritage Lottery Fund, that English Heritage was fully supportive of the Human Henge project. It demonstrated that we were not only prepared to offer staff time and to give financial support to fund mental health research at historic sites, but that we were also happy to offer our most important site to test the approach.

Mental well-being and the historic environment

Using archaeological sites and collections for recovery is, of course, not new. There have been many projects at historic sites in recent years and a number of excellent examples were presented at the Human Henge conference at Bournemouth University in 2018. Historic places are likely to have always played a role in well-being and recovery, connecting people to their surroundings and to where they have come from. Looking into the distant past, it has been suggested that Stonehenge was a place where people came together to meet and to be healed (Darvill and Wainwright 2009). It is a compelling argument that Stonehenge — especially its bluestones, that must have held enormous significance for those who brought them from the Preseli Mountains in Wales — retained a mythical, healing quality, remaining potent and valued for centuries after the circle was constructed.

Much more recently, the mental health benefit of time spent in the natural environment was widely recognized in the nineteenth century, and access to fresh air and open space was adopted as a new way to treat patients with a variety of conditions. Public funding poured into the construction of new asylums between 1800 and 1900, and most of them featured extensive grounds and gardens that were safe, accessible and often tended by patients as part of their treatment. In the aftermath of the First World War (WWI), there was a further shift in the wider community's attitude towards people with mental health conditions, and a growing understanding that anyone could be affected. Towards the end of the war, new approaches in the treatment of people with 'shell shock' were being explored. The benefits of access to the countryside and historic sites were recognized and used to help with the rehabilitation of WWI veterans (Cohen 2001).

Today there is a re-awakening of awareness around this approach. There is a renewed appreciation of the importance of access to the natural world as an aid to recovery for all conditions, not only to help those suffering from mental ill-health. In hospital design, there has been a move away from sterile and anonymous, artificially-lit spaces, where patients (and staff) have no connection with the natural world; in such an environment, they are sometimes not even aware of the time of day. One example is Horatio's Garden at the spinal treatment centre in Salisbury, completed in 2012. Its design incorporates the form of the human spine in its low limestone walls. The walls and multi-sensory planting create intimate spaces, but they also draw the eye outwards to the landscape beyond the garden. Patients' beds and other equipment can be moved into the garden, so some treatment can take place outside. There is also a large gathering space for events. The aim here is to treat the mind and the body, encouraging patients to feel connected to the world and not removed or excluded from it. With Human Henge we wanted to explore whether there was a benefit in making connections, not just with the natural environment and with other people; we also wanted to explore what additional benefits could be derived from spending time in an historic environment, helping people to connect with their own place in time.

The last 100 years

Before considering the impact of Human Henge on English Heritage I want to look back over the last 100 years at the ways in which sites in state care have been used to promote healing and well-being. I will consider how Stonehenge and other historic sites came into the guardianship of English Heritage, and how the horrific events of WWI changed attitudes — not only towards people with mental health conditions but also to historic sites and the way people used and valued them. The war left the nation traumatized by the brutality of the conflict and the loss of so many loved-ones. It shaped people's views of the past and it also influenced how historic sites were conserved and presented. These places took on a new role in the post war years, becoming places of order, tranquillity and peace in a shattered world.

As well as marking 100 years since the armistice at the end of WWI, 2018 is an important anniversary for Stonehenge. It is 100 years since local barrister Cecil Chubb and his wife Mary, gifted the monument to the nation in October 1918, having bought it at an auction in Salisbury in 1915 (Parkinson 2015). Prior to that, the site had been owned by local landowner, Sir Edmund Antrobus, who had been reluctant to carry out essential repairs or to put this nationally important monument into public ownership.

As we reflect on these two events a century ago, we can see how they are closely related. Under Sir Edmund Antrobus's custodianship, at the start of the twentieth century the monument was in a dangerous state of decay, with the stones propped up by timber supports to prevent further collapse. With the steadfast refusal of Sir Edmund to offer the site into the guardianship of the Office of Works, and constant wrangling with the archaeological community and proponents of the nascent conservation movement, efforts to save Stonehenge were at a standstill. Perhaps the only positive aspect of this, was that the lack of major archaeological intervention in the late nineteenth century may have saved the site from wholesale excavation, preventing the permanent loss of sub-surface archaeology (Fry 2014b).

In 1914 everything changed. The country plunged into WWI and soldiers who served on the Western Front endured some of the most terrible forms of warfare ever known. Spending regular tours of duty in the trenches and under the constant threat of shell fire, the men faced scenes of unimaginable horror and distress. Many are reported to have suffered from conditions known at the time as 'war neuroses' and shell shock that today would be categorized as Post-Traumatic Stress Disorder (PTSD). The scale of the war meant that it touched the lives of the entire population, not just those serving at the front lines. On the home front wives and families had to come to terms with the grief over the loss of so many loved ones. Everyone had to adapt to a changed way of life, with many veterans suffering from physical disabilities and psychological trauma for the rest of their lives.

Sir Edmund Antrobus's own son and heir was killed in action on the Western Front in 1914, a few months after the war had started. Sir Edmund's own death in 1915, possibly hastened by grief, led to the Amesbury Abbey Estate —including Stonehenge — being put up for sale. It was purchased by Cecil Chubb, who took a very different approach to Stonehenge.

During the war Stonehenge was surrounded by military activity, although it remained open to the public. Cecil Chubb, had directed that the admission price should be halved for serving soldiers and that the revenue from Stonehenge was to be donated to the Red Cross. In the closing months of WWI in September 1918, Cecil Chubb, aware of its national significance, decided to give Stonehenge to the nation (Daw 2013). In a ceremony at the site on 26 October 1918 to mark the event, Sir Alfred Mond, the First Commissioner of Works, expressed the gratitude of the nation and said:

> 'This ceremony takes place at a time which is perhaps a turning point in the history of our country. After four years of anxiety, toil, and peril we see at last the sun of victory shining over the horizon. It is a good augury. Our ancestor's hero worshipped the sun when it rose. We today can turn our eyes towards the sun of victory won so gallantly by the men who have gone out and fought and died for us'.
> (*The Times*, 28 October 1918).

Cecil Chubb's gift was a major turning point in the way that Stonehenge was protected and made accessible for the public. It set in train a programme of conservation for the monument and the surrounding landscape that continues today under the auspices of English Heritage and the National Trust. There is little evidence as to why Chubb decided to buy Stonehenge in 1915 or for his motivation to give it to the nation in 1918. We know that he was a local man, born in Shrewton, a village four miles west of Stonehenge. He attended the local village school and then Bishop Wordsworth's School in Salisbury, Wiltshire. He went on to Christ's College, Cambridge and became a successful barrister. Chubb was no stranger to the world of mental health. He met his future wife, Mary Finch, at a cricket game between his Bishop Wordsworth School and Fisherton House Mental Asylum, in Salisbury — then the largest private mental hospital in England. Mary's uncle owned the asylum and, after her uncle's death in 1905, the business and buildings were transferred to her along with a considerable legacy (Howe and Percy 2000). It was Mary Chubb's inheritance that allowed her husband to make the momentous decision to buy Stonehenge.

Both Mary and Cecil were closely involved in running the hospital. In 1924, financial problems with the Fisherton House Asylum resulted in the formation of a new limited company to manage it and the name was changed to Old Manor Hospital (Art Care 2018). Sir Cecil Chubb was appointed managing director of this company, Old Manor (Salisbury) Ltd, and left his law practice to concentrate solely on the management of the hospital. New wards were built in the 1920s to house former members of the armed forces suffering from PTSD. Later in the 1930s, Chubb's former home, Bemerton Lodge in Salisbury, was used as hospital accommodation for 'officer patients' and the 'hospital had two motor cars at the disposal of those who could afford it to make excursions in to the countryside' (Barham 2007). It seems likely that those excursions included trips to Stonehenge and to other historic sites nearby.

Heritage and mental well-being in the twentieth century

Chubb's involvement with the treatment of people with mental health issues as the owner of a private mental hospital, and his decision to buy Stonehenge, may be coincidental. However, it is interesting to speculate as to whether he would have made any connection at the time — and indeed, what he would have made of the way historic landscapes like Stonehenge are contributing to people's well-being one hundred years later. Likewise what would the senior staff in the Office of Works, who took over Stonehenge in 1918, have thought? Did they recognize at the time that historic sites could help people with mental health challenges? I believe that, even if it was not fully articulated at the time, they did appreciate the role that sites could play in recovery; not only for individuals but also in rebuilding the nation. The rapid development of the national collection of historic sites in the post war years, now cared for English Heritage, was a response to the personal grief and the horrors everyone faced during WWI and in the years that followed. This exercise was born of a political desire to rebuild Britain and to reinforce a sense of history, identity and pride in a 'fit country for heroes to live in'.

The monuments chosen to be saved, represented what were then thought to be the defining moments in British history. But there was more to it than that. People's lives had been shattered and the sites also provided peaceful places for contemplation, where visitors could look back to an imagined past when things were better, safer, and more ordered. In those post war years, Charles Peers was the Chief Inspector of Ancient Monuments from 1913 to 1933 (Fry 2014a). He created order from chaos, turning ruined and dangerous sites into controlled and safe spaces, with neatly clipped lawns and carefully maintained structures — not dissimilar to the thousands of war cemeteries at home and abroad created by the Commonwealth War Graves Commission during the same period.

Ancient monuments played a practical role too in the post war recovery. As the war went on, the numbers of men suffering from PTSD continued to rise and new ways to treat them were explored. At Seale Hayne Hospital, near Newton Abbott in Devon, Arthur Hurst, who was a pioneer of using therapeutic landscapes, took men to the peace and quiet of the Devon countryside (Jones 2012). Men worked on the farm and were encouraged to use their creative energies as well as their physical abilities. The positive results showed that time spent outdoors, and involvement in activities such as gardening and crafts, could help shell-shocked men. Empowering the patient, tackling social isolation and diverting the mind, could help with recovery.

At a number of recently acquired historic sites, such as Rievaulx Abbey in Yorkshire, that came into guardianship in 1917, work began immediately after the war to stabilize the ruins and to open them to the public. The men recruited to work on clearing the sites were often veterans of the war and their skills acquired when digging trenches were put to good use in work such as stabilizing the buildings. Men with disabilities were also recruited under the King's National Roll Scheme, set up to encourage employers to take on disabled ex-servicemen. By 1933, over 273 monuments had been taken into the care of the state — a phenomenal enterprise, breathtaking in its ambition. For those whose lives were broken by conflict, caring for historic places, strengthening and repairing them, was, I think, a precursor to Human Henge.

Further conflict followed, but after the Second World War (WWII), with increasing wealth, more leisure time and the widespread growth in car ownership, visiting historic sites grew in popularity. Although the benefits of getting out into the countryside became widely appreciated, the focus of the Ministry of Works was very much on building conservation and historical research, rather than consciously exploring or developing the impact that sites could have on mental health and well-being.

The history of English Heritage

Through the last quarter of the twentieth century, there was a change in approach to the management of historic sites in the guardianship of the state. There was a dramatic shift away from central government control and a new focus on the commercialization of historic places, resulting in the development of the heritage industry. This was led by museums, historic houses and charities such as the National Trust. In 1984 a new body called English Heritage was created, to advise on and care for the nation's historic environment. From the outset, the organization's ambition was to be outward facing and responsive to the needs of the public.

In recent years English Heritage has separated from government control. In 2015, following a fundamental change, we became the English Heritage Trust; a new charity set up to run the nation's collection of historic properties. With our new freedom as a charity, independent of government, our ability and desire to engage with millions of people is now greatly strengthened. We have identified four major priorities for the new charity under the headings of: Inspiration; Conservation; Involvement; and Financial Sustainability. Although he might not have used the same language, Sir Charles Peers and his fellow heritage pioneers would certainly have understood the sentiments. But there is a difference now; a shift in emphasis in our work, with a renewed focus on what we can do for people, so that they continue to support us.

English Heritage and Human Henge

It was against this background of change, in the early years of the new charity, that Sara Lunt and Laura Drysdale from the Restoration Trust approached me with an idea to use Stonehenge to engage with people who are socially excluded and have mental health problems. I was immediately excited about it. I had worked with them both before and I knew that they would deliver something outstanding.

The original idea developed into Human Henge — a journey of ten weekly walks for a facilitated group of local people with mental health issues, accompanied by archaeologists and musicians, and culminating in access to the stone circle at Stonehenge. The programme ran successfully at Stonehenge and then at Avebury for 52 local people. The participants were all clients of the Richmond Fellowship, an organization commissioned by Wiltshire County Council and Avon and Wiltshire NHS Partnership Trust to provide mental health services. The project partnership comprises the Restoration Trust, the National Trust, Bournemouth University, the Richmond Fellowship and English Heritage, with funding support from the Heritage Lottery Fund (HLF).

Although relatively small in scale, with a limited sample of participants, this was a big idea. As an aspirational project, with an ambition to highlight an aspect of cultural heritage management not fully developed or rigorously researched before, it was something that English Heritage was very keen to support. Given that it was innovative and had the capacity to contribute to our new corporate goals as a charity, I was hopeful in gaining the support of our Chief Executive,

Kate Mavor. She warmly welcomed the initiative, which gave me the green-light both to put some cash funding into the project to support the first HLF bid, and to give the project free reign at Stonehenge. We were also able to provide English Heritage staff support on the ground from Catherine Snell, the Stonehenge Education Officer. Kate Mavor has continued to support the project and when I asked for some feedback she responded by saying:

> 'You know I love this project and I highlighted it at the staff conference last November because it was so good. That is the English Heritage we need!'

Having listened to the BBC Radio 4 Open Country programme (BBC 2017) about the project, Kate said:

> 'I listened to the whole programme last night and really enjoyed it. Very uplifting to think our site and its stories made such a difference to the health and wellbeing of the group. I am quite sure the same effect is manifest in lots of other places, albeit undocumented. This was great profile for our "involvement" piece, and I am sure people felt warmer towards us on hearing it'

She went on to say:

> '...make sure EH is name-checked in all the communications about the project so that people think to contact us elsewhere in the country for similar projects.'

Whilst it was important to have support at board level, it was critical for the project to be fully supported at the site. There was some apprehension amongst some staff members, mostly because they didn't know what to expect but also because the project was resource-heavy in terms of staff time and the use of space on site. The need for a private room to run the sessions was especially challenging, as the site has very limited space; the education room at the Stonehenge Visitor Centre is in high demand and booked up many months in advance. However we had full support from the site director Kate Davies, and any issues were quickly addressed. Our volunteers played a vital role too, ensuring the smooth running of the project and embedding it at Stonehenge. One volunteer, Chris Jessop, wrote a short piece in the English Heritage volunteers' newsletter, outlining his experience and helping to promote the project more widely in the organization. Vital in all of this were the professional and responsive contributions of Yvette Staelens, the Human Henge Co-ordinator, and Danny O'Donoghue, the Richmond Fellowship Locality Manager, who managed the project on site. Also essential were the energy and enthusiasm of the Stonehenge Education Officer, Catherine Snell. A large element of spontaneity was needed to create this first pilot project, and was provided by everyone involved.

Human Henge and the importance of collaboration

It was agreed at the outset, that it was essential to get good regional and national media coverage; we needed to tell people about the project, to raise awareness, and to promote discussion about mental health. As well as the partner organizations, the project's main funder, the Heritage Lottery Fund was also keen to ensure that Human Henge received as much media coverage as possible. PR for the project was sensitively managed by the English Heritage

Press Officer, Jessica Trethowan, who worked closely with the Human Henge team. We knew that the wishes of the participants took priority; some were happy to be filmed, interviewed and quoted in the media, whilst others did not feel comfortable being publicly identified with the project. The organizers also had to take account of safeguarding issues, such as taking and publishing of photographs and videos in the media and on websites.

Print and radio journalists, including BBC Radio 4's Open Country presenters, worked sensitively with the project team and the participants. As a result, their involvement was not seen as intrusive. In contrast, the regional TV news journalist and cameraman were felt to be disruptive in the session they attended at King Barrow Ridge. Although some participants were happy to be in the spotlight, others requested not to be filmed. Whilst the agreement to allow filming was discussed and agreed in advance with the participants, some felt anxious about the cameras even though they themselves were not filmed. A lesson was learnt here. At Avebury in the second pilot, we decided to exclude television coverage in favour of print and radio coverage.

Whilst the stone circle at Stonehenge and the group of sites at Avebury are in the guardianship of English Heritage, their ownership and management is complex, being divided between English Heritage and the National Trust. Both organizations are inevitably commercial rivals, dependent on visitors and other income-generating initiatives for their financial sustainability. They are also both careful to protect their brand identity and are often reluctant to take any risks. In this project, however, both organizations were focussed on the bigger picture and put aside any differences or rivalries to work collaboratively. The Human Henge project team, ensured that the wider Stonehenge landscape owned by the National Trust, and the stone circle itself, that is in the care of English Heritage, were treated as one. This collaboration has brought our two organizations together and whilst the commercial rivalries remain, the partnership has grown.

The project would not have gone ahead without the support of the Heritage Lottery Fund. We know that the project's focus on research and the potential development of replicable initiatives was a critical factor in the success of the HLF bid. Their focus is not only on the safeguarding of historic assets, but also on ensuring that their financial support leads to sustainable developments at historic places. They seek to promote systemic changes in the organizations responsible for managing historic sites, so that they become more outward facing and responsive to the needs of the public.

Conclusion

At Stonehenge, the Human Henge project team managed to balance the need to create a smooth-running and beneficial programme for the participants, against the complexities of managing a busy, sensitive archaeological site within a globally important landscape. The results so far are very promising. The initial research by Bournemouth University, and the responses from the participants, have shown that that engaging with historic landscapes does make people feel better, happier and more connected to other people. The response from our staff and from the public has been extremely positive. Human Henge has also made a lasting impact on English Heritage, by opening up a discussion about mental health in the historic environment.

The connection that people have with the past — where they have come from and where they are going to — is important for everyone; by using archaeological landscapes we can provide a bridge from modern times back into the past. What we have demonstrated at Stonehenge and Avebury, is that inviting people with mental health issues to engage with historic sites and landscapes in a structured way, can change their lives. It is tantalizing to consider the ways in which Human Henge might develop now, with its vision of making this approach part of mainstream treatment available to anyone with poor mental health. At Stonehenge there is a compelling argument that it has always been a place where people have come to be healed. Human Henge has shown that we can continue that tradition and that historic places have a role in today's society as a place to heal.

Bibliography

Art Care 2018. Salisbury Health Care History Project: Old Manor Hospital [Webpage]. Viewed 8 January 2019, <http://salisburyhealthcarehistory.uk/old-manor-hospital/>.

Barham, P. 2007. *Forgotten Lunatics of the Great War*. New Haven (CT): Yale University Press.

BBC 2017. Open Country: Stonehenge and Mental Health [Webpage]. Viewed 8 January 2019, <https://www.bbc.co.uk/programmes/b08md98n>.

Cohen, D. 2001. *The War Come Home. Disabled veterans in Britain and Germany 1914-1939*. Oakland (CA): University of California Press.

Darvill, T. and G. Wainwright 2009. Stonehenge excavations 2008. *Antiquaries Journal* 89(1): 1–19.

Daw, T. 2013. Stonehenge Handed Over [Webpage]. Viewed 8 January 2019, <http://www.sarsen.org/2013/10>.

Fry, S. 2014a. *A History of the National Heritage Collection. Volume Four: 1913-1931. The Ancient Monuments Branch Under Peers and Baines. Research Report Series No. 48-2014*. Swindon: English Heritage.

Fry, S. 2014b. *A History of the National Heritage Collection. Volume Three: Stonehenge. Research Report Series No. 47-2014*. Swindon: English Heritage.

Gosling, G.C. 2018. World War I Centenary. Lloyd George's Ministry Men [Webpage]. Viewed 8 January 2018, <http://ww1centenary.oucs.ox.ac.uk/body-and-mind/lloyd-georges-ministry-men/>.

Hawkes, J. 1967. God in the machine. *Antiquity* 41: 174–180.

Howe, T. and G. Percy 2000. *The Old Manor Salisbury, A Glimpse into the Past*. Salisbury: Salisbury Heath Care NHS Trust.

Jones, E. 2012. War neuroses and Arthur Hurst: A pioneering medical film about the treatment of psychiatric battle casualties. *Journal of the History of Medicine and Allied Sciences* 67(3): 345–373.

Parkinson, J. 2015, BBC News Magazine. The Man Who Bought Stonehenge – And Then Gave it Away [Webpage]. Viewed 8 January 2019, <https://www.bbc.co.uk/news/magazine-34282849>.

Chapter 11

People making places making people

Briony Clifton

Abstract

Since its inception over 100 years ago, the National Trust has acknowledged the importance of the places that it cares for and their influence on well-being. While supporting Human Henge at Avebury, we strove to balance the desire to support a smooth-running and beneficial programme for the participants, with the complexities we face as a busy, sensitive site within an internationally important landscape. Through welcoming Human Henge to the National Trust at Avebury, we hope to have made a positive impact by creating and facilitating a safe and comfortable environment in which the participants could contemplate this unique and special landscape.

Keywords: Avebury; Human Henge; National Trust; Prehistoric landscapes; Well-being

Introduction

The connection between landscapes and well-being has long been recognized by the National Trust. Indeed it was the holistic outlook of our three co-founders that was in large part the inspiration for the formation of the National Trust over 100 years ago. Human Henge, it seemed to us, was exactly the kind of project that our co-founders would have encouraged: a project that improves access to some of the country's most outstanding sites and monuments in two areas of real beauty and inspiration. An appreciation of the natural environment and the benefits this could bring to individuals was an early theme for the three founders. Seven years prior to establishing the National Trust with Sir Robert Hunter and Canon Hardwicke Rawnsley, Octavia Hill said, 'the need of quiet, the need of air, the need of exercise, and, I believe, the sight of the sky and of things growing, seem human needs, common to all' (Darley 1990: 290). Hunter, likewise, had an enthusiasm for the open air and turned the cogs on the new charity quietly and efficiently in the background.

As the National Trust developed in these early years, a key objective was providing access to countryside spaces for those who had none. In one appeal made by Hill to raise funds to acquire Gowbarrow Park, Ullswater in the Lake District, she said:

'A mile of lake shore, not to be cut off from the visitor by enclosure or garden but by which he can wander at will and hear the ripples breaking on the pebbles...valley, lake, mountain peaks, slopes of russet fern or heather, wood and stream and rocks, when spring sets the primroses in thousands on the banks of the stream, or autumn turns the wild cherry trees crimson, and the birches gold, when the storm sweeps over the mountains, or the summer sun streams among the trees... Is it all to be ours for our rest, refreshment and inspiration and handed on by us in all its beauty in perpetuity for the England that is to be?' (Darley 1990: 291)

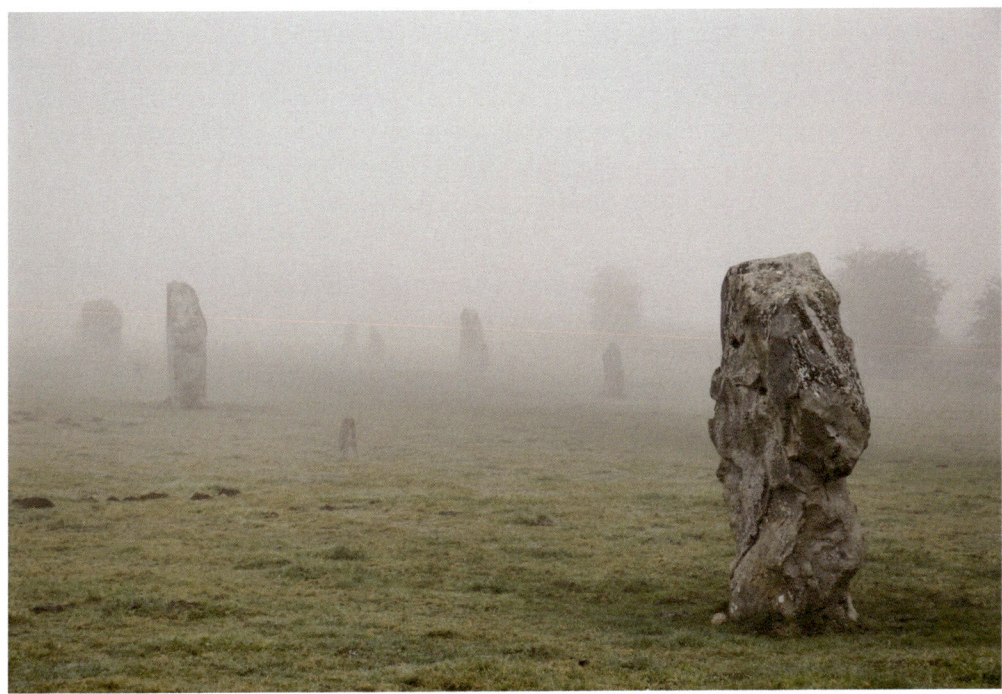

Figure 11.1 Avebury mist on the West Kennet Avenue. (©National Trust/Abby George)

Over a hundred years later, one Human Henge participant writes about their experience on a night walk along the West Kennet Avenue at Avebury, connecting the past, nature, and the sight of the sky:

> 'We ended the session walking back along the avenue toward the henge. Another person and I walked alone at the back. Being alone in the Avenue, surrounded by grey figures and misty fields, shrouded by the starry night sky, the atmosphere felt heavy. I was being transported back in time to a place of unfamiliarity and yet, at the same time, feeling strangely familiar? I looked up to the stars, the sky and the earth connected as one. I was being drawn in, into the briefest of glimpses of a cosmic plan. As I left the avenue behind, mist hung over the ground, the moon shone, stars twinkled, and all was still.' (Human Henge 2018a)

As a project that is a fresh, original and specific way of connecting landscapes, heritage and well-being, Human Henge was one way in which the National Trust could actively implement this fundamental and original root of the charity: the use of landscapes for well-being. Three groups have taken part in Human Henge. The first two groups spent their sessions in the Stonehenge landscape. Avebury, as the other half of the Stonehenge and Avebury World Heritage Site, was an ideal location for the third group of Human Henge participants.

This chapter has been written from the viewpoint of hosting Human Henge at the Avebury National Trust site. The first part discusses considerations around National Trust staff involvement and the background to choosing a safe and secure setting. The second part discusses some of the Human Henge session locations. It examines the specifics, challenges, requirements and sensitivity of location, and goes on to consider the benefits of full support from the National Trust property, together with future connection and involvement for participants.

Human Henge at National Trust, Avebury

Depth of local team involvement

The local National Trust team within the Stonehenge and Avebury World Heritage Site, was invited to join the Human Henge project at the launch in 2016, just before the first group was due to start their ten week journey. For the first two groups, Human Henge had its base in the English Heritage Stonehenge Visitor Centre Education Rooms and journeyed out into the Stonehenge landscape. This culminated in the final week with a special event inside the stones. The National Trust owns a significant portion of the Stonehenge World Heritage Site, including many of the major monuments, and took part in some of the sessions for Group Two, talking with the group members about our roles in nature, conservation and archaeology in the landscape.

When the Restoration Trust asked if Human Henge could bring a third group to Avebury, this meant a much greater involvement from the local National Trust team. Three National Trust members of staff led or co-led five of the ten sessions with Yvette Staelens. For two sessions, this increased involvement was a relatively organic process, where the author was already present and could discuss the background of the sites. Three sessions (Lockeridge Dene with Peter Oliver, Museum Collections with Dr Ros Cleal, and the clay workshop session with the author) were prearranged. Human Henge requires significant property support and enthusiasm in the form of location facilitation; staff and volunteer time is needed in order for the participants to have the best possible experience at these sites, and to gain an understanding of the work that goes into caring for these places.

Setting

One of the most important elements for us from the outset was to provide a dedicated space set aside at Avebury for Human Henge groups, that was safe, comfortable and consistent. It was also important to keep this initial place as unobtrusive as possible. The Education Room at Avebury was chosen as the primary base where participants, volunteers and organizers were to gather at the start and end of each session.

The Education Room has a small kitchen with a partition to a larger room. After discussions with a volunteer who had attended Human Henge sessions at Stonehenge, it was decided that the tea and coffee area needed to be opened up because it had previously formed a natural hub for the groups at Stonehenge. After adapting the refreshments layout, this indeed ended up being the case and became an important part of the morning and afternoon ritual and routine for members of the group.

The National Trust General Manager responsible for Avebury offered a dedicated member of staff who would be present throughout the sessions. This would maintain consistency for the

Human Henge participants and supporting staff, and for the National Trust team. As a Human Henge Board Member and National Trust co-ordinator for the project at Avebury, the author was chosen for this role. Before the Human Henge sessions began, the National Trust team realized the importance of consistency for all parties, and in having a familiar face for the group who is also accustomed to the workings and management of the site. It is essential to note here that this consistency aided and added to the smooth running of each Human Henge session from the point of view of the Avebury National Trust team. Therefore we hope to have made a quiet difference in the background of the Human Henge sessions.

The National Trust team at Avebury invested significant time in the project. With critical interest and support from management and vital individual staff and volunteer investment, the Human Henge project at Avebury benefitted from a range of facilities. Trust staff were able to pass on our own knowledge, appreciation and experience of working in, managing and understanding the National Trust sites at Avebury.

The landscape location

An important aspect of Human Henge is that it draws on specialists with site-specific knowledge. To this end, the author and two other National Trust staff members were asked to co-lead a Human Henge session. The sites and monuments at Avebury contain thousands of years of archaeology and include some thriving chalk grassland sites. The group visited Lockeridge Dene in the fourth week of Human Henge where Peter Oliver, the Area Ranger at Avebury, led a tour of the site. This site (and the similar nearby site of Piggledene) was

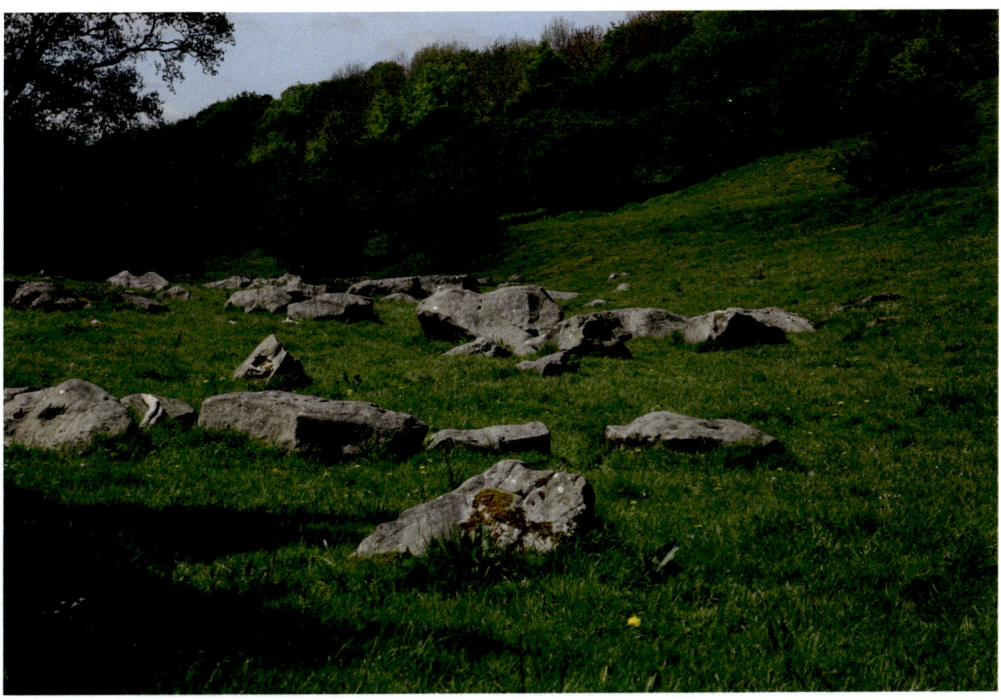

Figure 11.2 Sarsen boulders at Lockeridge Dene, Avebury. (©National Trust/Mike Robinson)

acquired by the National Trust in 1908 after a public appeal, and they were the first Wiltshire countryside sites purchased by the National Trust (NT 2018).

The Rangers care for these chalk grassland sites, and Peter discussed how certain species thrive here through the way the site is managed. He walked us through the lichen-rich sarsen 'boulder streams' that formed there over 30 million years ago and helped to shape the landscape that we see today - including the centuries during which many of these huge stones were broken up and removed to provide the building materials for local buildings. One participant described his thoughts as he walked through the dozens of sarsens speckling the fields:

> 'Personally, I have always found the stones owning a unique presence and awe within the landscape. Their feel, texture, patterns, the holes, the weathering, the lichen and the puddles, all owing to this uniqueness.' (Human Henge 2018b)

The museum archive

The wealthy archaeologist, Alexander Keiller, who inherited money from the family marmalade business, purchased Windmill Hill near Avebury in the 1920s. He carried out five seasons of excavations at the site, a Neolithic causewayed enclosure, and later sold the land to the National Trust. The artefacts recovered during these excavations, were gifted to the nation by his widow. The causewayed enclosure, a Neolithic monument constructed around 5650 years ago, covers the top of Windmill Hill (Darvill 2010: 99). It comprises three concentric rings of segmented ditches and banks, containing gaps (or causeways) in the rings. This monument

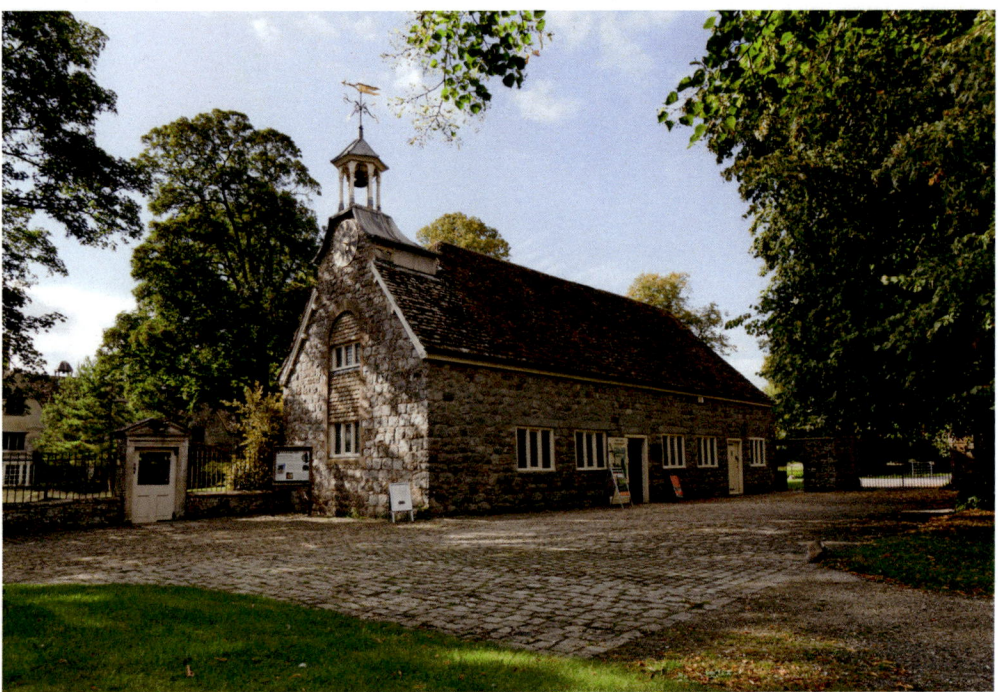

Figure 11.3 The Stables Gallery in front of Avebury Manor, Wiltshire. (©National Trust Images/James Dobson)

was probably not permanently occupied, but used seasonally as a place for gathering and exchange for around 300 years. The causewayed enclosure was Keiller's first excavation in England, taking place from 1925 to 1929. The Avebury and Stonehenge Landscapes have been subject to centuries of research, and the Windmill Hill excavation archive forms only part of the extensive body of knowledge about these areas. Throughout the ten weeks of the Human Henge pilot project, this knowledge was shared with the participants in practical, stimulating ways.

During the museum collections session, the Human Henge group looked at the pottery and flint collection from the Windmill Hill excavations in the 1920s. This took place in the Stables Store, one of the museum store rooms. It was led by the Curator of the Alexander Keiller Museum, Dr Ros Cleal, a specialist in British prehistoric ceramics who has worked for the National Trust for many years. This session had extremely positive feedback from the participants after it gave everyone a chance to see and handle the artefacts:

> 'Looking at all of the styles and patterns was fascinating. People later noted how they enjoyed being able to actually handle the pottery, as opposed to seeing it in books or behind glass. The hands-on learning brought people closer to the past, to the peoples who created this pottery. People started to think how it may have been. What the peoples may have experienced.' (Human Henge 2018c)

The special access for the Human Henge participants, alongside handling and discussing objects made thousands of years ago with Dr Cleal, made the session particularly special.

The clay workshop

The ephemeral aspects of life in prehistory were also discussed and explored throughout most of the sessions, but during two in particular. One full session, and part of the final session, explored the properties and experience of clay and working with our hands. These were creative sessions using material the participants had encountered before in in the Collections session. However, instead of fired clay, which survives as ceramic material for thousands of years, the group used the raw material. The clay was manipulated into sculpture or pottery and was left out in the open where the elements would make it disappear within a week. The author had led a similar clay workshop in the summer of 2017 with a group of veterans and serving military personnel who were taking part in an archaeological project in Wiltshire as a pathway to recovery. This was run by Breaking Ground Heritage and Operation Nightingale with Wessex Archaeology. The success of this workshop led the author to develop it for the Human Henge clay session, during which the properties of clay, pottery-making and firing, fashions and typologies of ceramics were discussed.

Working with clay can engage people's sense of focus and absorption. Any intricate work requiring concentration and the use of your hands, can provide a sense of calm focus. As an archaeologist, a fascinating aspect of working with clay and, significantly, not firing it, is the discussion it generated in the Human Henge group about life in the past and what is found in the archaeological record. The fleeting existence of an unfired pot or sculpture, left outside to the elements to become washed away into the mud, highlights how much of the past can never be uncovered and how much mystery there is left to dwell on.

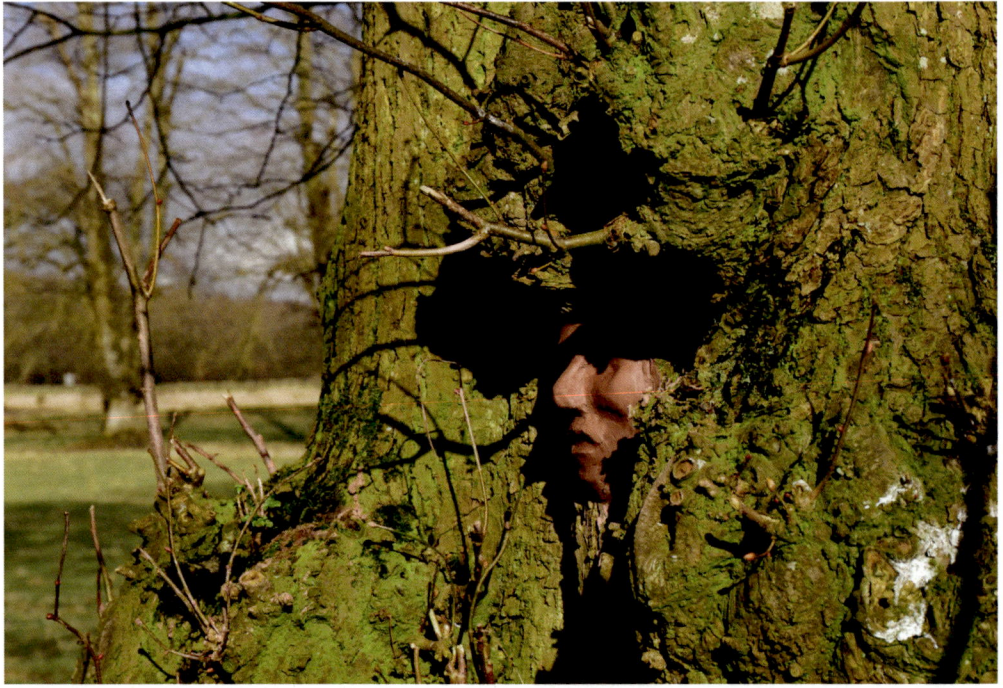

Figure 11.4 Clay sculpting workshop. (©National Trust/Abby George)

Specifics and challenges

Every place comes with its own stories, quirks and highlights, as well as external forces outside its control. The National Trust sites at Avebury and the wider landscape are acknowledged as special, internationally important places, specifically because of the extraordinary Neolithic and early Bronze Age archaeology. This does not only come in the form of the huge henge and stone circles, the atmospheric burial mound of West Kennet Long Barrow or the winding avenues of standing stone, but also in the concealed settlement sites with hand-crafted pottery and swathes of worked flint littering the soil beneath our feet. Besides all this, there are still so many secrets hidden beneath the topsoil, waiting to be uncovered. Although these sites have existed for millennia, they are also fragile and, in the case of the major sites, often busy with visitors.

Human Henge at Avebury took place once a week for ten weeks in early 2018, at a time when the weather was at its most dramatic and severe. This caused a few difficulties for the National Trust team at Avebury, with varying degrees of disruption for both the site and Human Henge. Avebury faced snow drifts, water damage and closures. And yet, with all this, the Human Henge participants, staff and volunteers remained patient and supportive of the team at Avebury. The incidents caused by unpredictable severe weather were important, as they were lessons in managing external interference with a Human Henge session. They taught the National Trust team how we could continue to support the project with the least disruption.

Despite the significance of turning these background cogs as smoothly and quietly as possible, a couple of buildings at Avebury were put out of action by the freezing weather. Consequently,

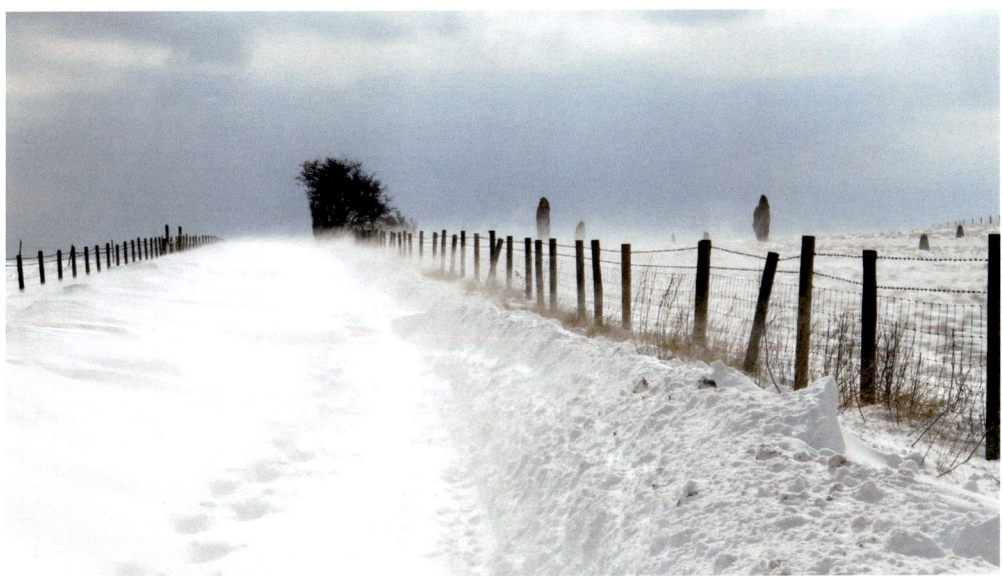

Figure 11.5 West Kennet Avenue and the road to Avebury in the snow. (©National Trust/Mike Robinson)

half way through the project, the Human Henge sessions had to be relocated away from the Education Room; the group's designated safe space. The author brought this challenge back to the team at Avebury; with some planning, we managed to secure a private staff room in an office attached to Avebury Manor which worked extremely well for the group.

Each site comes with its own day-to-day challenges and Human Henge comes with its own challenges, requiring resources and property support in order to run successfully. In addition, Avebury and the Stonehenge Landscape also have legal requirements to follow, with their Scheduled Monument and Listed Buildings designations, and other complexities. In the run-up to Avebury hosting and facilitating Human Henge, it was recognized by management that it was not enough to simply choose a staff member who works at the site, to become involved in the project. They needed to be prepared to be a part of the group, to care sincerely for the comfort of everyone in that group and to make every effort to achieve a positive and friendly environment; all of this, alongside maintaining responsible management of the sites.

After Human Henge for the Avebury team

The National Trust is a charity that depends on volunteers. People who, for whatever reason — be it the love of a specific site, the community created through volunteering, being outside, talking to the public, meeting new people, or for their own mental well-being — want to come and help us care for our sites. Recent research, where the National Trust worked with leading researchers and academics, has also demonstrated the significant beneficial connection between people and place, not only physically, but psychologically (NT 2017). The Volunteer Co-ordinator for the National Trust sites in Wiltshire is facilitating a pathway for Human Henge participants, which enables them to apply to volunteer with the National Trust should they wish to, either in the short term or in the future. In the final session, the author talked to the Human Henge participants about volunteering opportunities with the National Trust.

This had been discussed with the management team at Avebury, because the Trust wanted to help provide an additional step after the ten Human Henge sessions, offering participants the potential for continuity. This takes us straight back to the reason the National Trust supports the Human Henge project. We have acknowledged the importance of the places that we care for and the influence they can have on well-being for more than a century, and we will continue to support Human Henge and similar projects.

Conclusion

We can see analogies between the interests and guiding principles of the National Trust and the nature of the Human Henge project. These arise not only from the use of its landscapes and nature for well-being, but also from concepts of access and belonging; of landscapes to be shared with everyone (Waterson 1994: 45). Historic and, in the case of Avebury and Stonehenge, prehistoric landscapes, offer an additional depth; that of the human timeline going back millennia. The stories, ideas and emotions that these types of (pre)historic landscapes evoke, particularly to those who are already familiar with them (NT 2017), can help restore or inspire us. Places like these, especially if they carry meaning for a person, have been shown to benefit mental well-being, and contribute to feelings of security and peace (NT 2017).

By being a part of this project, the National Trust are continuing the pioneering vision of our founders whilst facilitating access for a new and original project which creates new emotional connections — or develops old emotional connections — to these unique sites. We were pleased to be able to welcome Human Henge to Avebury and the Stonehenge Landscape. We felt that offering our support and facilities to the project was worthwhile, both for the benefit of the participants visiting the sites and for ourselves as a National Trust property, learning from, and working with, Human Henge.

Bibliography

Darley, G. 1990. *Octavia Hill: Social Reformer and Founder of the National Trust.* London: Francis Boutle Publishers.
Darvill, T. 2010. *Prehistoric Britain* (Second edition). Abingdon: Routledge.
Human Henge 2018a. Avebury Session 6: West Kennet Avenue, night walk — 21 Feb 2018 [Webpage]. Viewed 22 October 2018, <https://humanhenge.org/>.
Human Henge 2018b. Avebury Session 4: Lockeridge Dene – 9 Feb 2018 [Webpage]. Viewed 22 October 2018, <https://humanhenge.org/>.
Human Henge 2018c. Avebury Session 7: Alexander Keiller Museum & Collections – 9 March 2018 [Webpage]. Viewed 22 October 2018, <https://humanhenge.org/>.
NT 2017. *Places that make us. Research Report* [Online document]. Swindon: National Trust. Viewed 21 May 2019, <https://nt.global.ssl.fastly.net/documents/places-that-make-us-research-report.pdf>
NT 2018. Lockeridge Dene and Piggledene [Webpage]. Viewed 22 October 2018, <https://www.nationaltrust.org.uk/lockeridge-dene-and-piggledene/>.
Waterson, M. 1994. *The National Trust: The first hundred years.* London: BBC Books and National Trust (Enterprises) Limited.

Chapter 12

'The archaeological imagination': New ways of seeing for mental health recovery

Rebecca L Hearne

Abstract

Participants in archaeology projects often mention archaeology's intensely real, deeply affecting, magical characteristics. Such overtly emotional dimensions are not commonly discussed or evaluated, due largely to their 'unscientific' and intrinsically qualitative nature. Expanding on what Michael Shanks termed 'the archaeological imagination' in his book of the same name published in 2012, this paper argues that the development of a subjective, emotionally and imaginatively meaningful relationship with the past, as experienced through an individual's own mental landscape, may provide a new insight as to why archaeology can be such a positive and uniquely beneficial tool within processes of recovery and well-being. This paper explores how the archaeological imagination manifests itself in individuals; it discusses how an archaeological 'habit of mind' can be developed, and how encountering the 'magic of the past' can catalyze emotional and intellectual processes that could contribute towards mental health recovery and well-being. The archaeological imagination is a fundamental component of what I would like to introduce as 'radical archaeology': archaeological practices in which social, emotional, and historical outcomes are weighted equally. If we are to implement the archaeological imagination into UK archaeological practice, then radical archaeology needs to win recognition as a new direction for traditional practice.

Keywords: Emotion; Imagination; Radical archaeology; Recovery; Social

Introduction

In this chapter I will talk about how archaeology makes us **feel**. I am interested in what makes people enjoy archaeology, and what keeps us coming back to it again and again. I want to know what happens to an individual's imagination, their thought processes, and their emotions while they are 'doing' archaeology. I will discuss how encountering archaeology can generate certain emotional responses in its participants, and how these emotional experiences might contribute to sustaining individual mental health and well-being, long-term. I believe that it is an individual's 'archaeological imagination' that allows them to experience the magical, emotion-rich side of archaeology, and that, furthermore, it is this imaginative process that makes archaeology an effective and unique therapeutic activity for individuals living with, or in recovery from, problems with their mental health.

Archaeological excavation is beginning to be recognized as a potentially therapeutic experience for individuals with mental health problems. Projects such as Past in Mind (Lack 2014), Operation Nightingale (Osgood and Andrews 2015), and Digability (Beauchamp et al. 2014) have in recent years employed archaeological excavation in collaboration with individuals who live with or are recovering from issues connected with their mental health. These projects have had positive results. Recognition of the archaeological process as 'therapeutic' is a recent development. Research is ongoing regarding the seemingly positive response overall of mental health to archaeology's constituent experiences (and see other chapters in this volume): these include outdoor exercise, teamwork, peer-to-peer support, building social networks, trust and hope, a sense of purpose, improving identity and self-esteem, purposeful and satisfying activity, and developing living skills (e.g. Carless and Sparkes 2008; Kiddey 2014; McEvoy et al. 2012). Contemporary mental health recovery models recognize these factors as positive contributors, advising their implementation into individuals' everyday lives (Jacob 2015; Regan et al. 2016.). These therapeutic characteristics are clearly not unique to archaeology. For example, surfing (Taylor 2013), singing (Shakespeare and Whieldon 2018), gardening and horticulture (Atkinson 2009), and dancing (Wilbur et al. 2015) have all been shown to similarly benefit mental health, and to harness many of the same beneficial aspects.

It is easy to take for granted the apparent causal relationship between the aforementioned aspects of archaeology and a positive impact on mental health. However, there is one key aspect of archaeological practice that is often neglected and which, I will argue, represents the processual relationship occurring between individuals and the past: one which determines how we experience archaeology both phenomenologically (i.e. subjectively through our embodied participation in the world) and **imaginatively**. The process of creating and interacting with the past in our own imaginations — the automatic, emotional response to, and generation of, imaginative past worlds and situating ourselves within them — is one aspect of the archaeological process that is unique, and can potentially contribute positively to mental health recovery and well-being.

I first discuss 'the archaeological imagination' as defined by Michael Shanks in his 2012 publication of the same name. I will then explore how the term can be profitably applied to the unique and subjective emotional encounter catalyzed by engaging with the remains of the past, and how these imaginative aspects are commonly marginalized within modern archaeology due to their highly personal, speculative nature. I lay out how the archaeological imagination is a 'habit of mind' that encompasses aspects of time, place, and personal identity, and how this unique combination can render archaeological practice 'therapeutic'. Finally, I introduce the concept of 'radical archaeology', explore what this might look like in practical terms, and discuss how adopting changes in traditional practice could facilitate the development of archaeological imagination and encourage mental health recovery and well-being.

The archaeological imagination

In his book *The Archaeological Imagination* published in 2012 Michael Shanks defines 'archaeology' not as a recreational activity, a subject of special interest or an academic degree course — i.e., a standalone activity divorced from the rest of the world and only optionally interacted with — but as an active experience that is all around us, happens to us every day, and provides the building blocks for much of the way in which we view society. This contemporary situating of archaeology — its location and embedding in culture — Shanks terms its 'actuality' (2012: 12). Although by no means the first to denote the concept of archaeology's cultural reflexivity, earlier works by Shanks, including *Experiencing the Past* (1992), and *Social Theory and Archaeology* (1987) and *Reconstructing Archaeology* (1992) with Christopher Tilley, began to set the scene for a recognition of the archaeological imagination as a distinct entity, without yet explicitly defining it. Others have explored how archaeology persistently infiltrates and influences our everyday lives, our culture, our politics and our senses of national identity, both consciously and unconsciously. This has been done through diverse analyses of poetry, historical writing, travel, and the preservation of artefacts — and human remains — in museums (e.g. Finn 2004; Sanders 2009; Wallace 2004).

Shanks' own definition of the archaeological imagination is not particularly easy to establish, and Paphitis (2013: 1–2) helpfully paraphrases it thus: it enables us 'to recreate the world behind the ruin in the land, to reanimate the people behind the sherd of antique pottery, a fragment of the past… a creative impulse and faculty at the heart of archaeology, but also embedded in many cultural dispositions, discourses and institutions commonly associated with modernity. The archaeological imagination is rooted in a sensibility, a pervasive set of attitudes toward traces and remains, towards memory, time and temporality, the fabric of history'. Shanks evidently intends to use the concept of the archaeological imagination as a vehicle for wider discussion of how archaeology is inextricably bound with contemporary culture. He suggests that archaeology is a mixture of, and contributor to, literature, pop culture, historical texts, material remains, antiquarian interpretation, philosophy, cultural geography, geology, photography, contemporary art, and social theory (Paphitis 2013; Shanks 2012). Shanks also briefly references other culturally influential ways of seeing, a pertinent example being the 'geographical imagination' (Harvey 1969; Prince 1962) that underpins much of Shanks' theory and which he describes as comprising '…responses to places and landscapes [with] sympathetic insight and creative understanding… [the] geographical imagination is a **habit of mind** that enables people to recognize the role of space and place in their own biographies' (my emphasis; Shanks 2012: 14).

The Archaeological Imagination provides a macroscopic view on how archaeology affects us every day. However, the text is somewhat of a 'theoretical and observational deluge' (Paphitis 2013: 2), rendering it challenging to locate the intention behind, or the purpose of, the archaeological imagination — or even the point of defining it. Shanks neglects to explore the possibilities of how the archaeological imagination might exist in a subjective, personal context. There is no attempt to explore what this might look or feel like for someone experiencing '…the pleasures and emotional dimensions of engaging with the material remains of the past' (Moshenska and Dhanjal 2011: 3). For example, examining the thoughts and feelings engendered by adopting an archaeological 'habit of mind' whilst participating in an excavation, visiting a museum, viewing a landscape, or engaging in some other means of intentional immersion in, or connection with, the past. By deconstructing and repackaging Shanks' archaeological imagination, we can begin to explore how the process might manifest itself individually — or phenomenologically — and how it encapsulates many of the key tenets of mental health recovery.

The magic of the past

The imaginative, emotional encounter commonly associated with the archaeological process has been variously described as invoking 'the magic of the past' (Holtorf 2005: 156; Shanks and Tilley 1992: 13), 'the rich sensual experiences associated with heritage' (Holtorf 2011: 13), 'enchantment' (Perry 2018), and 'the thrill' (Moshenska 2006: 91). Such terms refer directly to the imaginative encounter with archaeology; a feeling of awe, wonder, curiosity, and even 'magic'. Past in Mind, a Heritage Lottery Funded collaborative excavation project by the Herefordshire branch of the mental health charity Mind, reported thus: 'Several [participants] commented on the strong sense of a bond between themselves and the people whose houses, broken pots, and grassland they were handling. This is a common but under-acknowledged experience… Bridging the gap of centuries is a potent, almost tangible, discovery' (Lack 2014: 30).

Archaeology allows us to place ourselves in the past through the medium of creative and exploratory thought, catalyzed by encounters with its material remains. It allows us to imagine who our predecessors were, what they wore, how they looked, sounded, smelled, moved, and spoke. Something that is ordinarily so unknowable as to be alien — the direct, sensual experience of living in the past — is made tangible by its material presence. It encompasses what Moshenska has called 'the archaeological uncanny' (2006); the uncovering of that which should have remained invisible. Archaeological discovery, speculation, and imagining give us a thrill of something unusual in the mundane. They help us to practise storytelling, indulge in creative analysis of the past (Roberts 2000), and allow us to narratively make sense of our life experiences. We find new relationships or connections between ourselves and the world around us (Bierski 2016) through '...the knowledge that this unfamiliar geography is also part of ourselves' (Sawday in Moshenska 2006: 95).

Because such subjective, emotional experiences of archaeology are 'unscientific' and not easily described and compared, and because they in themselves do not further our objective knowledge of the past, they have become dispensable to the archaeological process. A traditional view of archaeology comprises excavation, classification, the display or archiving of artefacts, and report writing: practical activities that contribute authoritatively to our knowledge of past societies. Career archaeologists certainly still experience the archaeological 'habit of mind'; they are, however, dissuaded from pursuing it. Praetzellis describes encountering the past emotionally as a commercial archaeologist: 'It is a very personal thing, and it will not usually find its way into the report because I feel that it is too impressionistic. It just ain't Science' (1998: 1). Notwithstanding such perspectives, if it could be demonstrated that 'the magic of the past' can not only deepen our emotional attachment to the past, but also contribute towards better mental health and well-being, it might no longer be so glibly discredited.

The archaeological imagination and mental health recovery

The archaeological imagination can be classified as a 'habit of mind' that might be developed over time and with practice. It describes a way of seeing the world with archaeological eyes. This definition expands on Shanks, who, possibly unintentionally on his part, explains the archaeological imagination as being experientially ubiquitous and actively shaping cultural production, but simultaneously divorced from the individual. I would rather introduce the archaeological imagination as more generally describing the creative and emotive thought processes that occur when in the presence of archaeological material, in whatever form is of significance to the individual. In my experience of community archaeology projects, whether public-, university-, or developer-led, participants repeat, with reassuring regularity, some iteration of two key phrases: '...I'll never see a hole in the ground / a lump in a field / my garden in the same way again', and, 'I'm noticing things I never noticed before'. These two statements display the archaeological imagination in action: the world looks different (i.e. increasingly 'archaeological') once this habit of mind is activated. The archaeological imagination is a long-term investment; not something that is only experienced whilst participating in an excavation, but rather whenever the opportunity presents itself. These statements also indicate that the archaeological imagination is bound by time, place, and identity (i.e. situating oneself in an imaginary past as well as an imaginary future, and speculating on the sorts of physical places that might ignite the emotional process).

It has previously been suggested that archaeological practice is a form of 'dwelling-in-the-world' after theories put forward by Heidegger (Bierski 2016; Ingold 2000; Todres and Galvin 2010) that refer to the reflexive relationship between humans and the environment. This is characterized by 'a unity or integration with the world...becoming and transforming rather than simply residing' (Bierski 2016: 139); an 'ongoing temporal interweaving of our lives with one another and with the... constituents of the environment' (Ingold 2000: 348). By enabling participants to pay closer attention to their surroundings, kinesthetically engaging with, and sentiently noticing, features and landscapes around them, the archaeological imagination encourages 'attentive being' (Bierski 2016: 138). Arguably, this 'attentive being,' 'interweaving,' or 'dwelling,' involves particular ways of seeing and moving with intention through the world, and '...people can and do make sense of their experiences of mental health problems by contemplating and actively engaging with the world and its features' (Bierski 2016: 138).

Projecting forward through time (i.e. 'I'll never see so-and-so in the same way again') allows individuals to imagine their future, and relearn living in a different way. The narrative aspect of the archaeological imagination also provides a linear temporality within which individuals can bear witness to their own journeys from past, to present, to speculative future. Understanding imaginary, archaeological pasts may eventually assist in retelling one's personal stories differently, to oneself as well as others, as 'understanding one path helps navigate another' (Bierski 2016: 143). It may be that practising imagining the past makes it easier to imagine the future; one in which recovery and mental well-being are a distinct possibility. Todres and Galvin are reassuringly buoyant about mental well-being: '[The] deepest possibility of well-being carries with it a feeling of rootedness and flow, peace and possibility' (2010: 1), suggesting that well-being is feeling secure and at home in the world (dwelling) alongside the promise of future movement and change. Furthermore, imagination is posited as a safe space for personal experimentation. Historical accuracy and archaeological technicality are less important than the meaning derived from the imaginative experience, especially since so much of the past is utterly unknowable and therefore open to creative interpretation. The archaeological imagination could thus provide a vehicle for contributing towards individuals' re-ignited feelings of confidence, creative self-expression, and self-acceptance.

Imagination: Accessibility for all

There are as many different archaeological narratives as there are individuals experiencing them. Although archaeology as a discipline gives us material information about cultures, peoples, and trends in object creation and deposition, in imaginative terms it can only ever be a record of individuals: *someone* made such-and-such an object, and *someone* placed it in the ground. Every artefact, in its materiality, its use-wear patterns, or its depositional history, has its own story, to which each individual archaeological imagination will respond, generating a preferred, personally significant narrative. John Berger and Adrian Praetzellis sum it up between them: 'The past is never there waiting to be discovered, to be recognized for exactly what it is' (Berger 2008: 11) as, '...the site contains many potential stories... every one is a product of the archaeological imagination that pulls together historical and archaeological facts into an interpretation that is more than the sum of its parts' (Praetzellis 1998: 1).

Museums, living history centres, and other archaeological 'experiences' succeed in bringing the past evocatively and emotively to life. These include as the Jorvik Viking Centre in York, the London Mithraeum, Cardiff-based art and archaeology collective Guerrilla Archaeology, and Butser Ancient Farm in Hampshire, with their immersive displays, galleries and activities. Such institutions and groups achieve their success through the recognition that emotional experience renders the past highly accessible to all; anyone who can see, hear, smell, or taste 'the past' is able more immediately to imagine and understand it. Sensual accessibility, furthermore, requires no qualifying knowledge; significantly, historical accuracy is not a prerequisite for the archaeological imagination. It is this aspect of the emotional encounter that will cause complaint to undoubtedly arise from those sceptical of the archaeological imagination concept, or from those concerned about the substitution of feelings for facts. It is not a question of encouraging laziness or taking shortcuts (Praetzellis 1998); on the contrary, it is only by combining good archaeological practice with respect for human experience, that archaeology as a discipline can ensure its survival. As John Berger states in *Ways of seeing*, 'the real question is: to whom does the meaning of [the past] properly belong? To those who can apply it to their own lives, or to a cultural hierarchy of relic specialists?' (2008: 32). Now that archaeology's wider social applications are being recognized, we must become comfortable with the ambiguity and open-endedness that the archaeological imagination can provide, if we are to meet the requirements of archaeology's broader audiences.

It is becoming increasingly necessary to promote and explore the emotional side of the practice. We can legitimately promote subjective experience as an important and valid outcome of archaeological practice, and we can encourage and facilitate the experience of the archaeological imagination itself. Nevertheless, leaving room for, and promoting, the conditions under which every participant can experience the full emotional force of the discipline, would require a fundamental shift in the archaeological status quo.

'Radical archaeology': A new term for a key concept

'A characteristic of modern [archaeology] is to avoid... intimacies... burying the individual... that creates an unbridgeable distance between our own images of the past and the subjective and local intimacies of people's own lives as they were once lived' (Barrett 1994: 1). Though this description refers to historical individuals, it applies as well to the contemporary individual. By encouraging archaeology's commercialization we have justified the sidelining of the emotional encounter. Where developer-funded rescue projects work within financial and temporal constraints, emotional attachment is at best a hindrance, and at worst an unscientific weakness — 'melodrama over empirics' (Shanks 2012: 10). Commercially, the magic of the past must be ignored, and 'more often than not... individual investigators have accomplished this work through self-sacrifice' (McGuire 2008: 124). At present, much archaeology, even community-led, is still largely a spectator sport. Archaeology is rather like a play being performed by academics or commercial units to a public 'audience', resulting in 'shallow, passive consumption' by archaeological 'consumers' (Tilley 1989). These 'professional versus amateur' and 'scientific equals correct, sensual equals incorrect' hegemonies need to be dismantled in order for archaeology to be experienced subjectively and beneficially.

If we accept the omnipresence of the archaeological imagination throughout archaeological practice, future 'therapeutic' projects might be designed in ways that could potentially weight archaeological, emotional, and social outcomes equally; the symbiotic achievement of all three outcomes would be essential in determining such projects' success. In the light of outcomes equally weighted in this manner, I would like to argue for defining such projects as examples of what we might term 'radical archaeology'. Paolo Freire, in 'Pedagogy of the Oppressed' (1972), introduced the concept of radical pedagogy, in which he laid out democratic, person-centred education techniques that deal creatively with reality, and whose fundamental aim was contributing to social change and educating its students in conscientization, defined as 'learning to... take action against the oppressive realm of reality' (Freire 1972: 15). Key tenets of radical pedagogies are dismantling the student-teacher hierarchy, and an emphasis on individuals' understanding and transformation of the world through their interaction with it. This, I would argue, provides a workable parallel to mental health recovery models whose focus is on personal recalibration of understanding the world.

The definition of 'radical' in the *Oxford English Dictionary* is as follows: '(Especially of change or action) relating to or affecting the fundamental nature of something; far-reaching or thorough'. A radical archaeology approach, I would contend, should present truly democratic and inclusive person-centred methods that allow participants to take control of the past for themselves. In so doing, the nature of the traditional practice becomes transformed to suit the needs of more people. In effect, experiencing the past is made less capitalistic by focusing on the individual, the group, and the imaginative process, alongside good and responsible archaeological practice. The concept also leans heavily on the process of Participatory Action Research (Johnston and Marwood 2017; McGhee 2012), a democratic methodology likewise inspired by Freire's radical pedagogy. This aims explicitly for social change through community ownership of research, legitimizing indigenous knowledge, and rearranging the social structure of the knowledge production process (McGhee 2012).

'Therapeutic' projects, including the Human Henge project that this volume celebrates, have employed the creative arts — poetry, prose writing, song, or visual art — as a means of accessibly recording personal emotional responses to the archaeological world they inhabit (see also Beauchamp *et al.* 2014; Lack 2014); whether reflecting on personal experience of the past or reimagining past worlds in the present, all value the emotional encounter and treat individual narrative as valid. Archaeology projects could easily facilitate optimum conditions for the development of archaeological imagination within individual participants. This might be organized through workshops or briefings laying out the importance of the emotional encounter; through guided meditations; shared phenomenological experiences of the site and of finds; opening and closing ceremonies or meetings; discussion groups throughout the project focusing on subjective, imaginative experience; and/or art, writing, or other creative sessions to further explore emotional responses to the past. Furthermore, all participants, archaeologists, and staff should be encouraged equally to reflect creatively on their practice in ways significant to them. Conducting fieldwork that emphasizes and encourages the development of archaeological imagination would be a fascinating and rewarding exercise. What might the outcomes be if individuals were not only allowed but encouraged to relate emotionally to the past? Or if they were given the freedom to explore archaeology experimentally, to see what it could do for them?

Conclusion

When imagination evidently plays such a significant role in the archaeological process, we can no longer sideline it. We need to appreciate that people love archaeology in no small part because of its emotional dimensions. As professionals and practitioners we must therefore promote and facilitate archaeological practices that empower participants of all skill levels, qualifications, and regularity of engagement. The aim should be that all participants experience as much of this creative, imaginative process as possible. We need changes in practice that will allow for, and encourage the development and full experience of, the archaeological imagination. Those new to archaeology are often the most passionate, before professional conditioning and discipline subdue the imaginative impulse. Imagining what the past might have been like is a beautiful exercise; one that should be encouraged and facilitated, not dismissed. No single sector has the monopoly on interacting with the past, and no one body should proscribe how anyone else should or should not feel about it. The past is a common resource and we, as archaeologists, have a moral and social obligation to share our techniques in order to equip people with the tools for potentially helpful, long-term ways of interacting with it.

When individuals use their archaeological imaginations, they are experiencing the world as archaeologists; as active participants, fundamentally connected to the past. As Shanks has said, 'we are all archaeologists now' (2012: 21). The archaeological imagination might allow us to recontextualize our own experiences. It has the potential to help us rewrite our own narratives. It can help us see the world, and situate ourselves in it, in different ways. Bierski suggests that 'illness [emerges] as impairment, or the absence of awareness, and recovery the exercise of it' (2016: 141). By extension, the archaeological imagination may assist in recovering awareness through encouraging attentive being, and therefore contributing to mental well-being. Approached sensitively, the careful and progressive development of the archaeological imagination has the potential to encourage totality, coherence, imagination, and recovery. Dan Mouer (in Praetzellis 1998) states that a colleague once told him, 'we can't just dig sites and tell stories'. I would argue that the telling of stories, whether personal or historical, is the single most significant justification for archaeology's existence.

Acknowledgements

I am grateful to my PhD supervisors Dr Bob Johnston and Professor Brendan Stone of the University of Sheffield. Thanks to R Hearne for careful proofreading and enormously helpful editing. Thanks also to Professor Timothy Darvill and Dr Vanessa Heaslip for running the Archaeology and Well-being session at TAG Cardiff 2017, where the Human Henge project was first discussed, and for inviting my contribution to this monograph.

Bibliography

Atkinson, J. 2009. An evaluation of the Gardening Leave project for ex-military personnel with PTSD and other combat-related mental health problems. Unpublished report for Gardening Leave and the Pears Foundation, Glasgow University.

Barrett, J.C. 1994. *Fragments from antiquity: An archaeology of social life in Britain, 2900-1200 BC*. Hoboken (NJ): Wiley-Blackwell.

Beauchamp, V., R. Hindle and N. Thorpe 2014. '*Digability*': *Inclusive archaeology education project. Evaluation report* [Online document]. London: Workers' Educational Association. Viewed 3 December 2018, <https://digability.files.wordpress.com/2015/01/archie-report-master1.pdf>.

Berger, J. 2008. *Ways of seeing*. London: Penguin Modern Classics.

Bierski, K. 2016. Recovering mental health across outdoor places in Richmond, London: Tuning, skill and narrative. *Health and Place* 40: 137–44.

Carless, D. and A.C. Sparkes 2008. The physical activity experiences of men with serious mental illness: Three short stories. *Psychology of Sport and Exercise* 9: 191–210.

Finn, C. 2004. *Past poetic: Archaeology in the poetry of W.B. Yeats and Seamus Heaney*. London: Duckworth.

Freire, P. 1972. *Pedagogy of the oppressed*. London: Penguin Books.

Harvey, D. 1969. *Explanation in geography*. London: Edward Arnold.

Holtorf, C. 2005. *From Stonehenge to Las Vegas: Archaeology as popular culture*. Lanham (MD): Altamira Press.

Holtorf, C. 2011. The changing contribution of cultural heritage to society, in I. Vinson, C. Holtorf, B.E. Gustafsson and E. Westergren (eds.) *Museum international: The social benefits of heritage*: 8–16. Paris and Hoboken (NJ): UNESCO Publishing and Blackwell Publishing Ltd.

Ingold, T. 2000. *The perception of the environment: Essays on livelihood, dwelling and skill*. London: Routledge.

Jacob, K.S. 2015. Recovery model of mental illness: A complementary approach to psychiatric care. *Indian Journal of Psychological Medicine* 37(2): 117–119.

Johnston, R. and K. Marwood 2017. Action heritage: Research, communities, social justice. *International Journal of Heritage Studies* 23(9): 816–831.

Kiddey, R. 2014. Homeless Heritage: Collaborative social archaeology as therapeutic practice. Unpublished PhD dissertation, University of York.

Lack, K. 2014. *Past in mind: A heritage project and mental health recovery*. Hereford: Privately published.

McEvoy, P., O. Schauman, W. Mansell and I. Morris 2012. The experience of recovery from the perspective of people with common mental health problems: Findings from a telephone survey. *International Journal of Nursing Studies* 49: 1375–1382.

McGhee, F.L. 2012. Participatory action research and archaeology, in R. Skeates, C. McDavid and J. Carman (eds.) *The Oxford handbook of public archaeology*: 213–229. Oxford: Oxford University Press.

McGuire, R.H. 2008. *Archaeology as political action*. Berkeley (CA): University of California Press.

Moshenska, G. 2006. The archaeological uncanny. *Public Archaeology* 5(2): 91–99.

Moshenska, G. and S. Dhanjal 2011. *Community archaeology: Themes, methods and practices*. Oxford: Oxbow Books.

Osgood, R. and P. Andrews 2015. Excavating Barrow Clump: Soldier archaeologists and warrior graves. *Current Archaeology* 306: 28–35.

Paphitis, T. 2013. Review: The archaeological imagination. *Papers from the Institute of Archaeology* 23(1.2): 1–4.

Perry, S. 2018. 'The enchantment of the archaeological record': Paper presented to the European Association of Archaeologists Conference, Barcelona, 5–8 September [Blog]. Viewed 3 December 2018, <https://saraperry.wordpress.com/2018/09/06/enchantment-of-the-archaeological-record/>.

Praetzellis, A. 1998. Introduction: Why every archaeologist should tell stories once in a while. *Historical Archaeology* 32(1): 1–3.

Prince, H.C. 1962. The geographical imagination. *Landscape* 11: 22–25.

Regan, M., I. Elliott and I. Goldie 2016. *Better mental health for all: A public health approach to mental health improvement*. London: Faculty of Public Health and Mental Health Foundation.

Roberts, G. 2000. Narrative and severe mental illness: What place do stories have in an evidence-based world? *Advances in Psychiatric Treatment* 6: 432–441.

Sanders, K. 2009. *Bodies in the bog and the archaeological imagination.* Chicago: University of Chicago Press.

Shakespeare, T. and A. Whieldon 2018. Sing your heart out: Community singing as part of mental health recovery. *Medical Humanities* 44(3): 153–157.

Shanks, M. 1992. *Experiencing the past.* London and New York: Routledge.

Shanks, M. 2012. *The archaeological imagination.* Walnut Creek (CA): Left Coast Press Inc.

Shanks, M. and C. Tilley 1987. *Social theory and archaeology.* Cambridge: Polity.

Shanks, M. and C. Tilley 1992. *Reconstructing archaeology: Theory and practice.* London and New York: Routledge.

Taylor, J. 2013. Giving kids a break: How surfing has helped young people in Cornwall overcome mental health and social difficulties. *Mental Health and Social Inclusion* 17(2): 82–86.

Tilley, C. 1989. Excavation as theatre. *Antiquity* 63: 275–280.

Todres, L. and K. Galvin 2010. 'Dwelling-mobility': An existential theory of well-being. *International Journal of Qualitative Studies for Health and Well-being* 5: 5444–5450.

Wallace, J. 2004. *Digging the dirt: The archaeological imagination.* London: Duckworth.

Wilbur, S., H.B. Meyer, M.R. Baker, K. Smiarowski, C.A. Suarez, D. Ames and R.T. Rubin 2015. Dance for Veterans: A complementary health program. *Arts and Health* 7(2): 96–108.

Chapter 13

Prehistoric landscapes as transitional space

Claire Nolan

Abstract

In recent years museum research has generated a rich and sophisticated body of psychosocial theory to demonstrate how the symbolic capacity of museum objects can support people to achieve meaning, personal insight, and healing. Based on the psychoanalytic concept of 'transitional space' — the meaningful experience that occurs through imaginative engagement with cultural objects — this work offers a framework for understanding the therapeutic potential of the wider historic environment. Accordingly, this paper considers the concept of transitional space in relation to people's lived experience of prehistoric landscapes. Drawing on qualitative research recently undertaken in the prehistoric landscapes of Stonehenge, Avebury, and the Vale of Pewsey in Wiltshire, UK, it looks at how the significance of the age, form, and narratives of these places aid in the production of transitional space, and thus the realization of existential authenticity, personal growth, and healing.

Keywords: Existential authenticity; Historic environment; Prehistoric landscapes; Transitional space; Well-being

Introduction

Although there has been much research in recent years on heritage as a process to well-being, it is still not entirely clear how heritage assets in themselves directly impact well-being (Ecorys 2016; Neal 2015; Reilly *et al.* 2018). This may be due in part to the neglect of site and artefact materiality that Siân Jones (2010) has identified in recent constructivist approaches to the study of heritage experience. However, a notable exception to this rule is the corpus of museum-based research carried out over the past 20 years on the therapeutic power of heritage objects (see Annis 1994; Chatterjee *et al.* 2009; Dudley 2010; Froggett and Trustram 2014; Lanceley *et al.* 2011; Solway *et al.* 2016; Trustram 2013). Particularly illuminating, is the way in which some of this work has conceived of heritage artefacts as transitional objects (Froggett *et al.* 2011; Froggett and Trustram 2014; Lanceley *et al.* 2011; Solway *et al.* 2016; Trustram 2013).

Borrowed from the work of object-relations psychoanalyst Donald Winnicott, the concept of the transitional object has come to be used in museum contexts to denote the way in which heritage objects stimulate transitional or potential space; the 'intermediate area of experience' that occurs in the meeting between self and environment (Winnicott 1971). Based neither entirely in reality nor fantasy, the transitional space, can be understood (Bingley 2003) as a 'daydream-like' state of mind or being. Here, the individual draws on her inner experience to explore and play with the symbolic meanings and potential of external objects, in an imaginative way. Winnicott maintained that this 'creative apperception' of the world could facilitate new conceptions of self and environment. It was thus fundamental to the formation of self-identity and the foundation of a creative and meaningful life. Viewing culture as an inherited tradition — 'something that is in the common pool of humanity' that can be creatively re-imagined and interpreted by the individual — Winnicott proposed that cultural experience was transitional in nature, and that all cultural forms could be used as transitional objects (Winnicott 1971: 99).

Elucidating the transitional effects of cultural experience, Tania Zittoun (2013) explains that in their ability to capture the imagination, cultural objects and their symbolic meanings facilitate an immersive experience. She maintains that, in turn, this engagement encourages relaxation, respite from everyday life and offers people the freedom to live creatively. As a result, Zittoun suggests that the insights and affective qualities reflected in these meanings, enable individuals to contemplate and gain perspective on their own personal situations and potential. In this sense, transitional experience might be likened to the realization of existential authenticity; the freedom to be and express oneself, to see life from different perspectives, and to recognize one's unique existential possibilities (Steiner and Reisinger 2006; Yi *et al.* 2017). Zittoun (2013) asserts that, in their capacity to produce such effects, cultural objects assume the role of symbolic resources that can be drawn upon for the promotion of emotional well-being.

Employing object-relations theory to assess the therapeutic value of heritage objects, museum studies have shown that heritage objects too have the capacity to act as symbolic resources. This impact has been observed particularly in the way that the symbolic meanings of heritage objects help people to mediate personal issues and the effects of existential challenges, such as loss and terminal illness (Lanceley *et al.* 2011; Trustram 2013). Related effects encompass a sense of cultural inclusion or belonging to the wider cultural and collective frame of human existence that the artefacts represent (Froggett *et al.* 2011). In addition, Lynn Froggett and Myna Trustram suggest that, as heterotopic repositories of symbolic objects, museum galleries themselves act as transitional spaces for '…creative playing, symbolization and the management of transitions', and thus offer possibilities for 'authentic self-expression' (Froggett and Trustram 2014: 492).

In terms of its application to heritage, the concept of transitional space has hitherto been limited to museum-based studies. However, it arguably provides a valid artefact-oriented approach to understanding the social and well-being value of heritage assets in the wider historic environment. This is particularly pertinent to prehistoric archaeology, the public perception of which generally tends to be less well-understood (Last 2010; Waterton and Watson 2014). This paper reviews findings from qualitative research undertaken in Wiltshire to provide site-specific evidence of the ways in which individuals directly experience and interpret prehistoric heritage assets. Based on these results, the paper explores the validity of the transitional phenomena concept for prehistoric landscapes. It goes on to propose that these landscapes act as transitional places in their power to distance people from their everyday routines, engage their imaginations, and promote personal reflection, meaning, and insight. In conclusion, the prehistoric heritage landscapes discussed are posited as key symbolic resources for the realization of existential authenticity.

The empirical context

Situated in a mixture of chalk downland and greensand valleys, the Stonehenge and Avebury World Heritage Site (WHS), the Vale of Pewsey (Figure 13.1), and their surrounding landscapes in northern Wiltshire, are home to a dense concentration of prehistoric sites and monuments. Diverse in form and preservation, these antiquities span in age from the eighth millennium to the first century BC. Stonehenge and the Neolithic henges at Avebury, and Marden form the main focal points of the area. However, it also takes in a range of other lesser known sites and features, ranging from the Mesolithic through to the Neolithic, Bronze Age, and Iron Age, offering particularly rich potential for investigating public perceptions of prehistoric heritage.

The research discussed here comprised a series of semi-structured seated and walking interviews with residents of the study area. It also included three separate mindful heritage walks and corresponding group interviews in the Avebury landscape (Figure 13.2), with two groups of students from the University of Reading and a local community group. Participants were recruited via a mixture of snowball, convenience, purposive, and volunteer sampling. Between individual interviewees and

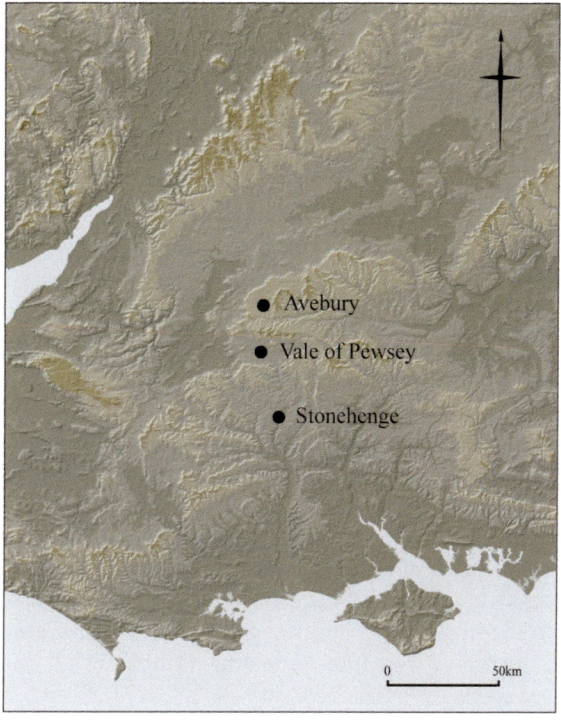

Figure 13.1 Location map of the study area. (Illustration by Elaine Jamieson. Contains Ordnance Survey data, Crown copyright, and database right 2015)

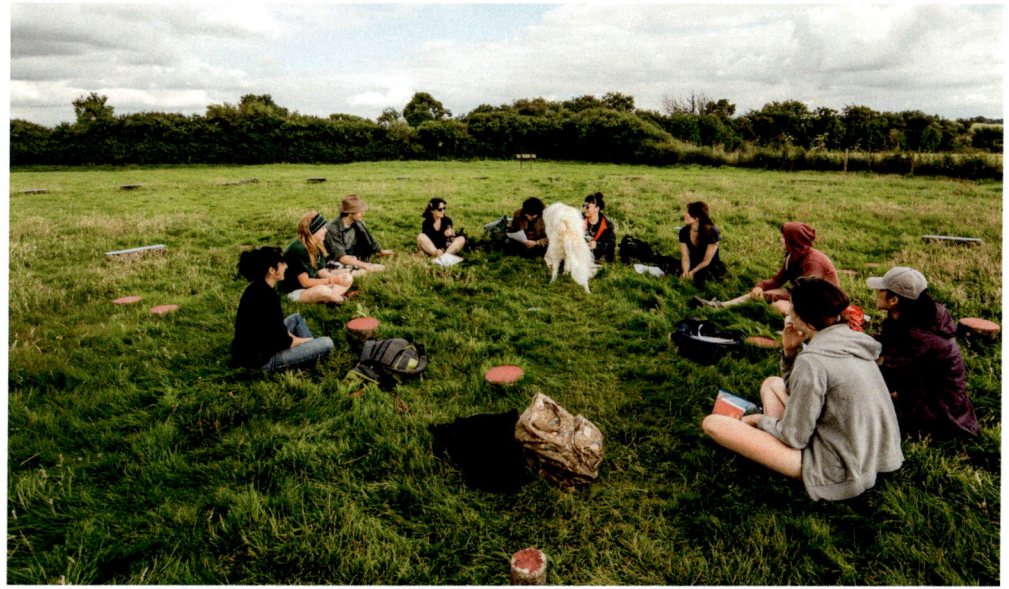

Figure 13.2 Research participants at the Sanctuary, near Avebury, Wiltshire. (University of Reading, used with permission)

groups, the study involved a total of 66 participants, 18 of whom were visitors to the area. The participant sample ranged from 19 to 87 years of age, with just under half aged 60 and over, and a quarter falling in the range of 18-29. In relation to gender, 38 participants identified as female and 28 as male. Five participants identified as American, Taiwanese, Turkish, South African, and European, with the rest of the sample native to the British Isles.

Alongside the interviews and group walks, participants were invited to create a reflective written or photographic account representing their personal experience and perceptions of the archaeology. All of the methods employed in the study were informed by phenomenological theory and practice drawn from mindfulness-based cognitive therapy (Williams *et al.* 2007), focusing-oriented psychotherapy (Gendlin 2003), landscape phenomenology (Tilley 1994), non-representational theory (Latham 2003; Lorimer 2005), and reflective lifeworld research (Dahlberg *et al.* 2011). This approach was chosen for its capacity to help participants reflect more deeply on their direct lived intellectual, emotional, and embodied experience of the archaeology.

Results

Participants discussed their experiences of the different sites and monuments within the landscape, both standing and excavated, as well as their responses to portable artefacts found in the area. They reported a range of positive effects, some of which could be described as transitional in nature. Following a thematic analysis of the feedback, these experiences were grouped under the category of 'existential authenticity', the sub-themes of which will be discussed in the sections below.

Imaginative playspaces

In his thesis on *Being and Time,* Martin Heidegger proposed that the level of conformity demanded by the mechanisms of daily life, prevents individuals from fully being themselves (Steiner and Reisinger 2006). He subsequently maintained that exclusive adherence to collective mores culminates in a failure to embrace one's unique existential possibilities, thus resulting in a loss of individuality (Steiner and Reisinger 2006). In their work on the role of heritage tourism in the promotion of existential authenticity, Xiaoli Yi and colleagues (2017) purport that heritage sites, in their capacity as heterotopic and culturally meaningful spaces, give visitors momentary freedom from conformity. Furthermore, they assert that this freedom ultimately enables people to rediscover their individuality, and to contemplate and interpret the world unselfconsciously in their own style. Comparable to the process which underpins transitional space, this description of existential authenticity resonates with Annette Kuhn's portrayal of cultural engagement as a kind of 'playspace' for the imagination that can be 'entered and left' (Kuhn 2013). Project participants frequently alluded to this type of in-depth imaginative engagement in relation to their experience of the prehistoric archaeology contained within the study area. As such, this feedback demonstrates how engaging with the symbolic meanings of prehistoric remains can create a transitional space where people can freely connect with, and express, their imagination and creativity.

The following quote, which describes a participant's day-to-day interaction with the site of Marden Henge in the Vale of Pewsey, provides a perfect example of how prehistoric archaeology and its obscure narratives creates a playspace for the imagination:

'And then if you start looking, your imagination starts going, especially out there [Marden Henge], like I said...thinking, now, I could be seeing people, I could be seeing this huge mound. Voices - I could be hearing voices, different dialects, probably, you know. And you're just making up this picture...of people, children, maybe it's a happy time there? A meeting place, a gathering place, like our families' barbacues in the summer, but just something different. But it doesn't seem to be a bad place there to me - if all this is going on, you know, this imagining that I am...' (Personal interview, resident, 60)

Another participant revealed how drawing on her individual creativity in this way to build a meaningful picture of past prehistoric landscape of Stonehenge, gives her respite from daily life:

'I think there's an element of, um, I think these days they kind of call it mindfulness, I guess? Where you just walk across, and you can see weird lumps and bumps, and you think, 'what's that? How's that work?'. And then you start scanning the rest of the landscape - you're trying to work it out in your head, what went where and trying to visualize stuff... so, I think when I go up and stand on the edge of the cursus, I play it out in my head again, and I look at the map, and I try and work it out all the time, and that takes your mind off of whatever else is going on.' (Personal interview, resident, 41)

Kuhn points out that certain types of cultural activities, such as viewing a film, can be so deeply immersive that the individual feels as though she is 'inhabiting' the 'spatio-temporal world' of the cultural object or medium (Kuhn 2013). This sensation was reported by a number of participants in terms of a sense of inhabiting the past. This phenomenon is exemplified by the following interview dialogue concerning one participant's experience of a mindful walk from Avebury Henge, along the stone rows of the West Kennet Avenue, to the Sanctuary, the site of a former Neolithic timber and stone circle:

Interviewer (I): And what did you think of the Sanctuary where we ended up?
Participant (P): Lovely. Walking up the hill to get to the Sanctuary, it was almost like a real sense of connecting with people who would have done that in the past. I really did actually feel that as I was going up.
I: Really?
P: Yeah. Much more open, yes, I could actually feel, sort of, a sense of belonging to the past rather than present.
I: Right, so you kind of went back, almost?
P: Yeah.
I: And how did that feel, what was that like?
P: It was actually really peaceful, sort of comforting feeling, to feel that I was actually part of that, and belonged to it. (Group interview, resident, 60)

Another participant reported a similar sensation of stepping back in time at the Iron Age enclosure at Martinsell (Figure 13.3), Vale of Pewsey:

'...coming up here and sort of connecting with this, you suddenly put three, four thousand years between yourself and those immediate worries in the present. And for me that's almost as good as travelling three or four thousand miles.' (Personal interview, resident, 57)

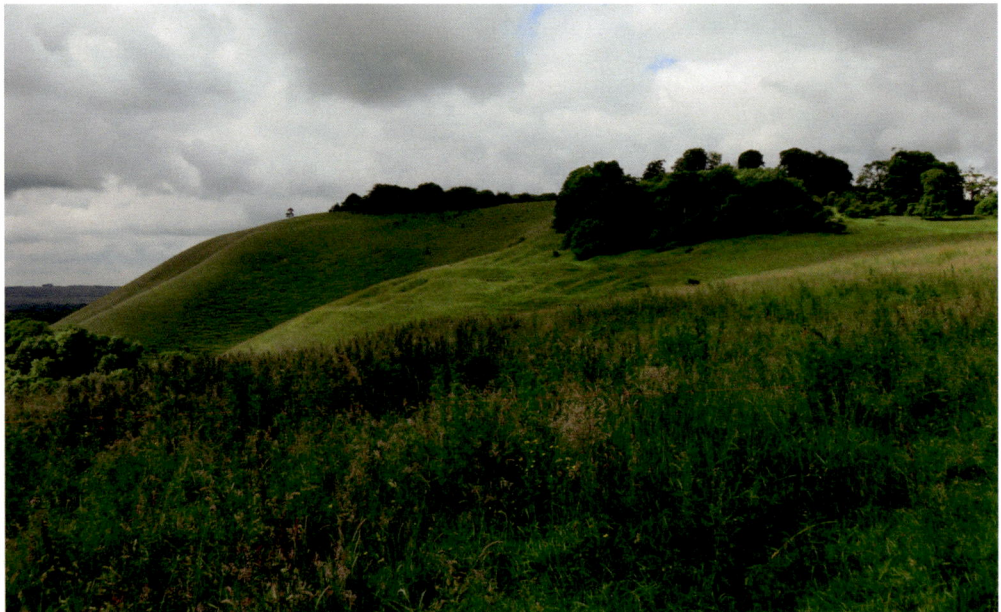

Figure 13.3 Martinsell Iron Age enclosure, Wiltshire. (University of Reading, used with permission)

These experiences indicate that the strong presence of the past evoked by certain sites, and the related images they conjure up, make these places seem to some like another world where they can go to escape everyday life. It could thus be said that engaging with prehistoric archaeology engages the imagination, allowing respite and space from everyday worries to live creatively.

Everyday creativity

Whilst imaginative engagement with the past may provide a source of respite, it is, as Phyllis Crème affirms in the case of the immersive power of film, '...more than "escapism"; it is life enhancing' (Crème 2013: 49). However, it is not just life-enhancing in the way that it prompts people to draw on their own creative capacity to imagine and connect with their environment. People also experience a sense of fulfilment and vitality when attempting to interpret the meaning of certain prehistoric sites, and solve the puzzle and mysteries they present.

Matthew Hills views this interpretative dynamic as a form of 'everyday creativity' where the individual is in a 'state of creative readiness'; playing with possible explanations in the hope of 'making new discoveries' and meanings (Hills 2013: 117). As one participant put it:

'...you look at all the theories on Stonehenge, of calculators, and moon things, and sun things. And now they say, 'no actually, it wasn't the summer solstice, it was the winter solstice'... And you think it's almost one of those open pallets that you can sort of colour with your own sort of [trails off], and then you can find all these things that can then justify what you think or make you rethink what you think.' (Personal interview, resident, 52)

Speaking of the prehistoric sites across the study area, a participant from the Vale of Pewsey revealed the sense of enlivenment this engagement affords:

'...when you're going back...thousands of years as opposed to a few hundred, that's mind blowing isn't it...and your brain can't work it out, but it doesn't stop it being fascinating and get the emotions going...' (Personal interview, resident, 70)

Another participant illustrated, in relation to the Avebury landscape, how this process gives him a sense of creative fulfilment:

'...it's about getting the information and then, kind of putting your own interpretations on it, and that kind of process, and then what you think it would be like...makes it more, enjoyable in a way...you actually are getting the information and then kind of using it for your own personal gain...' (Personal interview, resident, 20)

Essentially an exploration of cultural symbols and different world views, this type of imaginative engagement with prehistoric archaeology could be seen as a good example of how people draw on, rework and create their own meanings and enjoyment from the inherited tradition of the archaeological resource.

New horizons

The participant feedback indicated that the archaeology in the study area is also life-enhancing in the way that it continually enriches and renews people's experience of their everyday world. It opens up new dimensions to the landscape, both in the imagination and in the context of newly discovered sites and artefacts. This effect allows fresh conceptions of, and meaningful connections to, place, thereby presenting new possibilities for the individual.

Referring to the Iron Age/Romano-British enclosure and field systems on Parsonage Down, Salisbury Plain, a participant from the Stonehenge area described how encountering archaeology hitherto unknown to him has enabled him to appreciate the temporal dimensions of his environment. He discussed how this awareness has allowed him to see, experience, and relate to the landscape in a new light:

'...it's great, you know, when you go out there, like I said, when I went to the reserve – I've lived here for twenty-five years – and I found that little area, where those, the Celtic sort of field boundaries, village boundaries, and I'd never seen that before...And finding those stones, and thinking, you know, this might have formed part of the village...And that definitely enhances that sort of, you know, that sense of enjoyment out there...' (Personal interview, resident, 60)

This enjoyment is perhaps partly connected to the way in which — as one participant discovered at the henge enclosure at Durrington Walls, Salisbury Plain — the sense of past inhabitants helps to narrate the landscape and 'bring it all alive' (Personal interview, resident, 70).

Furthermore, this imaginative connection to past people adds another layer of significance to the landscape, thus creating new meaning in the life of the individual. Recounting his experience of finding a flint arrowhead while out walking in his local area, a participant from the Vale of Pewsey described the impact that such connections hold for him:

'...I picked an arrowhead up...And that whole anticipation and excitement, and when you held it in your hand, there was this thought that the last person that potentially touched that, was five thousand years ago. And just that thought alone was just so, so privileged, but uplifting, exciting.' (Personal interview, resident, 61)

The participant affirmed that the encounter, '...just really opened up the doorway to the area where I live, and that my dog walks can be quite meaningful, you see?'. He emphasized that, as a result, this connection to the past has given him '...a hobby with an in-depth meaning', as well as a new sense of self and purpose:

> 'And when something does that to you, you can't ignore, you don't ignore it...it opens up a door, and it opens up the avenue...but it's an avenue that you, you just feel compelled. You feel compelled that you want to pursue that, there's some, you know, it draws you - don't know why. Instinctive, that's why I said about instinctive - that's how I can explain the instinctive, and that's what I sort of get from it.'

Similarly, a lady from the Vale of Pewsey explained how, for herself and her husband, finding a flint axe has not only enriched their lives by imbuing their surroundings with meaning, but also by inspiring them to think about the wider world in different ways:

> '...you see beyond just what you can see... And I think that, for us, has enhanced our lives, because you get a better understanding, and you question - you wonder about things, which you wouldn't normally do because of you have this awareness that we've now developed, you know.' (Personal interview, resident, 70)

Kuhn describes the transitional space as '...a place from which objects appear' and thus one that broadens the individual's horizons (Kuhn 2013: 2). With regard to the experiences referred to above, this reading is reminiscent of the way in which awareness of the past dimensions of landscape can impact people. New objects or dimensions of place appear and in so doing, change or add to one's reality. They consequently mediate one's relationship to the environment and provide a new experience of the world, creating meaning and purpose in the process.

Liminal spaces

While the symbolic meanings of the sites discussed mark them out as transitional objects, their aesthetic agency and the affective states that this evokes for people, also contributes to this conception. Whether this comes as a result of feeling enclosed in a henge or being moved through the landscape in a linear fashion by ceremonial avenues, certain monuments cultivate a liminal atmosphere. This effect also creates the feeling of being in a heterotopic space where transitional experience and the possibility for transformation can occur.

This sensation of stepping into numinous space is well-described by a participant who, referring to Stonehenge, maintains that 'Being inside the henge is magical, almost like stepping inside a building, everything outside becomes insignificant' (Personal interview, resident, 45). Similarly, another participant reported that she and her husband view Avebury henge as an 'early cathedral' and that, 'Our sense of the circle is one of well-being' (Reflective account, resident, 64).

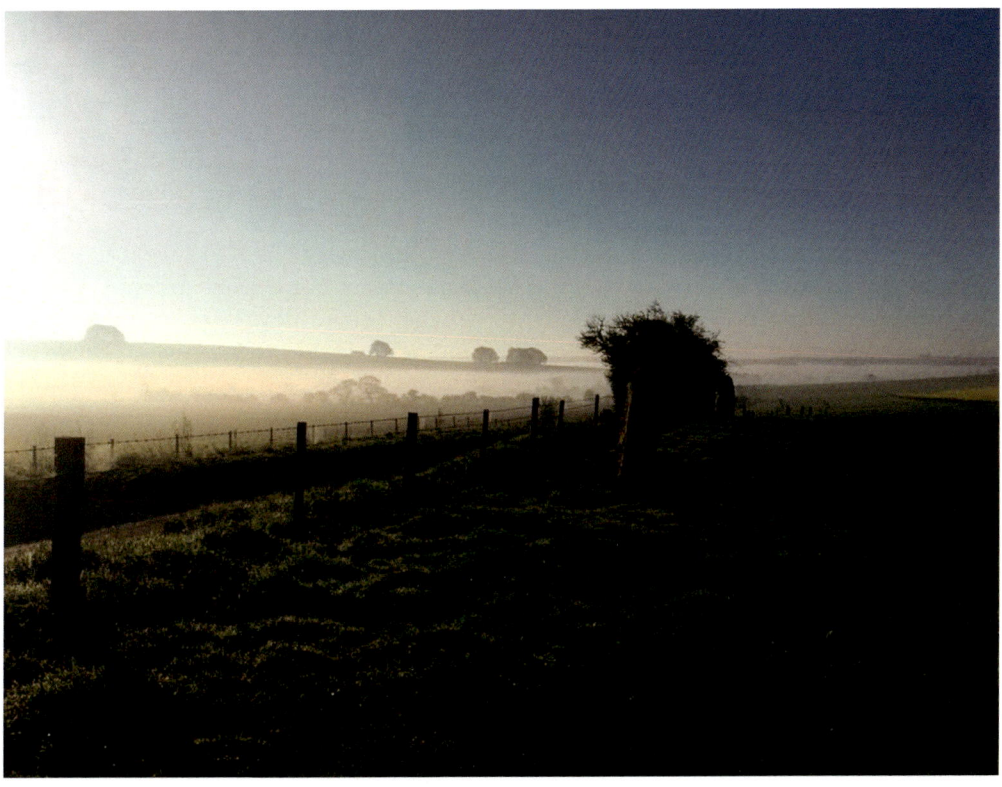

Figure 13.4 West Kennet Avenue, Avebury, Wiltshire. (University of Reading, used with permission)

The transitional nature of certain sites was also identified in relation to more linear features, as highlighted in the group interview extract below regarding a mindful walk along the West Kennet Avenue (Figure 13.4):

> Participant (P) 6: When we were going through those stones, the kind of long ones, rather than the circle, that felt like rather a different movement, if that makes sense?
> Interviewer (I): Right, yeah.
> P5: Yeah.
> P6: In the circle, it just felt like we were wandering, but that felt more -
> P2: Directional -
> P6: - like we were going somewhere.
> I: Yeah.
> P5: Yeah, 'you need to go this way - carry on'.
> P2: It's nice to have a mission. It makes you feel like you have a purpose. So you're just walking with purpose — it's nicer than just like aimlessly wandering round.
> P1: That's quite true, yeah.
> (Group interview, visitors, 22-30)

Likewise, another group member commented that, '…there's like a heightenedness as you walk through those stones' (Group interview, visitor, 23). Some participants reported that they experience a similar effect when walking through certain prehistoric landscapes in the area, likening it to a feeling of pilgrimage. As one student described his experience of walking from Avebury Henge to the Sanctuary:

> 'It's almost like guidance, essentially. Like a pilgrimage sort of like. It's like the "passing of man" or something. You know, that sort of, you're becoming something different or greater within your identity...' (Group interview, visitor, 21).

Akin to the idea of the museum as potential space, it appears that in some instances the sites themselves are experienced as transitional spaces that can be physically entered into and interacted with in ways that facilitate new understandings and expressions of self, creativity, and purpose. Thus, in essence, this experience supports Yi and colleagues' thesis that, '...architectural heritage helps tourists to develop the authentic-self and become more authentic, to escape their monotonous quotidian routines, and to pursue self-realization' (Yi *et al.* 2017: 1042).

Contemplation and resolution

It is perhaps a sense of liminality, combined with the imaginative process stimulated by the archaeology that gives people the license and space to think creatively. These influences enable individuals to reflect not only on the past and their surroundings, but also on personal issues. As Anthony Giddens clarifies in his work on existential authenticity, 'Creativity... means the capability to act or think innovatively in relation to pre-established modes of activity...' (Giddens 1991: 41). In the context of cultural experience, this manifests, as Zittoun (2013) points out, in the way the symbolic meanings of cultural objects enable people to gain perspective on their lives. This dynamic was reported by several participants, who described how they experience certain sites as places for contemplation and restoration.

Describing the feeling of support she gains from spending time in the Avebury landscape, one participant related, 'I find when I need to think or to clear my head, or just gain clarity about something troubling me, I go and sit by the stones...and I just feel it helps me somehow' (Personal interview, resident, 49). She revealed that when going through a particularly difficult period in her life, '...it was by walking around the stones at Avebury...that I came up with the answer one day...it simply was, just to be myself'.

Another participant from the Avebury area, who has lived with severe depression for over 40 years, has found that spending time in Avebury Henge has eased her symptoms. Attributing this effect to the spiritual energies she intuits within the henge, and the connection to natural cycles and ancestral foundations that it symbolizes for her, she asserted:

> 'It's sorted out my inner being. It doesn't get rid of all the stress, and I still live like everybody else does, with stress all around me. It makes me able to cope with it'. (Personal interview, resident, 62)

For others it is the age of the site that facilitates this contemplative process, as one lady expressed with reference to the Avebury landscape:

> '...just to be there [Avebury], and just to sort of, I suppose, get away from the problems that are here...I'll think through things, sometimes I get ideas, sometimes I don't, but it's still

good to do that…so, it seems that a lot of these old places pull me back, and I don't know why, but I want to go there, um, it feels good there, and I feel nourished there, which I don't always other places'. (Personal interview, resident, 52)

Similarly, a participant from the Vale of Pewsey reported that he derives 'a sense of sanctuary' from the symbolism of security mirrored in the age and scale of prehistoric sites in particular:

'At several points in my life…I have used prehistoric monuments as places of contemplation and reflection. On the first anniversary of the death of my mother, I went to Oldbury Castle [Iron Age fort a few miles west of Avebury] to be there and think of her at the exact time of her death. Months earlier, I had scattered some of her ashes on Martinsell. During the break up of my first marriage, I sheltered myself amongst the earthworks of Martinsell for several hours. And on numerous other occasions when wanting peace, I have found myself on one of the prehistoric monuments overlooking the Vale of Pewsey'. (Reflective account, resident, 57)

Zittoun (2013) argues that personal growth involves the use of cultural objects, in terms of their properties and narratives, as 'stand-ins' for specific relationships that are fundamental to the individual's sense of self, but which may be either absent or denied. In this connection, the above account also underscores how, for many people, certain monuments possess nurturing, stabilizing qualities, which establish them as suitable stand-ins for lost loved ones. As such, they help to mediate feelings of grief and allow what Trustram (2013) refers to as 'inner restorations'. This dynamic is visible in the case of another participant, who disclosed, '…when I come to Avebury, I remember my brother at a particular stone, and I stand with my back to

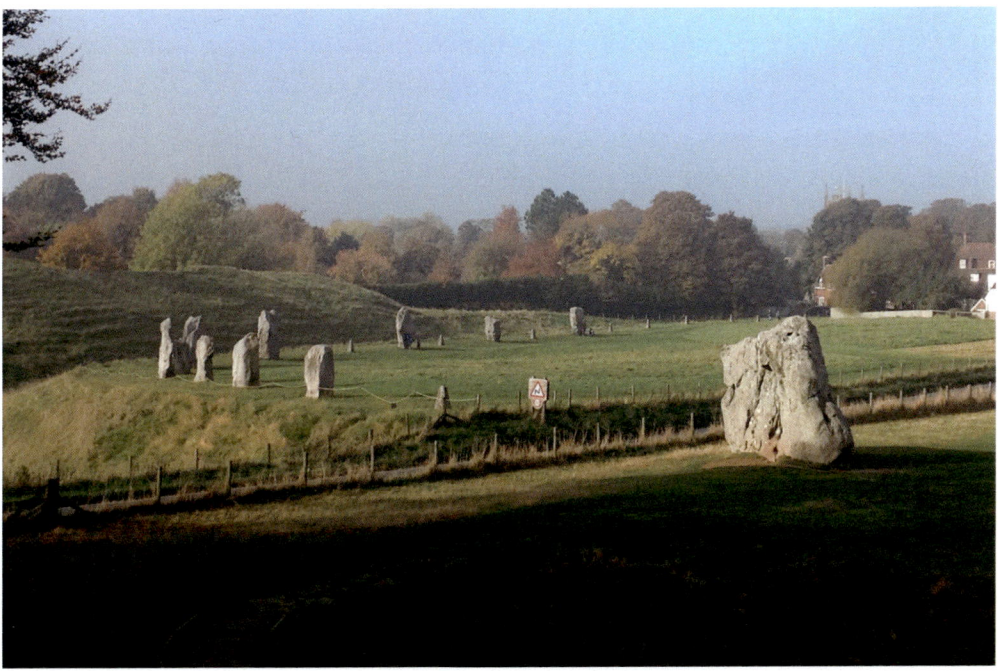

Figure 13.5 Avebury stone circle, Wiltshire. (Photograph by Claire Nolan. Copyright reserved)

the stone, and I think about him...' (Personal interview, resident, 70). He clarified that, 'that engagement is about...feeling in touch in my life', and that, '...I'd be lost without it, I think, that contact'.

Taking this feedback into account, it appears that the different qualities and symbolism of particular sites nurture and resonate in such a way that they enable people to contemplate and transform their perspectives on troubling issues and life events. As a result, this process helps people to regain balance within themselves.

Existential understanding

Many of the examples above illustrate the manner in which the symbolic meanings and agency of particular sites help people to experience and see themselves and the world differently. This form of creative living is a new mode of being, in and of itself. However, these meanings also afford fundamental existential perceptions which create additional possibilities for transformation and living more authentically. This is particularly noticeable in the way that certain meanings which people derive from the archaeology, allow them to gain insights into issues of meaninglessness, mortality, and anxiety. For some participants, this awareness gives them a sense of reassurance and hope.

Disillusioned with particular aspects of modern living, one participant described how he gains an appreciation for the simpler things in life, and thus greater meaning, through contemplating the subsistence narratives that Martinsell evokes for him:

'...you know, the person who dug this ditch, you know, what would a Barclaycard have meant to them, or, 5.4 per cent mortgage, you know? It just sort of puts things in perspective, that they were largely surviving. You know they weren't encumbered by all that slightly ephemeral stuff that we fill our lives with today'. (Personal interview, resident, 57)

Similarly enlightened by the potential narratives of the Avebury landscape, a participant currently writing a fictional piece on West Kennet Long Barrow, noted that:

'...I've had to think about things in all sorts of weird areas. And yeah, I think that, okay, if I just write a story set in the present day, I've had to think about humans and how they interact. If you write a Neolithic story, you've got to suddenly think about, not just that, you've got to think about so much more. So, it's really expanding my mind, and helping to make sense of things rather more.' (Personal interview, resident, 67)

Highlighting the importance of this increased perspective, he added, 'It's shaking us out of a complacent, Western view of the way things are and should be, this mind expanding'. Correspondingly, following a mindful walk in the Avebury landscape, one of the student participants reflected on how the monuments had prompted her to think differently about British attitudes to death:

'...you don't know if they had maybe a more healthier attitude to death. I don't think at the moment we've got a particularly great [trails off]...But then again, I don't think we like to talk about it, because I think we're scared of it. When, if you look at how they treated it centuries back, they were a lot more accepting.' (Group interview, visitor, 22)

In response, another group member remarked that she gained a sense of 'acceptance' of death through '...talking about mortality and landscape...'. (Group interview, visitor, 21). Participants frequently referred to the theme of mortality, particularly in relation to the way in which an appreciation of the age and continuity of the monuments gives them perspective on their place in time and life. This impact was noted by a lady from the Avebury area who observed that when she first moved to the area:

> '...what I found like walking round the circle, going down the Avenue, is it made me aware of the time of life, the passing time, especially when you see the stones and also, consciousness about death.' (Personal interview, resident, 60)

Evoking the Heideggerian notion that, '...human beings cannot authentically confront their concrete moments of existential choice until they grasp the full complexity or depth of their finitude' (Mulhall 2001: 138), she added, 'It's a reminder that, you know, you are only here for a short time...it's a reality check in some ways'. This awareness of choice was also emphasized in the following account given by a participant from the Vale of Pewsey, regarding his relationship to the age and permanence of the monuments in his local area:

> '...I don't tend to sort of like get really sort of frustrated or angry about things or really sort of like anxious about things because I tend to find myself just reflecting back to, 'well, we're just part of this long continuum of life in whatever form it is...' (Personal interview, resident, 54)

Illustrating the sense of well-being this outlook provides, he related, 'I sort of tend to find, I sort of look back to that perspective, just to balance things, you know, whether you get sort of het up or worried about things or angry about stuff, you sort of think, well it's pretty small in the scheme of things'. Gaining a similar sense of perspective through learning more about Stonehenge and the ingenuity of its design, a resident of the Vale of Pewsey conveyed:

> '...I find it reassuring in that it makes you think that for thousands of years we've, you know, found a way to at least come to terms with the problems. And, as I say, it's not as if the crises facing the world now, that we're the first ever intelligent generation, and you know, we can look back at history and see how people survived.' (Personal interview, resident, 54)

Furthermore, another participant from the Vale of Pewsey, inspired by the skill and competence visible in the construction of Stonehenge and other notable historic monuments, commented on how they fill him with a sense of possibility:

> '...if, as a civilization, we lost a whole lot of things - Stonehenge, Chartres Cathedral is another, Durham Cathedral is another ...that I personally think would be very sad, because ...they are examples of human ingenuity, industry, and in some cases religious significance, and...they are such amazing examples of what humankind can achieve...' (Personal interview, resident, 70)

Giddens maintains that the structures of late modernity are ill-equipped to help people answer and negotiate certain fundamental existential questions and challenges, thus making existential authenticity and security difficult to achieve (Giddens 1991). However, the above examples show how prehistoric archaeology can help people to gain perspective on, and solutions to, such matters. Perhaps in this sense it might be seen as a legitimate resource for mediating difficult life events and issues. As one participant suggested in the case of Stonehenge, 'Perhaps the purpose of the monument is to make us think and test us?' (Reflective account, resident, 52). This echoes David Lowenthal's (2015) conception of the past as a source of guidance. It also corresponds with Winnicott's (1971) understanding of culture as an inherited tradition, where the past is a source of possibility that can be drawn upon and reworked in innovative and individual ways.

Conclusion

The feedback here presented demonstrates, in the context of Stonehenge, Avebury, and the Vale of Pewsey, how engaging with the historic environment can provide transitional experiences conducive to the achievement of existential authenticity, possibility, and healing. In this sense, conceivably, this work serves to affirm or add another dimension to Lowenthal's claim that, '…the past is a route to self-realization; through it we become more ourselves; *better* selves, reinvigorated by our appreciation of it.' (Lowenthal 2015: 94). The research suggests that the transitional effects described are afforded variously by the embodied, affective, and sensory impact of the physical remains themselves, their temporal significance, and apparent narratives. However, in terms of the latter impact, whilst the themes discussed hold value for the wider historic environment, and can be applied to other periods, the relative incomprehensibility of the narratives conveyed by prehistoric archaeology arguably allows a particularly potent playspace for connecting with one's thoughts and imagination. As one participant put it:

> '…there are generally too many distractions in a church, temple or cathedral…Prehistoric sites, on the other hand, generally are not adorned with reminders of specific individuals or precise moments in time… Also, there is no demand for you to adhere to certain religious beliefs, or reminders of what awaits you if you do not, at least certainly not easily interpreted ones.' (Reflective account, resident, 57)

Moreover, it is possible that the age of the prehistoric remains, and the types of narratives associated with them, have the capacity to prompt existential thought in ways that perhaps the narratives of more recent heritage may not. Whilst the concept of transitional space is only one of many ways to assess the therapeutic impact of the historic environment, it does provide a theoretical framework and language useful for thinking about, and analysing, how and why individuals experience heritage assets therapeutically. Hence, this paper suggests that this framework can help to understand, and perhaps pinpoint and develop, some of the unique therapeutic impacts that the historic environment has to offer in respect of existential well-being.

Acknowledgements

Very special and heart-felt thanks to all the participants who contributed to the study and made it possible. I would also like to thank Jim Leary, Martin Bell, Joanna Brück, Rhianedd Smith, Hilary Geoghegan, Ruth Evans, Avril Maddrell, and Mwenza Blell for their support and guidance.

Bibliography

Annis, S. 1994. The Museum as a staging ground for symbolic action, in G. Kavanagh (ed.) *Museum provision and professionalism*: 21–25. London: Routledge.

Bingley, A. 2003. In there and out there: Sensations between self and landscape. *Social and Cultural Geography* 4(3): 329–345.

Chatterjee, H., S. Vreeland and G. Noble 2009. Museopathy: Exploring the healing potential of handling museum objects. *Museum and Society* 7(3): 164–177.

Crème, P. 2013. The playing spectator, in A. Kuhn (ed.) *Little Madnesses: Winnicott, transitional phenomena and cultural experience*: 39–51. London: I.B. Taurus.

Dahlberg, K., H. Dahlberg, and M. Nystrom 2011. *Reflective lifeworld research*. Sweden: Studentlitteratur.

Dudley, S.H. 2010. Museum materialities: Objects, sense and feeling, in S.H. Dudley (ed.) *Museum materialities: Objects, engagements, interpretations*: 1–17. London and New York: Routledge.

Ecorys UK 2016. Come as you are: Leave better. Scoping report for the evaluation of Quay Place. Unpublished report.

Froggett, L., A. Farrier and K. Poursanidou 2011. *Who cares? Museums, health and wellbeing research Project: A study of the Renaissance North West Programme*. Lancaster: MLA North West and Renaissance North West.

Froggett, L. and M. Trustram 2014. Object relations in the museum: A psychosocial perspective. *Museum Management and Curatorship* 29(5): 482–497.

Gendlin, E. 2003. *Focusing: How to gain direct access to your body's knowledge*. London: Rider Books.

Giddens, A. 1991. *Modernity and self-identity: Self and society in the late modern age*. Cambridge: Polity Press.

Hills, M. 2013. Recoded transitional objects and fan re-readings of puzzle films, in A. Kuhn (ed.) *Little Madnesses: Winnicott, transitional phenomena and cultural experience*: 103–119. London: I.B. Taurus.

Jones, S. 2010. Negotiating authentic objects and authentic selves: Beyond the deconstruction of authenticity. *Journal of Material Culture* 15(2): 181–203.

Kuhn, A. (ed.) 2013. *Little Madnesses: Winnicott, transitional phenomena and cultural experience*. London: I.B. Taurus.

Last, J. 2010. *English Heritage thematic research strategies: Research strategy for prehistory: Consultation draft* [Online document]. Swindon: English Heritage. Viewed 24 October 2018, <https://historicengland.org.uk/content/docs/research/draft-prehistoric-strategy-pdf/>.

Latham, A. 2003. Research, performance, and doing human geography: Some reflections on the diary-photograph, diary-interview method. *Environment and Planning A*35: 1993–2017.

Lorimer, H. 2005. Cultural geography: The busyness of being 'more-than-representational'. *Progress in Human Geography* 29(1): 83–94.

Lowenthal, D. 2015. *The past is a foreign country — revisited*. New York: Cambridge University Press.

Mulhall, S. 2001. *Heidegger and being and time*. London and New York: Routledge.

Neal, C. 2015. Know your place? Evaluating the therapeutic benefits of engagement with historic landscapes. *Cultural Trends* 24(2): 133–142.

Reilly, S., C. Nolan and I. Monckton, 2018. *Wellbeing and the historic environment. Historic England report* [Online document]. London: Historic England. Viewed 18 October 2018, <https://historicengland.org.uk/images-books/publications/wellbeing-and-the-historic-environment/wellbeing-and-historic-environment/>.

Solway, R., P. Camic, L. Thomson and H. Chatterjee 2016. Material objects and psychological theory: A conceptual literature review. *Arts and Health: An International Journal for Research, Policy and Practice* 7(3): 1–21.

Steiner, C.J. and Y. Reisinger 2006. Understanding existential authenticity. *Annals of Tourism Research* 33(2): 299–318.

Tilley, C. 1994. *A phenomenology of landscape*. Oxford: Berg.

Trustram, M. 2013. 'The little madnesses of museums', in A. Kuhn (ed.) *Little madnesses: Winnicott, transitional phenomena and cultural experience*: 187–200. London: I.B. Taurus.

Waterton, E. and S. Watson 2014. *The semiotics of heritage tourism*. Bristol: Channel View Publications.

Williams, M., J. Teasdale, Z. Segal and J. Kabat-Zinn 2007. *The mindful way through depression: Freeing yourself from chronic unhappiness*. New York and London: The Guilford Press.

Winnicott, D.W. 1971. *Playing and reality*. London and New York: Routledge.

Yates, C. and S. Day Sclater 2000. Culture, psychology and transitional space, in C. Squire (ed.) *Culture in psychology*: 133–134. Philadelphia: Routledge.

Yi, X., V.S. Lin, W. Jin and Q. Luo 2017. The authenticity of heritage sites, tourists' quest for existential authenticity, and destination loyalty. *Journal of Travel Research* 56(8): 1032–1048.

Zittoun, T. 2013. On the use of film: Cultural experiences as symbolic resources, in A. Kuhn (ed.) *Little madnesses: Winnicott, transitional phenomena and cultural experience*: 135–147. London: I.B. Taurus.

Chapter 14

Messing about on the river: Volunteering and well-being on the Thames foreshore

Helen Johnston

Abstract

Is volunteering in archaeology good for you? What impact does volunteering on the Thames foreshore have on people's reported well-being? The Thames Discovery Programme (TDP) has been running for ten years, and has trained over 700 volunteers as Foreshore Recording and Observation Group (FROG) members to monitor and record archaeology on the Thames foreshore. Drawing on recent work around volunteering, well-being, and emotional labour, this paper examines how spending time in the historic landscape of the Thames foreshore, is a key motivation for Thames Discovery Programme volunteers. The link between volunteering and a heightened sense of well-being, is increasingly being recognized. It has now started to influence policy and practice, through the development of models such as social prescribing in the NHS. This creates potential for new ways of working, and opportunities for involvement in archaeology. I will use our experiences at TDP Programme to explore the ways in which considering people's well-being in historic landscapes, can influence volunteer management practice and create new ways to work with communities.

Keywords: Community archaeology; London; River Thames; Volunteering; Well-being

Introduction

Is volunteering in archaeology good for you? This is a question that we have been wrestling with at Thames Discovery Programme (TDP) for some time. Recent research has demonstrated that in general, people who volunteer regularly have a greater sense of well-being than people who do not volunteer. This paper will draw on the experiences of TDP volunteers in order to explore the implications for archaeology of considering volunteers' well-being impacts.

Thames Discovery Programme

The Thames Discovery Programme is an award-winning community archaeology project. For the last ten years it has trained people to record and monitor the vulnerable archaeology on the Thames foreshore in Greater London. When the tide goes out it reveals London's longest archaeological site, with features dating from the Mesolithic to the twenty-first century. The archaeology of the foreshore is threatened by tidal scour, sea level change, and erosion. TDP Foreshore Recording and Observation Group (FROG) members regularly monitor the foreshore all year round, take part in volunteer fieldwork, conduct desk-based research, and assist with public outreach, a young archaeologists' club, and an oral history project.

TDP was initially funded by the Heritage Lottery Fund from 2008 to 2011; since then it has been hosted by Museum of London Archaeology (MOLA), and the project has continued to grow and evolve in this time. Since the project was founded, TDP has trained over 700 people in foreshore archaeology and recording techniques, and engaged with more through outreach activities. This work has introduced many Londoners to the rich archaeological landscape of the river foreshore for the first time, encouraging them to spend time in an environment that few people have visited. It has broadened people's understanding of the archaeology and history of London, and the importance of the river for the city's development and character.

Methodology

FROGs monitor 40 key sites on the tidal Thames in Greater London, stretching from Richmond in the west, to Erith, close to the Dartford Crossing in southeast London. There are several self-organizing FROGs, led by volunteers, who monitor a specific key site or group of sites in a local area, on a regular basis.

TDP runs up to three FROG Training sessions in the spring each year for people who want to start volunteering with the project. Through these sessions TDP trains around 40 to 80 people each year. From March to August there is a programme of fieldwork sessions at priority key sites, with volunteers working alongside TDP staff. (Figure 14.1) Throughout the year, the project delivers regular outreach activities for the general public in order to raise awareness of London's history on the foreshore. These activities include guided walks, family events, talks, and workshops, all supported by volunteers (Figure 14.2).

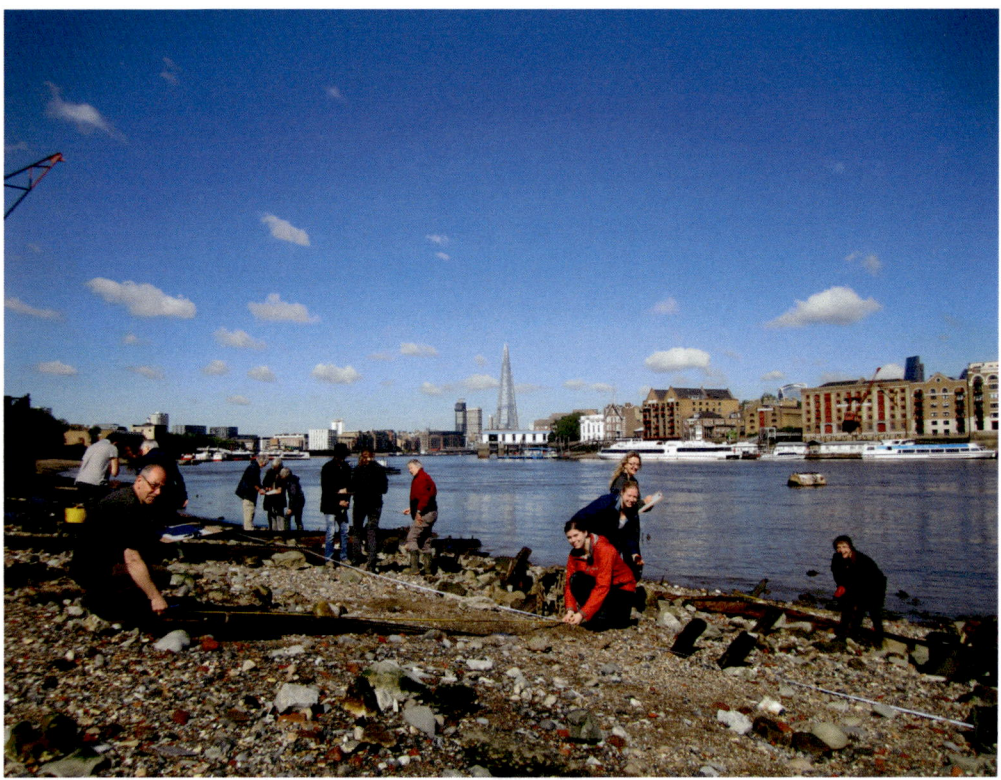

Figure 14.1 TDP volunteers recording post-medieval ship timbers reused in barge beds on the Thames foreshore in Rotherhithe, London. (Photograph by Helen Johnston. Copyright reserved)

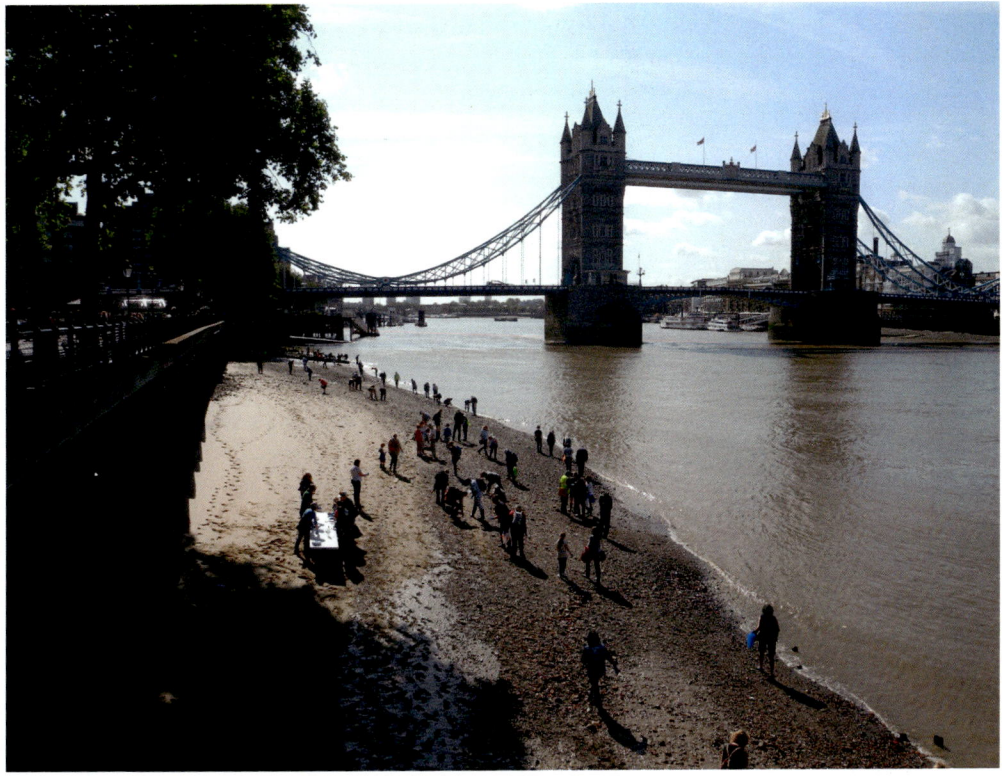

Figure 14.2 Participants at the Open Foreshore event at the Tower of London foreshore (Photograph by N. Cohen. Copyright reserved)

Key sites surveyed in detail by TDP include the Thames foreshores at Charlton, Greenwich, Rotherhithe, the Tower of London, and Isleworth. Features have been recorded dating from the Mesolithic at Vauxhall, through to evidence for twentieth century wartime bomb damage to waterfront properties and river defences along the length of the foreshore. Most of the sites have evidence for multi-period archaeology, including prehistoric peat deposits, Anglo-Saxon fish traps, Tudor palace river accesses, post-medieval shipbuilding and shipbreaking, and Victorian dock infrastructure.

Current projects

TDP is currently running two funded projects to broaden the project's reach and engage with new audiences. This funding allows the project to offer community activities at no cost to participants. The Older Londoners Project, funded by City Bridge Trust (2018), has been running since March 2016 and aims to engage Londoners aged over 75 with the archaeology of the Thames. The project has worked in partnership with older people's groups, including Parkinson's UK, The Alzheimer's Society, and University of the Third Age. It has delivered walks, talks, and workshops inspired by foreshore archaeology. The funding has enabled TDP to run object handling sessions and reminiscence sessions at residential care homes, and accessible riverside strolls for people who are not able to access the foreshore. A key part of this work is an oral history project, with trained volunteers interviewing people who have been visiting the foreshore for 20 years or more, in order to capture their experiences of the foreshore and the ways in which it has changed in recent memory.

Support from Tideway (2018), the organization delivering the Thames Tideway Tunnel, provides funding for work with schools and young people, as well as running a programme of public talks and workshops. The project has run foreshore archaeology sessions with schools, education and youth groups, and has worked in collaboration with organizations including Tower Bridge and the National Maritime Museum. A key part of this project is the creation of a young archaeologists' group, that enables eight to 18 year olds — known as TaDPoles — to take part in practical archaeological activities alongside adult FROG members. The community engagement strand of this project allows us to deliver four evening talks and four one-day workshops a year. These events are open to the public and are always well attended.

Volunteering and well-being

There have been several studies that have attempted to assess the impact of volunteering on well-being using a variety of methods and focusing on different population groups. Recent longitudinal studies in the UK have indicated that volunteering has a positive impact on well-being (Age UK 2017; Nazroo and Matthews 2012; Tabassum *et al.* 2016). In general, people who volunteer regularly appear to experience a greater sense of well-being than people who had never volunteered (Nazroo and Matthews 2012; Tabassum *et al.* 2016;). The link between well-being and volunteering varies across life course, and a positive association between volunteering and well-being begins from the age of 40 and continues as people get older (Tabassum *et al.* 2016).

In 2008, the New Economics Foundation (NEF), commissioned by the Government's Foresight project on Mental Capital and Wellbeing, developed 'five ways to well-being'; evidence-based actions that can be taken to improve personal well-being (NEF 2008). The five ways are:

- Connect
- Be Active
- Take Notice
- Learn
- Give

The five ways to well-being are often used as the basis for evaluation frameworks in order to measure well-being, and they can be used as a baseline to compare the well-being impact of different activities and life events, including volunteering. Nazroo and Matthews (2012), in a study commissioned by WRVS (the Women's Royal Voluntary Service, now RVS, the Royal Voluntary Service), found that volunteers had an improved sense of well-being compared to the general population, for each of the five ways to well-being.

When considering the data on volunteering and well-being, it is important to acknowledge that volunteers generally tend to be better off, in better health, younger, and still in work, compared people who do not volunteer; these are all factors that can contribute to an improved sense of well-being. However, when studies have adjusted for these different characteristics, they found that well-being impacts were still positive for each of the well-being indicators apart from social isolation, although the size of the impact was reduced (Nazroo and Matthews 2012; and see also Tabassum *et al.* 2016).

Evidence indicates that volunteering has a positive impact on well-being, across age groups and social and economic backgrounds. However, the extent of the impact changes depending on a range of factors and circumstances including age. The recognition of a positive link between volunteering and well-being, has led to volunteering being recommended as a route to maintaining or improving well-being, by policy makers, health care providers, and through the popular media. In October 2018, Prime Minister Theresa May launched the UK Government's first loneliness strategy that included social prescribing at its core, enabling GPs to refer patients experiencing loneliness to community activities, including volunteering, to improve their health and well-being (Prime Minister's Office 2018). The NHS Choices Moodzone website (2018), that provides practical information and tools to encourage people to look after their mental health, recommends helping others through volunteering as one of its ten 'Stress Busters'. It includes a page with advice and information on ways to give to others, including volunteering, to help with mental well-being.

Recent heritage volunteering projects have been developed with the aim of improving the well-being of participants. One successful example is the Inspiring Futures: Volunteering for Wellbeing ('if') project delivered by Imperial War Museum North (IWM) and Manchester Museum in partnership ten heritage venues in Greater Manchester, which ran from 2013 to 2017 (IWM and Manchester Museum 2018). This project provided a supported volunteering programme for people at risk of social and economic isolation. It included capacity building for staff in order to improve the volunteering support, and a structured programme to support people in their volunteering. The evaluation of the project demonstrated that taking part had a positive effect on the participants' well-being, that continued beyond the duration of the programme (Warby *et al.* 2017). The capacity-building and partnership-working between the heritage organizations has enabled them to increase aspects of their work. These include the support they are able to offer volunteers, the range of roles they offer, and the diversity of their volunteering team. This project demonstrates the significant social value and health benefits that can be delivered by volunteering programmes in the heritage sector and provides inspiration for similar projects in other organizations.

Well-being benefits of volunteering with Thames Discovery Programme

The Thames foreshore is a unique landscape; not wholly urban, but not wild. Being down on the foreshore, you see the city from a different perspective, in an environment that very few people have experienced. Although most of the foreshore is open to the public, many Londoners have never ventured down the access stairs and spent time there. Many assume that you need permission to go on the foreshore. Several of TDP's key sites are in the shadow of iconic monuments, such as Tower Bridge, the Shard, the Palace of Westminster (Figure 14.3), Canary Wharf, and the Old Royal Naval College at Greenwich. In addition, TDP volunteers have permission to access some of the few restricted areas, such as the foreshore in front of the Tower of London. Despite being in the Greater London area, the project also works in Thames foreshore locations with tree-lined banks and flocks of wildfowl; more rural environments, away from the hustle and bustle of the city. Running through the heart of the city, the

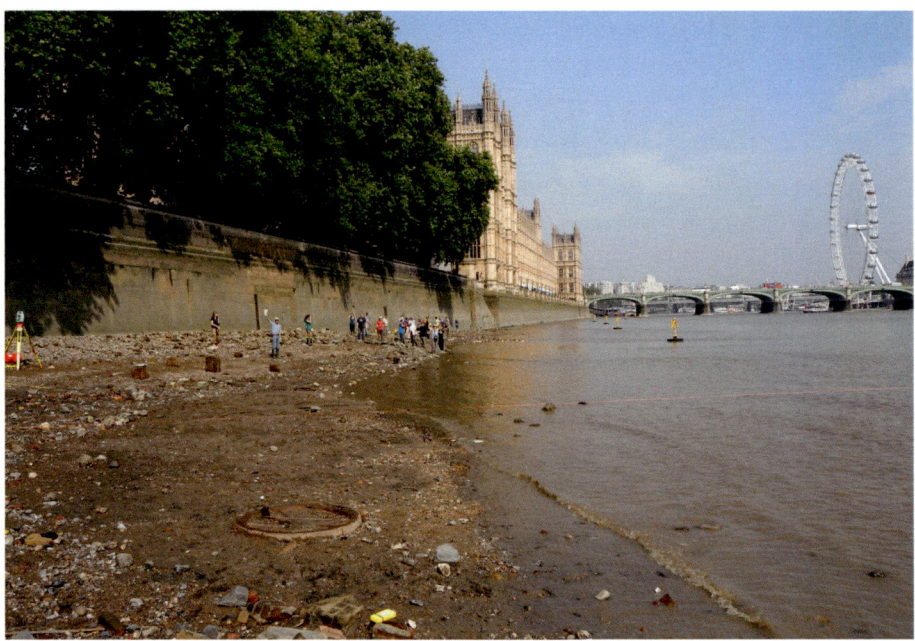

Figure 14.3 Recording WWII bomb damage to the river wall upstream from the Palace of Westminster, London. (Photograph by N. Cohen. Copyright reserved)

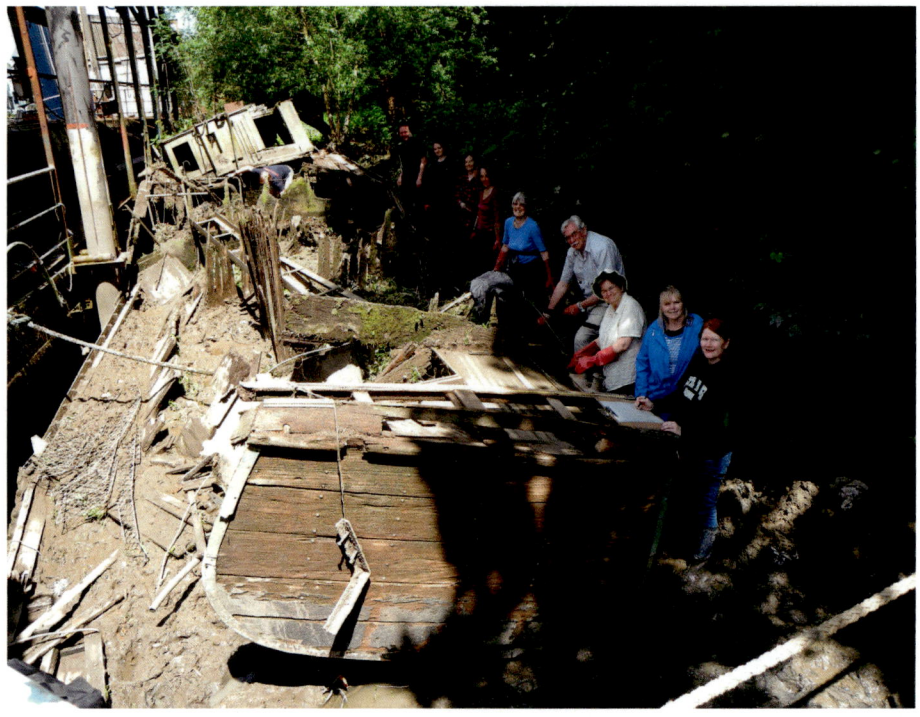

Figure 14.4 Volunteers recording a WWI Submarine Chaser in the mud at Isleworth, London. (Photograph by N. Cohen. Copyright reserved)

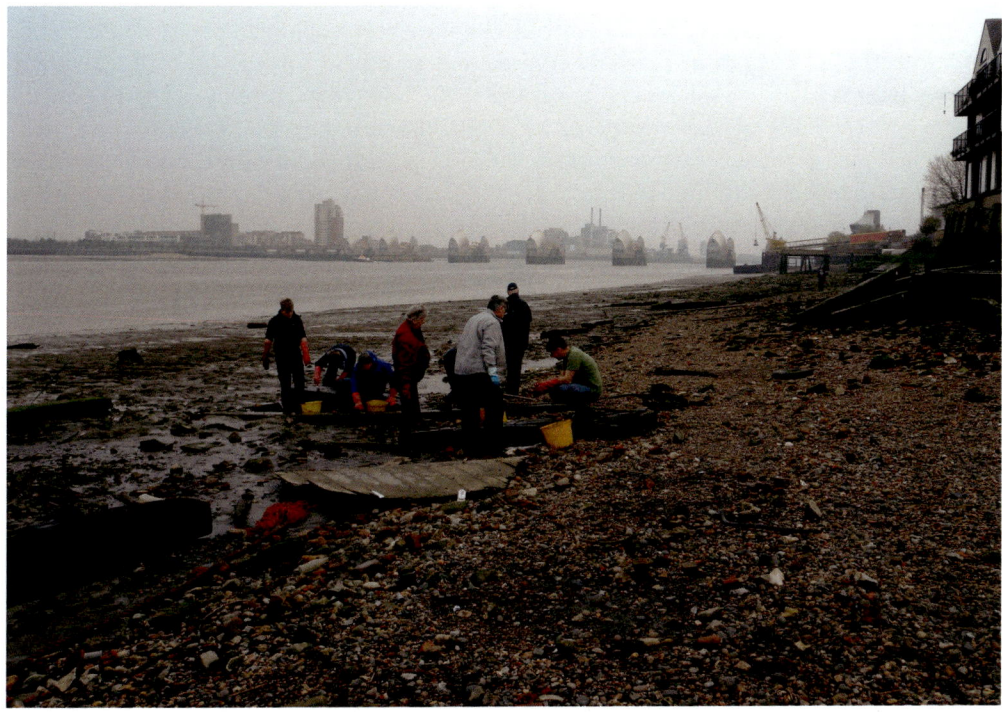

Figure 14.5 Working on the foreshore on a misty day at Charlton, London. (Photograph by N. Cohen. Copyright reserved)

foreshore, with its tides, mud, pollution, and unexploded ordnance, can be a dangerous and dirty environment that can be difficult to access (Figure 14.4). It is not always beautiful, but it is always atmospheric. It has captured the hearts of many people, not least TDP volunteers (Figure 14.5).

Since the beginning of the project, formal evaluation and anecdotal feedback from volunteers consistently mentions their positive relationship with the historic and natural environment of river as being a strong motivator for getting involved with the project and continuing to volunteer. These responses are often self-reported and unprompted. One example is the formal evaluation of the volunteering project at the end of the Heritage Lottery Fund (HLF) support in 2011. This did not aim to analyse well-being as such, yet several participants mentioned the well-being benefits they had gained from being involved:

'Nothing to do with the job, but my balance was shot; paddling around in the mud has improved it no end! The physio is delighted!'

'I have benefitted personally in many ways: my energy levels have been higher and the FROG/TDP initiative has motivated me and inspired me, and this relates to an increase in self-esteem and confidence and general health.'

'Social benefits of working with others who share a common interest.'
Bell (2011)

The well-being benefits of volunteering with TDP have been explored in more depth by Gray in a 2016 thesis, through in-depth interviews and an online survey with TDP volunteers. Although the study had a small sample size, Gray found that involvement with TDP seemed to have a positive effect on the five ways to well-being developed by NEF. The impact was found to be increased for older volunteers across all five indicators. As with the HLF Evaluation, volunteers independently cited the foreshore and the river as being significant factors in their motivations for volunteering and impact on their well-being:

'I find the river therapeutic and as an important part of my well-being want to learn more about it and give something back'

'I have always loved beach-combing and shores of any kind and I'm sure that without this aspect of being a FROG I would have opted for a more land-based activity'

'It's lovely, and I sit there sometimes and you could be anywhere. It's definitely the Thames. It makes me feel very London.'
Gray (2016)

Emotional labour and volunteering

Nazroo and Matthews (2012) demonstrated the importance of well-supported and well-run volunteer programmes for well-being. In the two years covered by the study, volunteers who felt appreciated had a significant increase in their sense of well-being compared to non-volunteers. However, there was no significant difference in the change in well-being between volunteers who did not feel appreciated and non-volunteers (Nazroo and Matthews 2012). Not all volunteering projects will have well-being benefits, and there is a risk that poorly-run projects may even have negative impacts on the participants' sense of well-being.

The well-being benefits of volunteering, particularly in historic landscapes, are intertwined with emotional connections to volunteering activities and locations. The implications of this for managing a volunteering programme, were explored in a research project by Green and Ward (2016) on behalf of the National Trust. This study argued 'that the management of volunteers is emotionally complex and demanding' (Green and Ward 2016: 31). At the National Trust, volunteers had a strong emotional connection to the place and the space where they volunteered; they were passionate about the properties where they volunteer, above and beyond the broader National Trust organization (Green and Ward 2016). The study identified this emotional connection as a potential source of tension, when volunteers felt that staff members they were working with did not recognize or share this emotional link. The study highlights the important emotional labour that volunteer managers undertake in order to manage this tension; work that is often unacknowledged and poorly-understood.

This study has implications that should be considered by anyone managing volunteers on archaeological projects that are frequently embedded in a specific place or landscape. These often set out to encourage volunteers and the local community to increase their engagement with, and sense of ownership of, an archaeological site or historic landscape. What support and training should people running archaeological volunteering projects receive, in order to ensure that they have the skills to manage the emotional labour this entails?

Conclusion: Implications for volunteering in archaeology

It is suggested that volunteering in archaeology should benefit the five ways of well-being identified by NEF: Connect, Be Active, Take Notice, Learn, and Give. The evidence from TDP indicates that this is the case, but that more studies are needed. Longitudinal studies, as were conducted as part of the Inspiring Futures project, should continue after the activities have finished in order to assess the long-term benefits. This would create benchmark data that could be used to compare the impact of different forms of involvement within archaeology, as well as the benefits of volunteering in archaeology compared to other sectors. However, there is a need for resources and support which allow projects to effectively measure impact and the social return on investment of volunteering on archaeological projects. This is currently lacking.

It seems evident that the historic environment is important for people's well-being and sense of place. It is a direct motivation for volunteering, but there is little consideration for the implications this can have on managing volunteering projects and encouraging community involvement. Many projects are short term, and there is little support and training on how to manage the emotional and social aspects of volunteering.

The Inspiring Futures project in Manchester demonstrated the value of carrying out targeted work in the heritage sector, with people at risk of social isolation. This type of engagement often requires investment and increased support for the staff and volunteers involved, and cultural change at the organizations where the volunteers are hosted. However, the project demonstrated that these efforts can provide a significant return on investment, both for the organizations and individuals involved.

As improving well-being is a priority for policy makers and health strategies, there are funding opportunities available for well-designed well-being projects. At a time when funding is becoming more focused, it is vital to look for new opportunities and consider ways in which income and funding streams can be diversified.

What next?

At TDP we are inspired by the anecdotal and more formal evidence from our volunteer evaluations — as well as the broader evidence base — that demonstrates the ways in which volunteering has a positive impact on well-being. More work needs to be carried out to measure the impact on personal well-being of volunteering with TDP, building on the work of Gray. It is also necessary to examine the broader social return on investment of the project. We are currently looking to secure funding to support people at risk of social isolation in exploring the archaeology of the Thames and the foreshore environment, working in partnership with mental health organizations, and developing the evidence-base for the well-being impact provided by volunteering in archaeology.

Acknowledgements

The author would like to thank MOLA for hosting and contributing financial support to Thames Discovery Programme, the Heritage Lottery Fund for financing the creation of the project, and various other funding bodies for generous support including: City Bridge Trust,

Tideway, the Port of London Authority, Tower Bridge, MBNA Clippers, English Heritage, UCL Public Engagement Unit, Historic Palaces and the Crown Estate (Marine Stewardship Fund). The final thanks goes to the hundreds of Thames Discovery volunteers who have contributed their time to monitor and record the fast eroding archaeology on the foreshore; the project would not exist without them.

Bibliography

Age UK 2017. *A summary of Age UK's Index of Wellbeing in Later Life*. London: Age UK.

Bell, N. 2011. Evaluation of the Experience of the FROG Volunteers in the Thames Discovery Programme. Unpublished report prepared for the Heritage Lottery Fund.

City Bridge Trust 2018. City Bridge Trust [Website]. Viewed 29 November 2018, <https://www.citybridgetrust.org.uk/>.

Gray, S. 2016. Is Being a FROG Good For You? An Examination of the Well-being Benefits of Taking Part in Public Archaeology, with an Emphasis on Older People. Unpublished MA dissertation, University College London.

Green, A-M. and J. Ward 2016. *To what extent is the management of volunteers similar or different to the management of paid staff within the National Trust? A commissioned study by the National Trust 2013-2015* [Online document]. Leicester: University of Leicester. Viewed 29 November 2018, <https://www2.le.ac.uk/departments/business/images/research/work-and-employment/a-report-of-the-findings-from-the-national-trust-project>.

IWM and Manchester Museum 2018. if: Volunteering for Wellbeing [Website]. Viewed 29 November 2018, <http://volunteeringforwellbeing.org.uk/>.

Nazroo, J. and K. Matthews 2012. *The impact of volunteering on well-being in later life: A report to WRVS*. Cardiff: WRVS.

NEF 2008. Five ways to wellbeing: The evidence [Webpage]. Viewed 29 November 2018, <https://neweconomics.org/2008/10/five-ways-to-wellbeing-the-evidence>.

NHS 2018. NHS Choices moodzone: Ten stress busters [Webpage]. Viewed 29 November 2018, <https://www.nhs.uk/conditions/stress-anxiety-depression/reduce-stress/>.

Prime Minister's Office 2018. Prime Minister Theresa May launches government's first loneliness strategy. Press release [Webpage]. Viewed 29 November 2018, <https://www.gov.uk/government/news/pm-launches-governments-first-loneliness-strategy>.

Tabassum, F., J. Mohan and P. Smith 2016. Association of volunteering with mental well-being: A lifecourse analysis of a national population-based longitudinal study in the UK. *BMJ Open* 6(8), viewed 29 November 2018, <https://bmjopen.bmj.com/content/6/8/e011327>.

Tideway 2018, Tideway [Website]. Viewed 29 November 2018, <https://www.tideway.london/>.

Warby, A.G., D. Garcia and A. Winn 2017. *Inspiring futures: Volunteering for wellbeing final report 2013-2016: Social return on investment* [Online document]. Manchester: IWM and Manchester Museum. Viewed 29 November 2018, <http://volunteeringforwellbeing.org.uk/wp-content/uploads/2017/03/IF_VOLUNTEERING_FOR_WELLBEING_REPORT_2013-16_SROI_IWM.pdf>.

Chapter 15

Between the Barrows: Seeking a spirit of place

Christopher Howard Elmer

Abstract

This chapter describes the Between the Barrows project, a community archaeology programme run by the University of Southampton and based at Harmony Woods, near Andover, Hampshire, which is managed by the Andover Trees United charity. This project seeks to engage a wide range of local community members, some of whom are actively suspicious of, or even hostile to, the project and, occasionally, other participants and community groups. The aim is to bring the community together and instil a greater appreciation of the natural and historic environment. The methods of engagement and the archaeological activities are described, together with the ways in which their impacts on participants were measured and evaluated. Building on the experience of the Between the Barrows project, a range of concepts are explored including the ideas of 'gifts', 'sense of place', and 'spirit of place'. The ways in which these have proven beneficial to project participants are explained, and how they might be applied in order to improve well-being for the participants in this and future projects, is discussed. The ongoing Between the Barrows project has resulted in increased community cohesion and a better — and sometimes deeper — connection to place for participants. It is anticipated that future project activities will build on these positive well-being impacts.

Keywords: Community; Engagement; Gift; Spirit of place; Well-being

Introduction

In Marcel Mauss's work *The Gift* (Mauss 1990) he writes about the Polynesian concept of the 'hau'; the spirit of the object and the spirit of the place. For objects that contain this spirit, the material components have a life and a multiple relational meaning. In their lives, they journey across space and time, often as exchanged gifts, but they are always seeking to return to their place of origin (Mauss 1990:15). Humans have equally complex relationships with place, and for many, whether they are new arrivals to a place or long-term residents, a connection with landscape and the deep history of their locality can offer surprising and potentially therapeutic or healing outcomes (Helm 2015:190; National Trust 2017).

I encountered one such place as part of a project I co-created in 2016, that centred on a tract of land between two very different communities. The project formed an element of my research into collaborative archaeology practice as part of my PhD (Elmer 2017a) and this chapter draws on some of the illustrative and textual material that resulted from this research.

Project Background

The site in question lies close to Andover in Hampshire and comprises a 44-acre (17.8ha) field purchased from the Trinley Estate by Hampshire County Council in 2011. The land is managed as a planting estate to enable the creation of urban woodland by a charity known as Andover Trees United (ATU). The charity has set aside a 12-acre (4.8ha) section of the estate which is known as Harmony Woods. The area is surrounded by low fencing, and is to be planted by the

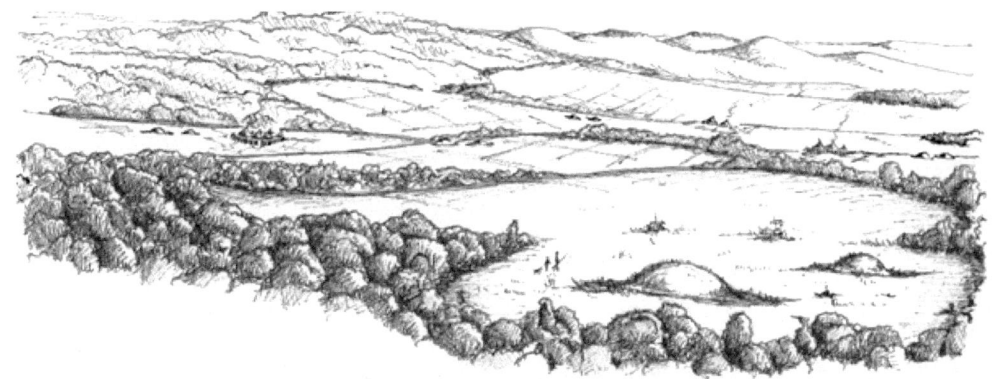

*Figure 15.1 The Harmony Woods site reimagined during the Bronze Age.
(Artwork by David Hopkins. Reproduced by kind permission)*

community. This activity is led by children who often come as part of organized school visits. By 2017 over 5000 trees had been planted in the Harmony Woods site as part of the charity's aspiration to provide community engagement with the local natural environment (ATU 2018).

The Between the Barrows project (Elmer 2017a: 289-307; YouTube 2016) was initiated in 2016 to build on this aspiration. It sought to provide local schools and community volunteers with a chance to engage with the landscape across a wide disciplinary spectrum, integrating natural history and archaeology with creative responses as part of a structured visit to the site. The 2016 community dig lasted for two weeks in May, and was focussed on the site of a proposed pond. After consultation with the County Archaeologist, (whose interest in the site had led him to create the drawing reproduced in Figure 15.1), the pond location was selected to sit between two ploughed out barrows, one of which was located in the Harmony Woods tree planting area. The project continued in 2018 with a ten day community excavation close to the pond site.

When the Harmony Woods project was first described to me I naively imagined a landscape imbued with the presence of the past and perhaps, in some mysterious way through the physical remains, offering a connection with the prehistoric communities who had once lived there. In reality I encountered a windswept rise with a solitary steel container, some rows of newly planted saplings and, significantly, a complex local community response to the site (Figure 15.2).

The nearby housing estate, the Augustus Park estate, that lies to the southwest was still being built. However, phased occupation meant that many residents already lived on the edge of the Harmony Woods planting site. The estate residents used the newly developed sports ground as well as the adjacent fields to walk dogs and, for young people especially, to escape the adult oversight of the built estate. To the east of the Harmony Woods site, accessible via a wooden gate and then a tree lined hollow way, sits the village of Enham Alamein. This is a typical Hampshire village in appearance, but is owned in large part by the Enham Trust. Since WWI the Trust has offered purpose-built accommodation for disabled veterans, and has more recently been involved in supporting adults with a broad range of disabilities (Hampshire Life 2017).

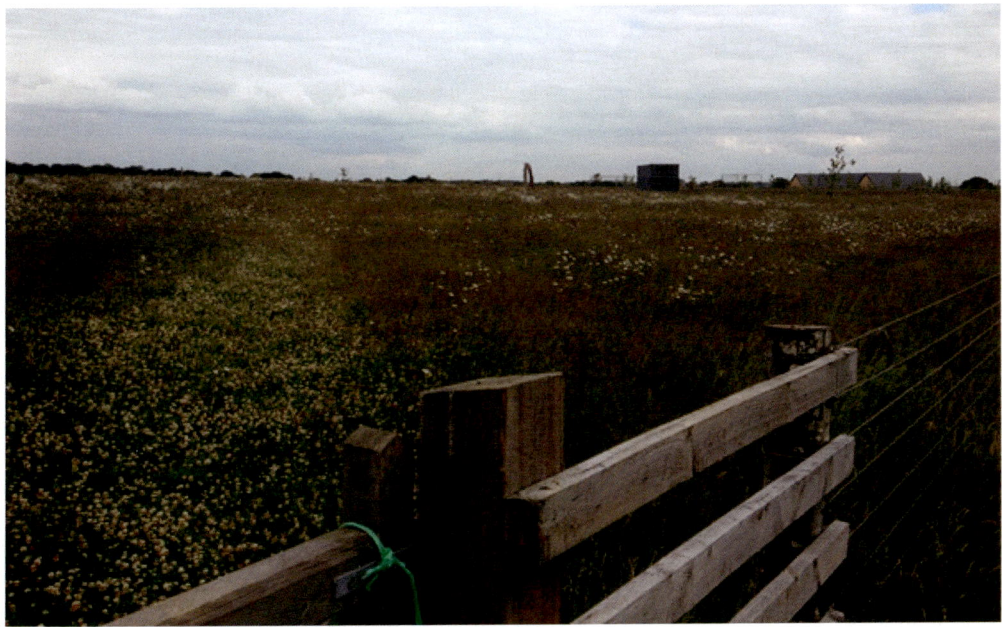

Figure 15.2 The Harmony Woods planting site with the sports pavilion in the distance. (Photograph by C. Elmer 2016. Copyright reserved)

Disruption and community dissonance

The Harmony Woods site separates these two very distinct communities. Anecdotally, the land managed by the charity was seen as a territorial separator; a barrier between the two communities, who rarely either mixed or acknowledged the special historical and natural potential of the site. More disturbingly for the ATU volunteers, some elements of the community resented the 'control' imposed on their access to the woods despite provision of mown walkways and clear entrance points. Those people perhaps assumed that the fencing and gateways erected around the Harmony Woods planting site were actually constraining their access to land that bordered their houses, land that they perhaps perceived as belonging to the local community.

Locally-based volunteers on site had mentioned these perceptions through their conversations with neighbours, and the volunteers frequently referred to these underlying resentments as well as incidents during which, by 2016, young people had begun to deliberately enter the site at night and vandalize property. This culminated in the frequent illicit late-night use of the site to make fires and gather socially, as well as the destruction of the wooden 'bothy' that had been built to provide a shelter for school groups. Litter, including broken bottles and remnants of wood fires, became, and continue to be, a problem for the site. One of the key concerns for developing a programme of engagement with local schools, centred around challenging this behaviour and attempting to inculcate valuing behaviours and positive attitudes to the land. In offering local residents and schools the opportunity to participate in excavating and exploring the Harmony Woods site, it was hoped that the project would provide a 'sense of place' for the participants; a deeper understanding of the area's history and natural history, creating a sense of connection and appreciation. This would, in turn, provide protection to the environment. It was also hoped that by bringing two communities together, the project would begin a process of 'healing', whereby the land became a bridge rather than a barrier between the two communities.

The 2016 excavation, therefore, balanced activities between those days that offered local community involvement and those that offered structured school activity. Volunteers from the local community were invited to support the excavation from the start, with de-turfing and physical labour, monitored by myself and three other (at the time post-graduate) colleagues from the University of Southampton Archaeology Department. Portaloos were provided and gazebos erected, whilst water was transported in containers from the nearby sports pavilion. The University team opted to camp on site over the entire fortnight, primarily to assuage fears of vandalism, but also to establish a 'presence' on site that led to many evening time conversations with dog walkers and young people, explaining the project, inviting support and building a sense of trust with the community.

The 2018 excavation followed the same approach, but there were ongoing incidents that demonstrated the mix of emotions around the site. A3 posters pasted to fence posts advertising an event-filled open day were torn off the posts and scattered across the site. On two occasions, the access gate for vehicles was found to have been padlocked shut from outside, excluding emergency vehicle entry and access, and bolt cutters were needed to break the locks. On one evening, a group of youngsters entered the site and had to be challenged as they began to make a fire close to the new wooden education building; they eventually moved on, but subsequently created a disturbance at the sports pavilion and the police were called.

Developing 'community conversations'

There are no quick fixes in community archaeology. However, the programme of activity did create 'community conversations' around the site, whether formally invited through adverts in the local press calling for volunteers, or more informally managed through talking about the project with dog walkers and the local residents who visited whilst set up for the excavation was in process. This prompted an influx of volunteers who signed up to work on the excavation, with over 40 local residents, from both the Augustus Park estate and Enham Alamein village, volunteering to work assigned shifts during the 2016 season. Many returned to support the 2018 season. Similarly, in both years, seven primary and secondary schools from the local area, who were targeted using email contacts and face to face visits, registered their interest. The schools were provided with a multi-disciplinary activity session, in which pupils participated in the dig (Figure 15.3), explored the tree planting area, and created their own art works representing the site. Mixing disciplines was deliberate and seen by schools as a positive cross-curricular offering. The core focus on the historic dimension of the site, alongside the natural history elements, allowed the project to reconceptualize the site for all participants as a multi-sensory, multi-disciplinary, meeting ground for members of the two separate communities.

Impact measures and generic learning outcomes

The community response was captured through anecdotal evidence, with the researcher acting as an embedded participant (Davies 2008), as well as through a more formal meaning

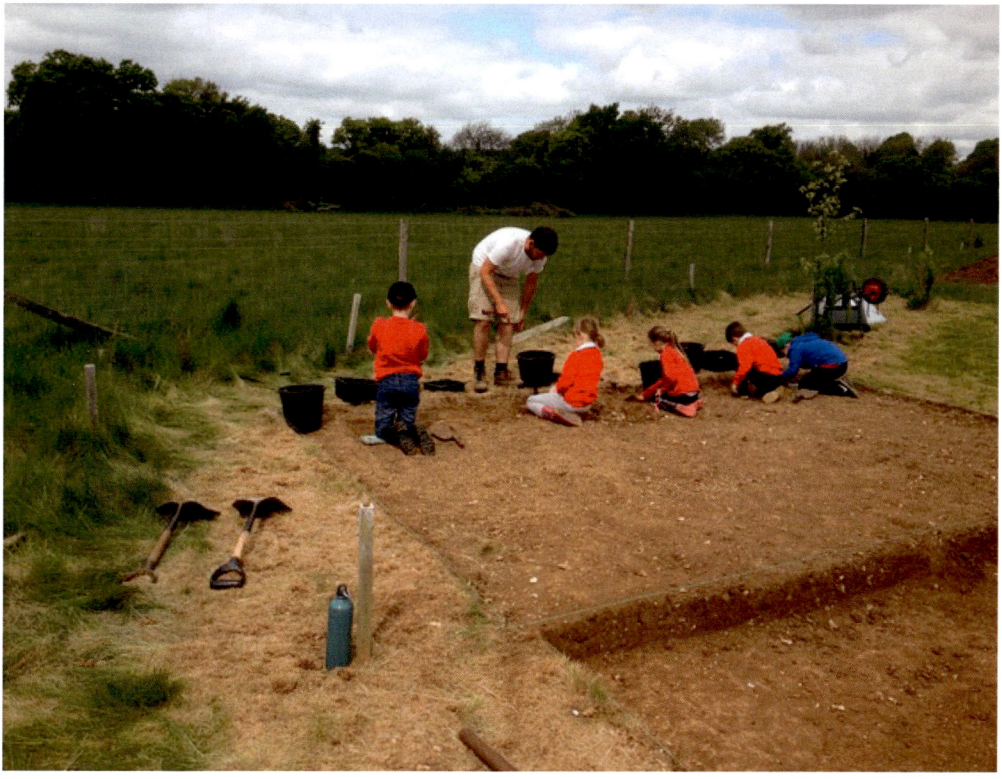

Figure 15.3 School children excavating the 2016 trench. (Photograph by C. Elmer. Copyright reserved)

mapping exercise in which participants were asked to respond to the phrase 'Between the Barrows'. The school responses were also captured through a formal process of evaluation (Elmer 2017b), including teacher post-visit questionnaires and the use of 'memory clouds' (Figure 15.4) for pupils.

All of this summative evaluation data was categorized using a heritage industry generated evaluation tool, the Generic Learning Outcomes (GLOs), developed by the University of Leicester for the Museums, Libraries and Archives Council (MLA). Although the MLA no longer exists, the evaluation tools are now available on the Arts Council webpages (Arts Council England 2014). GLOs examine responses to engagement with arts and heritage through five key categories:

- Knowledge and understanding
- Skills
- Attitudes and values
- Enjoyment, inspiration and creativity
- Activity, behaviour and progression

The GLOs offer a useful tool for understanding learning, but they can also play a role in measuring well-being as they prompt reflection on personal health, physical activity, and

PUPILS: YOUR MEMORY CLOUD

This is what I remember from visiting the archaeologists

(You can draw pictures in the memory cloud as well as write words)

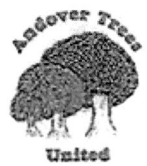

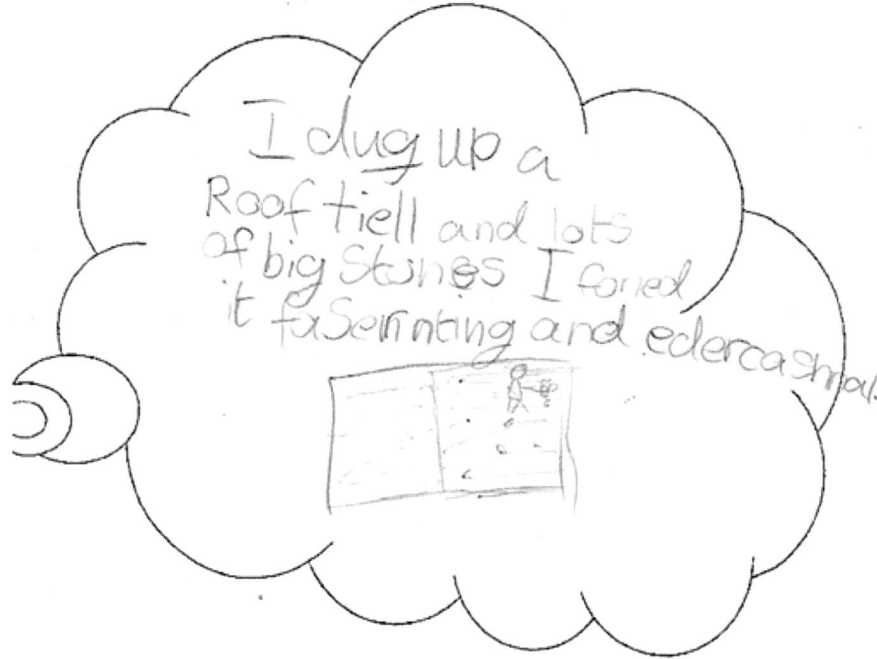

Now write down two words that you think best describe what you did with the archaeologists (e.g. exciting, boring, funny)

WORD 1   WORD 2

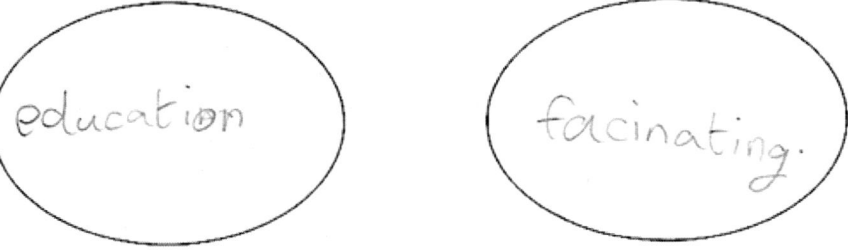

Figure 15.4 Example of a completed memory cloud. (Illustration by C. Elmer. Copyright reserved)

social interaction. These are all factors that the Mental Health Foundation suggest offer us insights into people's state of well-being (Mental Health Foundation 2018).

The project outcomes were also examined through the lens of John Holden's work on cultural value (Holden 2006). This equates intrinsic, institutional and instrumental values with interest groups that fall within the public, professional, and political domains respectively. According to this model of cultural value, the political constituency is most concerned to prioritize instrumental value, measured through tangible targets and outputs. The public and professional constituencies are more likely to seek the intrinsic, experiential benefits of a project or activity.

The schools response

This predicted disparity in prioritized values seemed to be reflected in the analysis of the data that emerged from the project (Elmer 2017a: 289–307). The school children's responses to the site, when compared to the teachers' responses, showed a clear contrast in prioritized values. The teachers — the professional constituency in Holden's terms — were most concerned to realize the curricular relevance of the activity, and to demonstrate the instrumental and institutional benefit this conferred. However, the participating pupils — the public constituency — showed an intrinsic motivation and connection with the activity.

In effect, the value of the visit lay primarily in an emotional and enjoyable connection with the past. This held some knowledge benefit, but for pupils helped to develop real-world skills and for teachers provided an insight into the significance and importance of archaeological evidence. The experiential value of the visit for the pupils fitted much more into an identity-making frame of reference, whereas the teachers' viewpoint encompassed learning established truths about the past and reinforcing notions of historic significance.

The community response

The local community volunteers offered their feedback on the project in 2016 and 2018 at celebration events designed especially to capture their responses. Written statements were supplied on sheets that asked participants to respond to the phrase: 'Between the Barrows'. These demonstrated a common motivation to engage with the process of archaeology on site, to develop skills linked to archaeological excavation and recording, and a desire to gain or validate knowledge and understanding about the history of the area. Typical responses included phrases such as:

> 'It was interesting to see the archaeological process and to participate. Getting immersed in it. I was involved in an archaeological dig a long time ago. The completeness of it was worthwhile, the way of setting it out/planning it.'

> 'I've always been interested in archaeology, always watch the Time Team. I wanted an opportunity to have a go. I didn't know who was going to be here, but I wanted to offer my physical skills. The enthusiasm of the digging team was great-the archaeologists helped us to get involved.'

'I understand the process and it was fascinating to see the passions of the diggers and youngsters, the leaders prepared to camp and show their passion. It helps you to grow, you really are doing it for real.'

'I was interested in the orientation of the barrows and the roads-old tracks and droveways.'

'It was not like I was expecting, I wasn't expecting so much hard work. It helped me to understand archaeology and to experience the community as a volunteer, working together.'

The community voice was also aligned with the school pupils' desire to seek the inspirational, experiential, and identity-making benefits from participation. The responses mentioned the immersive nature of the activity and the passions of the diggers and youngsters, as well as the socially bonding benefits of working together. Many of the responses fell into the 'attitudes and values' GLO, demonstrating a sense of revelation and reconnection with a known landscape. Typical responses here included the role played by the University postgraduates in supporting the excavation:

'Experts helped to guide, it was about right, time to ask and answer questions and to learn about the site.'

'Talking to the dig team helped to understand the significance of the barrows and local area and other sites around here.'

In effect the volunteers, (the public constituency), were seeking the whole raft of outcomes that can be categorized as learning outcomes using the GLO model. These range across gaining knowledge and understanding, acquiring skills and expressing future intentions for positive learning behaviours, to participating in transformative experiences in relation to personal attitudes and values. They also highlight the desire for a meaningful, enjoyable and intrinsically rewarding experience, as predicted by John Holden in his values model of cultural engagement; the success of the project was in part because the project partners, the professionals, were able to align their own values to this approach.

Between the archaeology

The University team were keen to provide a high-quality learning experience that also created an opportunity to examine project impacts. The partner, ATU, and the participants, sought an experientially focussed project design, but also demonstrated an epistemological stance that sought the 'truth' in relation to the deep history of the site. The University team were perceived as 'experts' helping to reveal these hidden truths about the site but also, by their very presence, were deemed to confer significance to the site. Although this contrasted with the researcher stance (that the site was open to multiple interpretations and uncertainty), the primary focus on the 'public' experience as opposed to a 'professionally' successful outcome in terms of archaeological data meant that the atmosphere on site was conducive to positive social and experiential outcomes. Despite the underlying epistemological variance, the partners and participants both adhered to a pedagogy that focussed on the intrinsic value of the site.

As the excavation progressed we were aware that, from a professional standpoint, we were excavating a reasonably uninspiring trench. My colleagues felt that we should re-label the project 'Between the Archaeology'. However, at the same time I realized that even though the community excavation failed to detect any archaeological features of significance (although plenty of worked and struck flints were found) the participants were not overly concerned. In fact, they delighted in finding artefacts and then problem-solving the identification of worked or struck flint, working together, and at the same time connecting with their locality. There was a sense that they were learning skills and improving their understanding of their locality, but also that something deeper was going on. There were 'qualities of engagement' that moved the experience beyond a range of specified learning outcomes, and which seemed to hint at a connectivity with the past and the landscape that held a deep emotional and even 'spiritual' resonance.

Viewing the land and the past as a gift

The objects and landscape seemed to be being offered up as a gift as the past was being revealed, and participants were actively creating a connection with the landscape and the objects they were encountering. The 'experts' were perceived as offering their experience and time for free — another form of gift — and the relationship with volunteers grew from a mutual understanding that the project was intrinsically motivated. This notion of gift, it seems to me, resonates with many public perceptions of heritage and nature. Where an intrinsically motivated connection with landscapes and past places is formed, including through projects that seek to examine well-being benefits, there also lies a tension with the increasingly instrumentalized and commodified practice that underpins the management of our heritage. (Elmer 2017a; Hewison 2014; Hewison and Holden 2014).

This connectivity, so frequently expressed by participants in the Between the Barrows project, could be said to tap into the notion of 'spirit of place' (Marsden 2014). In this, the benefits of participation go beyond the development of a skills and knowledge-based competency, and the experience moves from engaging in an enjoyable learning activity in a socially welcoming atmosphere, into impacts that could be categorized as spiritual self-reflection.

Morris Hargreaves McIntyre, a heritage research consultancy, have developed a model of museum visitor motivation that examines museum visiting in terms of four key motivations (Morris Hargreaves McIntyre 2005). These demonstrate that visitors will sometimes seek a spiritual and emotional connection with the heritage on display, as well as a more commonly-sought intellectual and social reward (Morris Hargreaves McIntyre 2005: 9–10). The categories are offered as a hierarchy of motivation, with spiritual and emotional motivations the least common, but nevertheless evidenced by many people who engage with museum displays. The response of many participants in the Between the Barrows project suggest these spiritual and emotional connections with the locality were being realized, often through a connectivity with a distant past:

> 'I've always known this area was full of archaeology, that's interesting and to actually meet it, gives a perspective about what it means to live in a place. There's not a lot of continuity in modern society, in a sense of where we are from, particularly Andover where people move in, but an understanding of that continuous history is good.'

'I felt a strong connection with the people from the past, the traces of activities made the whole thing come alive. The sense of place was enhanced, you could relate this open field to human activity, it made a connection for me. The activity of the dig released something special.'

'It's not just about artefacts, there were birds singing here 3000 years ago just as they are now. Connection with the human activity you were digging, our fields and woods are not just blank spaces but places where communities lived in the past.'

Seeking a spirit of place

The project has led me to think about how this connectivity might be enabled, and also to postulate on the well-being benefits accruing from this. How do we provide the best possible opportunity to seek the spirit of place?

My reading has taken me into realms of research that some would classify in the category of pseudo-science or romanticism. However, writers who have tried to explore this concept of a 'spiritual' connection with place do offer worthwhile points for exploration. William Blake's fourfold vision (Rose 1964) suggests an approach to therapeutic engagement with heritage; mixing the purely rational and material with an aesthetic and spiritual connectivity. This has inspired several more recent writers who have made comment on therapy, the human experience, and the links between scientific rigour and a more spiritual aesthetic (Bateson 1972; Freeman 2012; Palmer 2017).

Rupert Sheldrake (2017) has speculated on the relationship between science and spirituality. He lists the mental well-being and health benefits of 'reconnecting with the more than human world' (Sheldrake 2017: 68-70) and offers strategies which, in many ways, are mirrored by the public engagement approaches developed in community archaeology projects such as Between the Barrows. Sheldrake's list captures many of the stated or observed 'qualities of engagement' that became apparent as the two communities at Harmony Woods came together to excavate the site.

Sheldrake mentions the importance of 'meditation' and the application of 'mindfulness' through repetitive physical and mental routines as one route to improving mental health (Sheldrake 2017: 37–40). Archaeological excavation, particularly when combined with working in outdoor environments, can often lead to periods of meditation and self-reflection, providing a form of physical activity that is repetitive and focussed, but rarely boring. Taking this a step further, it could be argued that, on occasion, the development of a physical and intellectual competence in the process of excavation can lead to what Mihály Csikszentmihalyi calls a 'flow' experience; a life affirming and positive affect that can also include group affects enabling group cohesion (Csikszentmihalyi 1990: 190-1).

Intriguingly, the concept of 'gratitude' — seeing the past as a gift — is postulated by Sheldrake to be one of his key requirements for reconnecting with the spiritual. In his view, gratitude as an emotion has discernible well-being benefits (Sheldrake 2017: 56-7). The comments from participants in the Between the Barrows dig, offered a view of the landscape and the past as a gift and also saw the expert support and leadership as a form of gift that created a social bond. The well-being outcomes that could be nurtured through presenting projects in this way, rather than as commodified transactions, might be worth exploring. Also the very notion of perceiving and interpreting the relationship with past landscapes as a gift.

Another of Sheldrake's requirements for seeking a spiritual connection with place, is formed by 'relating to' plants and nature, (Sheldrake 2017:100) that is often, though not always, another feature of working in the landscape. This connection with place is reinforced through becoming aware of the 'presence of the past', promulgating a sense of place that is especially powerful when linked to historic sites and artefacts (Sheldrake 2017:111–2). The 'convergence' of disciplines, evidenced in the activities offered by Between the Barrows and many other similar projects, links landscape with heritage and nature in a manner that breaks the disciplinary boundaries imposed by school or university curricula. It also suggests a need for improved interdisciplinary practice as a means to form successful well-being outcomes. This can be achieved through the construction of more effective collaborations at intra- and inter-organizational levels in order to provide the impetus to break the rigour-relevance gap that often hinders research-led partnerships (Dillon *et al.* 2014; Elmer 2015).

Sheldrake writes about providing opportunities for communities to connect with the past through 'rituals' (Sheldrake 2017:112–3). This calls for behaviour that could be linked to religious forms of ceremony, but may also be extended to enacting structured socially engaging activity that includes some form of celebration or ceremony. The Between the Barrows project enacted this during its celebration evenings, when recognizing the support of all volunteers and thanking the organizers for their input. Others have made this connection between archaeology and ritual; Vitor Jorge for example talks about the notion of excavation as performance and writes about it in terms of a ritual activity (Jorge 2008: 77).

Controversially, one could argue that, in a sense, the intrusive and unwelcome activities of some residents who use the site to gather and drink around temporary fires itself demonstrates a type of ritual; a rite of passage, with a youthful connection to the land under the night sky. Indeed, Sheldrake goes on to talk about 'sacred groves' and trees acting as bridges between land and sky (Sheldrake 2017: 101–5). How far were the volunteer diggers aware of the site's status as a Bronze Age cemetery, aware of the saplings and trees that surrounded them, and equally aware of the subtle metaphors suggested by the physical reality of the landscape past and present? At the most extreme, could it be argued that, in some sense, the daily visits to the site reflect Sheldrake's idea that people need to see some journeys in life as 'pilgrimages'; a means to connect them with a landscape or place that holds a special significance for them? The notion of pilgrimage as a sublime and healing journey, but not necessarily linked to a religious faith, has been touched upon most recently by the travel writer Guy Stagg (2018). His book *The Crossway* details a pilgrimage taken as a means to cope with mental illness by way of a walk towards recovery.

This idea of physical therapy also informs another of Sheldrake's contentions that 'dance, music and song' (Sheldrake 2017: 136–49) are key to unlocking this sense of spiritual experience. I would take this analysis a step further and draw on current models used to examine visitor experience and interpretive strategies in museums. These can assist with understanding, and also reinforcing, the notion that we can contrive an emotional and even spiritual response to place by allowing for multiple channels of response. Thinking about multiple intelligences

(Gardner 1986; 2006) would be a useful way of planning for these multiple responses. So, dance yes, but also provide opportunities for storytelling, creative art, problem-solving, and so on.

It seems to me that the search for a spirit of place is essentially a reflection of a personal sense of well-being and competence. Any project seeking to enable personal connections with place requires an approach that is rooted in individual meaning-making and an epistemology that acknowledges relative truths. This can be challenging for people (and organizations) that are uncomfortable with uncertainty. Again, drawing on museum sector thinking, the desire to offer individually relevant and meaningful experiences has led many practitioners to apply the principles outlined by George Hein (1998), in his work on constructivism and museum learning. Constructivism challenges certain established pedagogic and epistemological approaches to learning. It focuses on the individual as a learner, providing multi-sensory active engagement constructed through negotiation with the learner (Copeland 2005). In many ways, constructivism offers a model for validating the more esoteric assertions offered by Sheldrake. We know that actively engaging through learner-focussed projects can deliver positive outcomes (Arts Council England 2014; Butler 2017; Chaterjee 2008; Falk and Dierking 2007; Kolb 1984), and the opportunity to provide these projects through cross-disciplinary, convergent philosophies, allows for multi-sensory and emotionally rewarding experiences. The notion of gratitude is also important here. How can we provide activities that are negotiated and perceived as 'gifts'? And how does this concept fit with contemporary well-being and heritage management practice?

Sense of place and spirit of place

Despite a heavily promoted health and well-being agenda (APPGAHW 2017; Arts Council England 2014), heritage organizations are becoming increasingly instrumentalized (Elmer 2017a). Their need to deliver on income and 'usage' targets, so vital to justifying funding, has meant that the intrinsic value of heritage has become less successfully celebrated (Hewison and Holden 2014: 9). The value of heritage is often measured against quantitative outcomes. Even where an emotional component is recognized, as with the 2016 Taking Part survey (DCMS 2016), it is scored against a financial value. Despite this, notions of 'sense of place' play a distinct role in contemporary government agendas (World Economic Forum 2017). Well-being studies, such as the Arts and Humanities Research Council funded 'Sense of Place: Exploring Nature and Wellbeing through the Non-Visual Senses' project (AHRC 2018), and the National Trust commissioned *Places That Make Us* (NT 2017), frequently highlight the importance of sense of place as a medium for delivering meaningful and therapeutic public engagement with heritage.

This idea of 'sense of place' and its relation to heritage has been explored in the past through the 'Sense of Place, Historic Environment and Social Capital' project (Graham *et al.* 2009). This suggested that by 2009 little work had been done to link the three areas under scrutiny. This is still very much the case. The report's authors did however demonstrate that clear links can be made between a sense of place and social capital, describing the latter as 'a term which refers to benefits in terms of wellbeing, good health and civil engagement which are generated through the interactions between people' (Graham *et al.* 2009: 3). Significantly, the authors point out that social capital is expressed in different forms. 'Bonding' capital provides an exclusive, intra-group transaction, as opposed to 'bridging' and 'linking' capital generated through links between different groups. The report concludes with a call to action, a desire to see the development of new methodologies that explore the inter-relationship between historic environment, sense of place and social capital.

In many ways, the Between the Barrows project attempted to explore these interconnections, developing benefits in terms of individual and community well-being, and attempting to build bridging and linking capital between two juxtaposed but very different communities. It proved difficult to demonstrate that this form of community bridging had occurred, and I believe it will take several years of activity to get close to seeing this process in action. However, the feedback from the project revealed personal connections with the landscape and the past, suggesting that for some, a strong sense of place was formed to the degree that one could argue some participants sensed a 'spirit of place'. The bridging and linking capital manifested itself as a form of gratitude, and this sense of social capital and the nature of the gift seemed to also link into a perception of the historic and natural environment as a gift; a gift from nature and a gift from the past. This suggests to me that the exploration of 'gift' as a concept could provide the elusive interconnectivity for future studies on sense of place, social capital and historic environment.

Conclusion

The evaluation methodology for the project took its inspiration from heritage industry evaluation techniques. It relied on a project plan that accepted a dilution of professional authority, where the experiential and social outcomes were prioritized above the 'hard science' to be provided through archaeological excavation. This is not to say that professional standards or expectations were compromised, but it did require a reassessment of resources, including the additional time and energy needed to work responsibly with schools and community groups. Benefits such as well-being and therapeutic potentials have been tentatively acknowledged, but will be even more thoroughly evidenced as the project continues. The desire to explore these further has led me to a point in my own active planning where I have become aware of the need to apply a number of key principles in my community engagement work. These include the need to proactively engage in community conversations, employ constructivist philosophies and seek connectivity across landscapes and timescapes.

Ultimately, the community responses garnered through evaluation of the Between the Barrows project revealed a clear connection with place. Indeed, an almost 'spiritual' experience was described in some instances, where the environment comprising (in Sheldrake's terms) a 'more than human' landscape, but including a presence of the past, seemed to enable connection with a deeper sense of place. In terms of the healing agenda, members of two very divergent communities met and worked across this landscape during two seasons of excavation, School children from the local area took part in activities in a location that had previously been open to vandalism and abuse. The project is incomplete, but plans are being made to continue with the excavation over the next few years. It is hoped that, as the project continues, a more rigorous approach to understanding notions of sense of place and perhaps even spirit of place can be employed. This can be achieved through developing project methodologies that call on sense of place, social capital and historic environment research, enabling research outcomes that demonstrate the interrelationship between these concepts, and enhancing the community and individual well-being of all of those living around the Harmony Woods site.

Bibliography

AHRC 2018. Sense of place: Exploring nature and wellbeing through the non-visual senses [Webpage]. Viewed 5 December 2018, <https://gtr.ukri.org/projects?ref=AH%2FR009678%2F1>.

APPGAHW 2017. Creative health: The arts for health and wellbeing [Webpage]. Viewed 5 December 2018, <http://www.artshealthandwellbeing.org.uk/appg-inquiry/>.

Arts Council England 2014. Inspiring learning for all [Webpage]. Viewed 5 December 2018, <http://www.artscouncil.org.uk/about-ilfa-0>.

Arts Council England 2018. Arts culture and wellbeing [Webpage]. Viewed 5 December 2018, <https://www.artscouncil.org.uk/how-we-make-impact/arts-culture-and-wellbeing>.

ATU 2018. Working together to create woodland for the benefit of all [Website]. Viewed 5 December 2018, <https://www.andovertrees.org.uk>.

Bateson, G. 1972. *Steps to an ecology of mind.* New York: Ballantine.

Butler, T. 2017. Museums 2020 column. The Museums Association [Webpage]. Viewed 5 December 2018, <http://www.museumsassociation.org/campaigns/museums2020/m2020-tony-butler>.

Chaterjee, H. J. (ed.) 2008, *Touch in museums: Policy and practice in object handling.* Oxford: Berg.

Copeland, T. 2005. Constructing pasts: Interpreting the historic environment, in A. Hems and M. Blockley (eds.) *Heritage interpretation*: 83–96. London: Routledge.

Csikszentmihalyi, M. 1990. *Flow: The psychology of optimal experience.* London: Harper & Row.

Davies, C.A. 2008. *Reflexive ethnography: A guide to researching selves and others* (Second edition). Abingdon: Routledge.

DCMS 2012, *Taking part: The National Survey of Culture, Leisure and Sport Adult and Child report 2011/2012.* London: Department for Culture Media and Sport.

Dillon, C., N. Bell, K., Fouseki, P. Laurenson, A. Thompson and M. Strlic 2014. Mind the gap: Rigour and relevance in collaborative heritage science research. *Heritage Science* 2(11): 1–22.

Elmer, C. 2015. Lego and zombies: Finding the perfect heritage partner. *Journal of Museum Education* 36: 51–2.

Elmer, C. 2017a. 'A Sustainable Feel': Heritage, austerity and the pedagogical predicament. Unpublished PhD dissertation, University of Southampton.

Elmer, C. 2017b. 'How did it go?' Evaluating success for archaeological educators and other group leaders, in M. Ritchie (ed.) *Outdoor archaeological learning. An outdoor learning resource for teachers for excellence level 2*: 71–73. Edinburgh: Forestry Commission Scotland.

Falk, J.H. and L.D. Dierking 2007. *In principle, in practice: Museums as learning institutions.* Lanham, Maryland: AltaMira.

Freeman, D. 2012. *Art's emotions: Ethics, expression and aesthetic experience.* London: Routledge.

Gardner, H. 1983. *Frames of mind: The theory of multiple intelligences.* New York: Basic Books.

Graham, H., R. Mason and A. Newman 2009. *Literature review: Historic environment, sense of place and social capital. Commissioned for English Heritage.* Newcastle upon Tyne: International Centre for Cultural and Heritage Studies. Newcastle University.

Hampshire Life 2017. The remarkable story of Enham Alamein [Webpage]. Viewed 5 December 2018, <http://www.hampshire-life.co.uk/out-about/places/the-remarkable-story-of-enham-alamein-1-5249478>.

Hein, G.E. 1998. *Learning in the museum.* London: Routledge.

Helm, D. 2015. *Natural capital: Valuing our planet.* New Haven: Yale University Press.

Hewison, R. 2014. *Cultural capital: The rise and fall of creative Britain.* London: Verso.

Hewison, R. and J. Holden 2014. *Turbulent times: The prospects for heritage. A provocation.* London: Heritage Lottery Fund.

Holden, J. 2006. *Cultural value and the crisis of legitimacy.* London: DEMOS.

Jorge, V.O. 2008. Archaeological excavation as ('artistic') performance: Dissolving some unnecessary boundaries between art and science for the sake of knowledge, in. J. Thomas and V.O. Jorge (eds.) *Archaeology and the politics of vision in a post-modern context:* 76–100. Newcastle upon Tyne: Cambridge Scholars Publishing.

Kolb, D.A. 1984. *Experiential learning; Experience as the source of learning and development.* New Jersey: Prentice Hall.

Marsden, P. 2014. *Rising ground: A search for the spirit of place.* London: Granta.

Mauss, M. 1990. *The gift: The form and reason for exchange in archaic societies.* London: Routledge.

Mental Health Foundation 2015. What is wellbeing, how can we measure it and how can we support people to improve it? [Blog]. Viewed 5 December 2018, <https://www.mentalhealth.org.uk/blog/what-wellbeing-how-can-we-measure-it-and-how-can-we-support-people-improve-it>.

Morris Hargreaves McIntyre 2005. *Never mind the width feel the quality. Museums and Heritage Show research report* [Online document]. Manchester and Worcester: Morris Hargreaves McIntyre and The Museums & Heritage Show Ltd. Viewed 5 December 2018, <https://mhminsight.com/files/never-mind-the-width-Tw57-68-5093.pdf>.

NT 2017. *Places that make us: Research report* [Online document]. Swindon: NT. Viewed 5 December 2018, <https://www.nationaltrust.org.uk/documents/places-that-make-us-research-report.pdf>.

Palmer, H. 2017. Fourfold vision in practice: Data, theory, intuition and the art of therapy. *Human Systems* 28 (1): 21–39.

Rose, E.J. 1964. 'Mental forms creating': 'Fourfold vision' and the poet as prophet in Blake's designs and verse. *The Journal of Aesthetics and Art Criticism* 23(2): 173–83.

Sheldrake, R.S. 2017. *Science and spiritual practices.* London: Hodder and Stoughton.

Stagg, G. 2018. *The crossway.* London: Picador.

World Economic Forum 2017. Special Address by Theresa May, Prime Minister of the United Kingdom [Online video]. Viewed 5 December 2018, <https://www.weforum.org/events/world-economic-forum-annual-meeting-2017/sessions/special-address-by-theresa-may-prime-minister-of-the-united-kingdom>.

YouTube 2016. Between the Barrows archaeology dig 2016[Online video]. Viewed 5 December 2018, <https://www.youtube.com/watch?v=dBt9YRMaN_o>.

Chapter 16

The Roman Baths: A place of recovery

Paul Murtagh

Abstract

A Roman bathhouse near Glasgow, Scotland, was the site chosen to trial a project called Recovery through Heritage (RtH). This provided a convenient archaeological case study through which to explore ideas of historical well-being, demonstrating the benefits that archaeology can bring to recovery work. The project was run with partners— Phoenix Futures a charity that supports individuals with alcohol and drug problems; and Northlight Heritage — as part of the Clyde and Avon Valley Landscape Partnership (CAVLP) supported by the Heritage Lottery Fund (HLF) and Historic Environment Scotland (HES). It piloted a project that worked with service users to design a heritage trail, enhance archaeological sites and help out on archaeological digs, focusing on the Roman bathhouse at Strathclyde Park, Motherwell, North Lanarkshire, Scotland. A range of activities resulted in the successful completion of the project, including positive outcomes for the service users, the wider community, and ourselves as practitioners. This paper outlines the ways in which the Recovery through Heritage project developed, describing the archaeological and recovery outcomes achieved, the problems and challenges that were encountered, and how these were overcome. The paper also explores the ways in which current archaeological theory influences the delivery of community focused heritage projects, and how theory is deployed in daily professional practice.

Keywords: Assemblage; Emergent; Process; Outcomes; Recovery

Introduction

This paper outlines the processes and methodologies developed during a trial project delivered as part of the Clyde and Avon Valley Landscape Partnership (CAVLP) called: Recovery though Heritage (RtH). The project was developed alongside Phoenix Futures, a charity that works with individuals with drug and alcohol problems, and focused on the development of a heritage trial in North Lanarkshire, Scotland. Participants were engaged in trail development, historical research, archaeological site enhancement, and path maintenance. By the end of the year-long project a heritage trail had been completed; this was one of the key output milestones for the HLF-supported programme. It will, however, be argued here that, whilst this output was important, it was the process and associated outcomes of the project that had a more important and lasting impact — for well-being, for the participants, and for the historic environment.

Additionally this paper will explore how current archaeological theory influences the delivery of both this type of project and daily heritage practice. It will be argued that by recognizing our current theoretical frameworks within which we as practitioners operate, and the ways in which they can be deployed in our daily professional practice, we can begin to approach our work in new, exciting, socially engaged ways. The case study outlined in this paper in particular allows us to explore how projects and project outputs, such as the heritage trails, in fact emerge from a series of relationships between humans and non-humans. These take the form of archaeological sites, paths, vegetation, tools and equipment, software packages, funding bodies, project frameworks and method statements, project partners, service users, archaeologists, and landscapes.

The Clyde and Avon Valley Landscape Partnership

Recovery through Heritage formed part of the Local Landscape Heroes project, itself part of the Clyde and Avon Valley Landscape Partnership Heritage programme, delivered by Northlight Heritage for the CAVLP. CAVLP was a major five year HLF-funded programme that ran from 2013 to 2018. Itdelivered70 projects, with the CAVLP Heritage programme, supported by Historic Environment Scotland (HES), delivering seven of these projects. Northlight Heritage was one of ten partners in the Landscape Partnership. This also included North and South Lanarkshire Councils, Central Scotland Green Network, New Lanark World Heritage Site, The Rural Development Trust, RSPB Scotland, Scottish Natural Heritage, Scottish Wildlife Trust, and Clydesdale Community Initiatives.

The Landscape Partnership area focused on the Clyde and Avon Valleys, located just southeast of Glasgow, Scotland, and was based around four key themes; to conserve the built and natural heritage of the area, to increase community participation and landscape connection, to improve access to and learning about the landscape and heritage, and to provide new training opportunities in local heritage skills (CAVLP 2011).The partnership is also aligned to the Scottish Government's Strategic Objectives for a 'Wealthier and Fairer, Smarter, Healthier, Safer, Stronger and Greener' country(Scottish Government 2018). All HLF-funded Landscape Partnerships are designed to deliver to the European Landscape Convention (HLF 2007: 3).

The Local Landscape Heroes project celebrated the people that had shaped or been inspired by the Clyde and Avon Valleys, from artists to farmers, both historical figures and those who continue to change or be inspired by the landscape today. The idea of the project was that it should focus on celebrating the lives of ordinary people, rather than famous historical figures. Working with volunteers and groups that would not normally engage in archaeology and heritage, the aims of the Local Landscape Heroes project were to:

- Undertake archive research on the people and places relating to Local Landscape Heroes;
- Involve volunteers in a programme of fieldwork to identify, record, assess and understand archaeological sites and the historic environments;
- Inform future archaeological strategies, enhance the protection and understanding of the landscape, and the sites within it and contribute to HER enhancement data; and
- Share and celebrate the significance of people and historic environment which contributes to the perception and character of the landscape of the CAVLP area.

When designing the project it was envisaged that there would be two key outcomes. The first was to help form greater understanding and appreciation of the ways in which people have shaped the character and perception of the Clyde and Avon Valleys. The second was to broaden intellectual and physical access to the heritage of the Landscape Partnership area. There were also two key outputs for the project: an exhibition; and the Local Landscape Heroes Heritage Trail.

Alongside volunteers recruited from the local area, the key audiences for this particular CAVLP Heritage project were people and groups that would not normally engage with, or have access to, archaeology and heritage. One group that we approached to participate in the project was Phoenix Futures, a charity supporting people with addiction problems. Phoenix Futures run a number of support initiatives across the UK, including their Recovery through Nature (Hall

2004) programme. This programme connects people using their services with nature, to aid in their recovery by working as part of a team on practical conservation projects in settings across England and Scotland. Research carried out by Phoenix Futures demonstrated that participants in Recovery through Nature (RtN) programme had:

> '…improved retention in treatment by 55 per cent and its participants are 44 per cent more likely to successfully complete their program compared with those who do not do RtN. Indeed, initial in-service analysis noted a 10 per cent improvement in physical and emotional health for those who took part in RtN. Service users have self-reported rediscovering themselves through nature and having increased motivation for recovery and a developed sense of self- worth, self-confidence, and self-awareness'. (Aslan 2016: 94)

By aligning our project to this already successful programme, we piloted RtH. This aimed to explore how archaeology and heritage could be used to help with recovery work, within the framework of the Local Landscape Heroes CAVLP project and with an objective of creating a heritage trail. Phoenix Futures have been working in this part of Scotland for a number of years, carrying out general environmental conservation activities as well as delivering enhancements to historical and archaeological sites and features. There has been particular focus around the garden and designed landscape of Dalzell Estate, Motherwell. This is a public park owned and operated by North Lanarkshire Council, and part-managed by RSPB Scotland who manage the adjacent Baron's Haugh Nature Reserve. Working with the Countryside Ranger Service and RSPB Scotland, Phoenix Futures have been helping enhance many of the historical features of the designed garden and landscape, including the preservation and enhancement of sections of a ha-ha wall, and the erection of a notice board explaining this important landscape feature to visitors. In addition, vegetation was cleared back from other parts of the estate so that the original landscape futures could be seen more clearly.

To Phoenix Futures, the North Lanarkshire Countryside Rangers, and the RSPB wardens — as well as our other nature focused partners in the Landscape Partnership — this kind of site enhancement is solely seen as a part of traditional ecological conservation work. However, by considering the natural and historic environments in a more holistic way, and in particular as assemblages of people, places, and things (Deleuze and Guattari 2004), we have the opportunity to refocus traditional understanding of such conservation work. The view becomes one that perceives both natural and cultural heritage as indistinguishable parts of a symbiotic relationship, contributing equally to the character of our landscapes. By approaching the landscape and its conservation in this way we can potentially better engage and work with natural heritage charities, new audiences, and groups of people who would not normally show interest in the historic environment. Furthermore, it allows us to deliver on wider national historic environment and archaeology strategies such as *Our Place in Time* (The Scottish Government 2014) and the *Scottish Archaeological Strategy* (HES 2015). These focus on not only the preservation and understanding of archaeological sites and landscapes, but also on specifically on sharing and celebrating archaeology for everyone.

The process

Setting up such a project takes time and involves a significant number of meetings, emails, and phone calls. Establishing a working partnership with another organization requires trust, skill, a bit of luck, and a lot of flexibility and compromise. The partnership that we struck up with Phoenix Futures emerged from a series of relations that were already established through the Landscape Partnership and its delivery partners, but it was also established through seeing mutual opportunities to deliver each of our organization's aims, objectives, and outcomes.

Before we settled on a programme of work, we had a series of onsite discussions with the various stakeholders. These concerned the project's aims and objectives, the desired outputs and outcomes, and how these could be aligned with the Phoenix Futures RtN programme. The outcomes and outputs also needed to align with the needs of the North Lanarkshire Ranger Service and the green spaces they manage. We decided that the work would initially concentrate on the enhancement of the Roman bathhouse in Strathclyde Park, Motherwell, North Lanarkshire. This site is a Scheduled Monument, excavated in the 1970s (Keppie 1981; RCAHMS 1978: 119–121 (No.250) and fig. 73), and partially reconstructed in the 1980s in a slightly different location because of the threat of rising flood water from the nearby man-made loch. The baths lie down slope from a Roman fort (Maxwell 1975; RCAHMS 1978:121), one of several in the area forming part of a network of Roman military bases used during the invasion of Scotland during the Antonine period of the mid-second century AD. Before the project took place, the bathhouse had fallen into a state of disrepair and was a common site of vandalism and antisocial behaviour. Trees and vegetation grew across much of the site, and

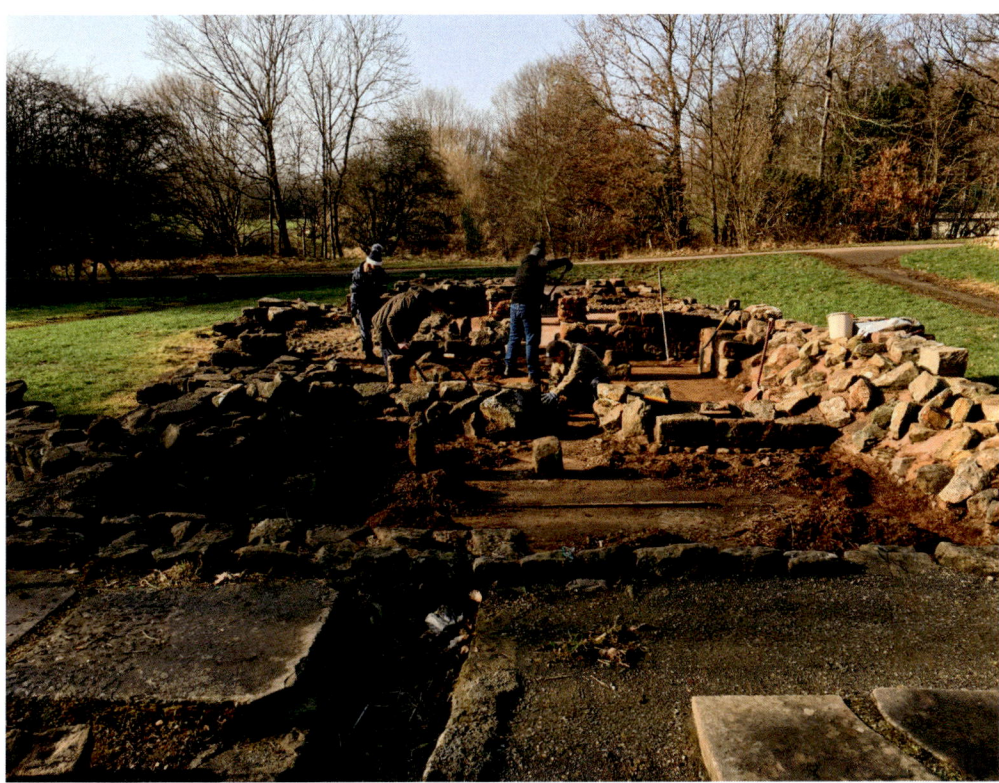

Figure 16.1 Participants from Phoenix Futures replacing fallen stones at the Strathclyde Park Roman Bathhouse. (Photograph by Paul Murtagh. Copyright reserved)

many of the walls had been damaged. Despite this, it was still actively used by local schools as a place to engage pupils in learning about the Romans. In addition to the site enhancement work, we envisaged that the participants would also take part in workshops in the local archives to identify important local people and historical sites that could be used to help inform the heritage trail. In addition, it was anticipated that they would participate in trail design workshops. However, the activities that emerged were not quite what we originally planned and did not necessarily align with our original project design.

Over several weeks, we cleared the bathhouse site of vegetation and rubbish, gathering up all the fallen stones and re-mortaring a number of them back into their original positions (Figure 16.1). During this time we also started to discuss the idea of the heritage trail with service users, how their work could contribute to such a thing, and what that would mean to them. Building on these conversations we began extensive walks across the landscape, exploring what the service users thought a heritage trail should look like, where it should go, what areas it should or should not include, how many sites or points of interest should be included, and how we would communicate the route to the public. The potential routes initially focused on the sites and places that the group had enhanced over the years around Dalzell Estate, and also looked at many of the archaeological sites in the area. By walking these routes, we came across several places, sites, historical features, and paths which the group found interesting or thought worthy of inclusion in the trail. We also identified a number of sites and paths needing further enhancement work, such as vegetation clearance and path maintenance.

During this time we also undertook a research session at the local library archives. The aim of this session was introducing the service users to online archaeological and historical research, and to start them considering the Local Landscape Heroes who would be celebrated within the trail. Unfortunately, this last element of the project did not work well. We had envisaged that the service users would be more involved in the research element, but it quickly became clear that this was not going to be possible due to the skillsets and educational history of the majority of the group. Many participants had secondary school-level academic experience which had either been negative for them or had not included a requirement for research. Many had limited IT skills which hampered their ability to access, organize, and present information. Whilst one or two of the participants enjoyed this aspect of the work, many were visibly —and indeed vocally—frustrated with this workshop; as might be imagined, this was not a fun or positive element of the project. However, this was not the fault of the service users; it was very much a problem with the design of this element of the project and the way it was structured. It can be argued that in general, as archaeologists, many of us are trained within further and higher academic institutions to think and practice in a particular way. Here, formal research and research processes are seen as important elements of a coherent and successful project. It is also a practice that many of us enjoy and do not consider daunting. However, within a community setting, particularly when working with audiences who have a range of abilities and previous experiences, this rather academic approach is just not suitable. The problem was compounded in that one of the main aims of the project outlined in our project method statement was specifically to broaden intellectual access to the heritage of the area. Our funders therefore expected us to deliver to this, and we were under pressure to carry out the project in a particular way. In the end, this element of the project did not emerge the way we had envisaged and it was unfortunate that many of the service users did not feel able to participate in this element as much as they might have. Given more time and a clearer structure, this element may have worked. However, due to commitments made to funders, specifically the need to produce an output on time and to a required standard (so that we could be paid), this was not possible. In the end it was left to our team to carry out much of the research element of the project.

Despite the issues encountered, the service users continued to enjoy the site enhancement work, particularly around the bathhouse, as well as along the trail itself and many of the paths in the area. Towards the end of the process, with the route and the sites established, our Digital Heritage Assistant began to design the leaflet and the trail markers. They took ideas and suggestions from the service users, some of whom engaged in a design sessions with us. Throughout this time John, the Phoenix Futures facilitator and project manager, managed the atmosphere of the sessions. He already had strong relationships with the service users, having spent a lot of time with them on a regular basis. He gave them stability in the sessions and made it easier for us to work with the group. The trail was officially launched in early December 2017 by the Lord Provost of North Lanarkshire, with the service users, local schools, funders, and press all in attendance (CAVLP 2018).

An emergent trail

Focussing on the process we went through in the creation of the heritage trail, helps to demonstrate how the trail in fact emerged from a series of relationships. Our relationship with the sites as we encountered and worked on them, the landscape as we walked, explored and negotiated it, between the service users and the work that they carried out, and our knowledge and experience as archaeologists and facilitators. This kind of emergent creative process is something conceptualized by new materialist ideas that see non-humans, such as objects or landscapes, as active agents in the production of relations and not merely as their outcomes (Conneller 2011; Harris and Cipolla 2017: chapter 8). The trail, as an assemblage of people, places, and things, emerged from the ways in which we and the service users engaged with non-human agents as we encountered them and entered into relations with them, through what Bennet (2010) would call 'the vibrancy of matter'. Bennett also suggests that:

> '...this is not a world of subjects and objects, but one of various materialities constantly engaged in a network of relations. It is a world populated less by individuals than by groupings that shift over time'. (Bennet 2010: 20)

This allows us to see how through 'the engagement of people and materials, with specific properties, memories and experiences that each of them bring, can lead to the emergence of new kinds of assemblages' (Harris and Cipolla 2017: 143), and that the vibrant agency of places, landscapes, and objects actively produce and help create new assemblages—or in this case, a heritage trail.

At the beginning of the process, we did not plan for the trail to go along a particular route, or for any particular sites along the route to be included in it. Instead, the trail emerged from our engagement with the sites as we enhanced them and worked on them, and as we walked across the landscape along paths and routes, encountering interesting places along the way. Their agency affected our choices, decisions, and process of work, meaning that we entered into, or formed, active emerging relationships with each other — we therefore

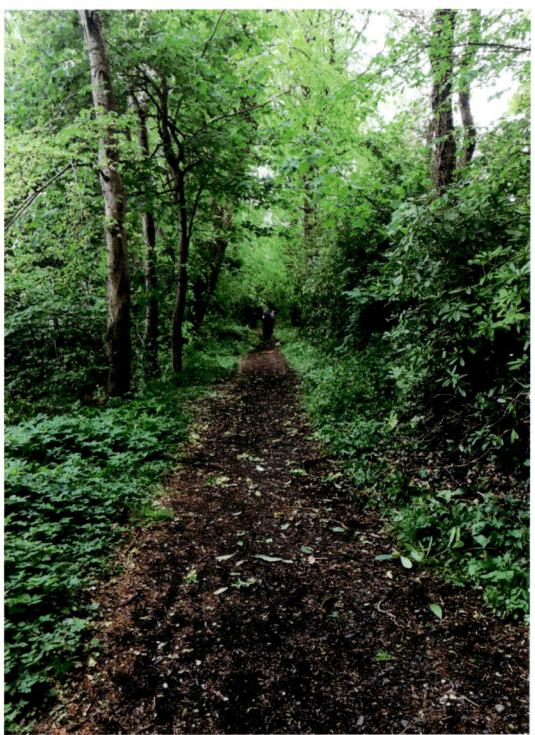

Figure 16.2 The trail emerging as we clear vegetation from the path. (Photograph by Paul Murtagh. Copyright reserved)

formed an 'assemblage' of service users, archaeologists, archaeological sites, paths, trails, and landscapes (Figure 16.2). It was through these emergent relations — between human and non-human co-creators — that the trail materialized or was assembled in the way it did, taking its particular form.

This emergent creative process is very much at odds with the way a heritage project would typically and consciously be carried out, and its outputs created. This reflects not least the framework within which the majority, if not all, community heritage and archaeology projects take place. Here, the measure of success is through the outputs created and the number of people engaged. Instead, this paper demonstrates an alternative process. It shows that by approaching a project in an open way, with co-creation between archaeologists, participants, and non-human elements at its core, a new methodology or form of practice can emerge. A methodology that sees the process itself and its outcomes as being the most important elements of a community project. For us, these were about connecting people to landscape, increasing physical and intellectual access to the heritage of the Clyde and Avon Valley, and about helping people with recovery.

Outcomes for Participants

People with drug and alcohol problems are usually treated by society in less than positive ways. They are often characterized as a homogeneous group of weak-willed, unsuccessful, people who are dangerous wasters and not worth much in social terms. The reality is that these individuals, who have had some difficult life histories often tied to mental health problems, can be supported to recovery. By working with Phoenix Futures we were able to help their service users engage with heritage and archaeology in a meaningful way. This was a positive experience for them as individuals, but it has also left a legacy for the historic environment though the better interpretation and management of a number of archaeological and historical sites. As a result, the wider public can now enjoy and experience it in more informed and positive ways (Figure 16.3).

A small quantitative survey about the project was undertaken with the service users, the results of which demonstrated the positive impact of the project and how well it was received by each of the participants. Evaluation also took the form of interviews, some of which can be

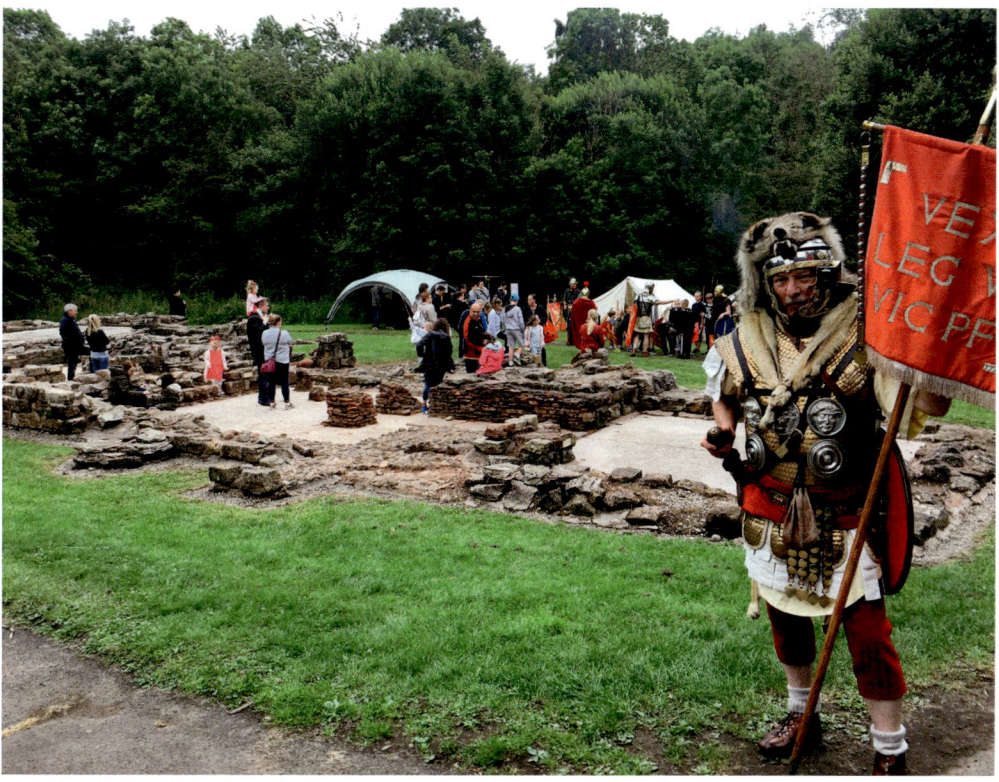

Figure 16.3 A public engagement event at the Strathclyde Park Roman bathhouse with members of the Antonine Guard. (Photograph by Paul Murtagh. Copyright reserved)

viewed online (CAVLP Heritage 2017). These demonstrate very powerfully the benefits that an archaeological and heritage project can bring to a recovery programme. When asked about the project and how it benefitted them, all of the responses were positive. One service user, Derek, stated that:

'I've learnt new skills …working to put a bit back into the community' and that he had 'worked in a team and that's helped.'

Another service user, Roy, said that:

'It's a great programme we're on because: A, it keeps you busy; and B, we've learnt a hell of a lot … I've got into things like archaeology…. it's really interesting and you just don't know what's on your back door and that's educating my grandsons so the spin off benefits are really good, plus the people you get to meet.'

These responses portray some of the more general outcomes of the project, including skills development and team working which are often seen as being important indicators of a successful engagement programme. However, some of the other outcomes were identified by the service users as being of equal importance. These centred around the social aspects of the project, such as meeting people and talking to each other. This was also reflected on a follow up project in 2018 when Phoenix Futures service users took part in excavations as part of the Northlight Heritage and University of Glasgow fieldschool. Again feedback from the service users was very positive. However, one of the most striking points was made by the Phoenix Futures coordinator Kenny, who said that:

> 'The benefits of this kind of work is phenomenal and it's a brilliant motivator for people. There are service users here that are socially isolated and whose social skills are poor but without prompting they are talking to students and interacting really well. That is a huge positive for that person.'

The highlight for Kenny was not the fact that the service users had learnt different skills, or been involved with archaeology or created a heritage trail; it was more that the service users were having a good time, and that they were socializing with each other as well as the students and other volunteers on site. It is significant that this kind of outcome can be achieved for an individual who might have social anxieties or other mental health problems. It highlights the positive impact on a person's well-being that can arise from working on an archaeological site or engaging in a heritage project. However, it also highlights quite powerfully that even this kind of small improvement in an individual's well-being is a major outcome for the project. This is a lesson for us as non-specialists in recovery or social work.

In terms of recovery, the work we carried out was only a small part of a much larger programme and journey that the service users are on, and a larger and longer term RtH project would have to be carried out to evaluate the effectiveness of such an approach. However, both Derek and Roy were positive about the impact that the project had on them. Derek stated that:

> '…it's definitely helped with the recovery side of it, and that's what it's all about. Getting people out, talking and working together and putting a wee bit back into the community … it's been good for me.'

Their views of archaeology in general were rather mixed, however. Roy was very positive and would recommend it to others, but Derek was a little more balanced. Asked if they 'would recommend archaeology to others?', Derek said:

> 'Oh aye, I'd give it a try, I enjoyed it, I'm not into doing these kind of things but I gave it a try and I enjoyed it, it was good … but I wouldn't like to do it for a living!'

Whilst our evaluation of the project allowed us some insights into the impact of the activities and their effectiveness in terms of promoting recovery, it remains rather limited because of the small size of the survey and the fact that the project was only a pilot. Further phases of RtH would have more robust monitoring and evaluation methodologies in place, so that the impact of such a project on people's lives could be properly measured. However, it is hoped that the evidence laid out here is useful as a guide for other practitioners, and that it demonstrates the ways in which the RtH pilot was worthwhile project that would benefit from funding to expand it in the future.

Conclusion

It is an irony of sorts that the site chosen as the focus of our RtH pilot project should be a Roman bathhouse. Roman bathhouses were public spaces; places where citizens shared publicly in bodily processes, enforcing an idea of the equality of the body (Fagan 2002: 213–214). After removing their clothes, bathers would usually undertake physical and mental exercise. After exercise, bathers would move through the hot rooms leading to the cold plunge pool, while oils would be used to cleanse the body (Fagan 2002: 10). Thus, a visit to the baths entailed exercise and rejuvenation for both the mind and the body; for the Romans, baths were linked to wider concepts of well-being (Bergdolt 2008: 77–79; Rotherham 2012: 22). The baths were regarded as restorative and therapeutic, with regular attendance seen as part of maintaining or recovering good health. The Strathclyde Park Roman Baths were a site of social and bodily equality that helped users maintain both mental and physical health. They were places of recovery, well-being, and transition: a fitting place to pilot our RtH project.

This paper has outlined the ways in which heritage projects can be influenced by current archaeological theory. Specifically, it has demonstrated the ways in which new materialist ideas are able to influence socially engaged heritage projects delivered with non-traditional audiences that have co-creation at their core. As such they recognize the importance of a range of co-producers, both human and non-human. It has also demonstrated that the process of co-creation is the most important element of such a project, and that aspects such as the archaeological or heritage outputs are secondary to the outcomes that might be reached for people and place. By approaching the RtH pilot project in the way we did we were able to test different methods of co-creation and be flexible in our approach to the changing circumstances — not least the ways in which we worked with the service users, responding to their needs and restrictions. More work needs to be done in order to develop the RtH approach. In particular, more should be done to analyse its long term effectiveness through longitudinal data sets, and the ways in which it can complement existing recovery strategies. Given the positive responses to the pilot project it is hoped that this work can continue in the future.

Acknowledgments

I would like to thank all of the service users from Phoenix Futures who took part in the project, especially Roy and Derek who agreed to help make the film that formed part of the presentation at TAG 2017. John from Phoenix Futures helped throughout the project, from its inception to the launch of the trail; it was inspiring to work with him and see his passion for recovery work. Hannah Cobb, Oliver Harris, and Gavin MacGregor helped me think through my ideas on theory and critical heritage practice and Gavin commented on an earlier draft of the paper. All of their comments and advice is very much appreciated. The project was funded by Historic Environment Scotland and the Heritage Lottery Fund.

Bibliography

Aslan, L. 2016. A qualitative evaluation of the Phoenix Futures Recovery through Nature Program: A therapeutic intervention for substance misuse. *Journal of Groups in Addiction & Recovery* 11(2): 93–108.
Bennett, B. 2010. *Vibrant matter: A political ecology of things.* Durham (NC): Duke University Press.
Bergdolt, K. 2008. *Wellbeing: A cultural history of healthy living.* Cambridge: Polity Press.
CAVLP 2011. *Clyde and Avon Valley Landscape Partnership landscape conservation action plan* [Online document]. Hamilton, Lanarkshire: CAVLP. Viewed 7 January 2019, <https://issuu.com/cavlp/docs/cavlp_lcap>.

CAVLP 2018. Local landscape heroes: Phoenix Futures trail, Motherwell [Online video]. Viewed 7 January 2019, <https://www.youtube.com/watch?v=o-kYuEjapS8>.

CAVLP Heritage 2017. Recovery through heritage [Online video]. Viewed 7 January 2019, <https://www.youtube.com/watch?v=bh7ETkQfk4k>.

Conneller, C. 2011. *An archaeology of materials: Substantial transformations in early prehistoric Europe.* London: Routledge.

Deleuze, G. and F. Guattari 2004. *A thousand plateaus: Capitalism and schizophrenia.* London: Continuum.

Fagan, G.G. 2002. *Bathing in public in the Roman world.* Ann Arbor: The University of Michigan Press.

Hall, J. 2004. *Phoenix House Therapeutic Conservation Programme: Underpinning theory. English Nature Research Reports. Report Number 611.* York: English Nature.

Harris, O.J.T. and G.N. Cipolla 2017. *Archaeological theory in the new millennium: Introducing current perspectives.* London: Routledge.

HES 2015. Scotland's archaeology strategy [Website]. Viewed 7 January 2019, <http://archaeologystrategy.scot>.

HLF 2007. *Landscape partnerships, application guidance* [Online document]. London: HLF. Viewed 7 January 2019, <https://closedprogrammes.hlf.org.uk/lp_application_guidance.pdf>.

Keppie, L.J.F. 1981. Excavation of a Roman bathhouse at Bothwellhaugh, 1975–76. *Glasgow Archaeological Journal* 8: 46–94.

Maxwell, G.S. 1975. Excavation at the Roman fort of Bothwellhaugh, Lanarkshire 1967-8. *Britannia* 6: 20–35.

RCAHMS 1978. *The Royal Commission on the Ancient and Historical Monuments of Scotland. Lanarkshire: An Inventory of the Prehistoric and Roman Monuments.* Edinburgh: RCAHMS.

Rotherham, I.D. 2012. *Roman baths in Britain.* Stroud: Amberley Publishing.

Scottish Government 2014. *Our Place in Time — The Historic Environment Strategy for Scotland.* Edinburgh: Scottish Government.

Scottish Government 2018. Strategic objectives [Webpage]. Viewed 7 January 2019, <https://www2.gov.scot/About/Performance/scotPerforms/objectives>.

Chapter 17

'The People Before Us' Project: Exploring heritage and well-being in a rapidly changing seaside town

Lesley Hardy and Eleanor Williams

Abstract

Illuminated in Folkestone's Creative Quarter stands the text-sculpture 'heaven is a place where nothing ever happens', encapsulating, some commentators note, the ennui of seaside towns. The words are, however, deceptive — Folkestone is evolving rapidly, partly fuelled by funding to regenerate through the arts. Whilst many are embracing this surge of creative development, such change can inevitably lead to anxiety and feelings of alienation for others. In June 2017 a small team from Canterbury Christ Church University, Kent, led a ten-day community graveyard survey at the Church of St Mary and St Eanswythe in the heart of historic Folkestone. The experience and outcomes were revealing — and at times unexpected — offering insight into both the significance of this 'hidden' place, and also the importance of small-scale heritage projects such as this for communities in transition. Immersing — not imposing — ourselves in the daily life of the site also provided a platform for communication with the many individuals and groups who have taken ownership over it, some of whom face significant social challenges. This paper will discuss some of our experiences and project outcomes, and reflect on the potential importance of historical sites such as these — and our uses of them — for well-being.

Keywords: Churchyard; Community project; Folkestone; Graveyard survey; Regeneration

Introduction

The Church of St Mary and St Eanswythe once commanded an impressive position in the landscape, occupying a high point on Folkestone's eastern headland. Situated on the Bayle — Folkestone's historic centre — it is prominent from the sea, and a landmark from the ancient road that winds to the town from Dover. Depicted by Turner and Constable, the church stood as a beacon — a visibly integral part of the town's identity (Figure 17.1). Now, except by sea, it is all but invisible, concealed by the modern town. On the face of it, it is a place forgotten, with its network of churchyard paths providing convenient cut-throughs to the modern town. Despite its central location, in many ways it is set apart; the churchyard, where heritage encounters nature, offers refuge from the busy urban centre but also provides a 'concealed' space for antisocial behaviour including vandalism, drinking, and drug dealing. For certain community members it has a reputation as an unsafe place, with some expressing nostalgia for how it used to be. From the outside, however, one can miss — or undervalue — the significance that this historic place holds for many people, in countless different ways. Its antiquity resonates throughout the site and beyond; it is both part of the everyday, but also distinct and special.

Our own relationship with this place developed in June 2017 when we ran a ten-day graveyard survey, 'The People Before Us', ahead of the launch of an 18-month Heritage Lottery Fund (HLF) community project led by Canterbury Christ Church University. 'Finding Eanswythe' is exploring the 'life and after-life' of the town's patron saint, a seventh century AD Kentish

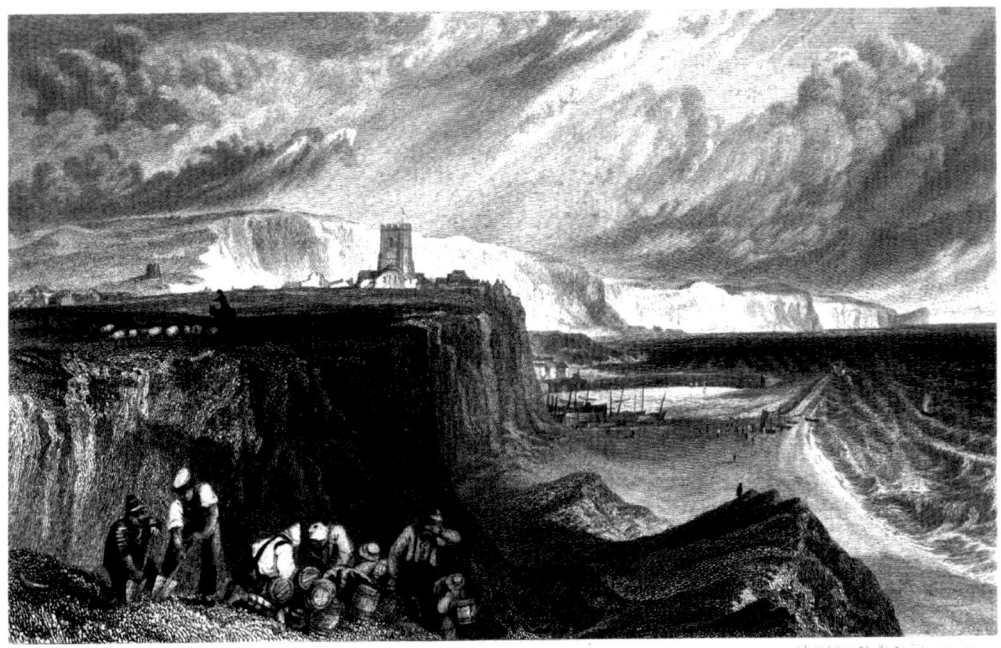

Figure 17.1 Folkestone, 1826, after Joseph Mallord William Turner (1775-1851), purchased 1988. (Photograph courtesy of Tate London, 2019. Copyright reserved)

princess whose relics, it is believed, survive within the church. The purpose of the broader project, however, was not purely to learn more about the history and heritage surrounding Eanswythe, but also to understand the meaning and significance of early heritage for a place in transition — one in which the community's connection and awareness of the past has been broken by extensive urban development. Folkestone is a complex place. Ancient, and significant over centuries (Coulson 2013), its identity has undergone radical re-inventions, arguably leaving a legacy of social division and community tension.

At the outset, 'The People Before Us' graveyard survey was envisaged in a fairly conventional sense. The churchyard is under threat from deterioration and vandalism; memorials have been toppled, broken or graffitied. Litter and drug paraphernalia (kept at bay through the perseverance of volunteer church wardens) collect around particular meeting points. Identifying and recording conservation and environmental issues was thus one of our main purposes. We also aimed to support the local history of the site, and to start building awareness for the larger HLF project. Events and experience, however, led us to somewhat different — but also more valuable — outcomes. Our formal activities and informal interactions with a wide range of people who use — and inhabit — the place, offered insights into the importance of the site itself, and people's perceptions of it. This paper will discuss some of these experiences and outcomes, but it will also reflect on wider questions that arose. In particular, it will consider how places such as the churchyard of St Mary and St Eanswythe — these essentially overlooked 'pockets' of heritage space — could offer significant benefits to people's well-being. This is both in terms of their importance and meaning in their own right, and as valuable and accessible places to engage a diverse range of people in small-scale community heritage projects.

Folkestone: A place in transition

> '…a feeling of sadness creeps over the mind, that a place once so goodly, with its five churches, should, being gradually consumed by the sea, have sunk into poverty and obscurity, and be left, in the days even of its revived prosperity, without a historian or a history' (Mackie 1856: 1).

Like much of Folkestone's history, the Church and churchyard of St Mary and St Eanswythe are both central and overlooked. The current building dates to the twelfth century AD and is the most recent in a series of church buildings on, or near, the site associated with the saint. The early history of these foundations is obscure, but documentary records trace the location of a minster at Folkestone to before AD 716 (Richardson 2013: 70). Centuries earlier, the town was the site of important Iron Age and Roman activity; it developed as a vital point of contact with the continent, and as an affluent and prestigious holding throughout the Middle Ages and into the seventeenth century AD. This history is written in the landscape, archaeology, history and built environment of the town, for those who can read such signs. Antiquarians such as Leland, Camden, and Lambarde visited Folkestone (Hardy 2013), noting it as a place of deep antiquity where the remains of the past could be daily found (Camden 1607) and the bones of religious stuck out from the ancient churchyard — 'a morsel too hard for the teeth of time to consume' (Philipot 1659).

Such a vision would be almost impossible to most visitors today. The town's early history is largely subsumed under development and Folkestone now appears almost exclusively Victorian or Edwardian. Walking down the modern high street you can easily miss the entrance to the Bayle. The reasons for this are worth noting. From the mid-nineteenth century, investors led by the landowner Lord Radnor oversaw a planned transformation of the town into a luxury health resort, largely for rich tuberculosis patients (Arnold 2013). By the 1880s, Folkestone had become a prosperous place as described by H.G. Wells in his novel 'Kipps' (1905). Written into this planned urban landscape were significant social divisions. Postcards show Edwardian ladies promenading along spacious walkways; these were privately policed and inaccessible to the poor and to the numerous migrant workers of the town. Most of these people lived in cramped, older housing in Folkestone's east end, under the shadow of the ancient headland of the Bayle and its church. These patterns of changing identity were not simply about the visibility of the past but about the triumph of new identities, closely linked to economic growth. This erasure of the early history of the town has been somehow consolidated by recent enthusiasm for its nineteenth and twentieth century identity; a fondness for past affluence stands almost in defiance of the town's serious economic decline, beginning with the closure of the harbour in the 1980s. Folkestone Harbour Ward, where the church is located, suffers from nationally high levels of deprivation (KCC 2015) and its roads of comfortable villas are sub-divided into flats, many of which show signs of deterioration.

More recent changes have added another layer of identity to the town. Since the 1990s, property development and contemporary arts have been combined with the aim of increasing visitor numbers and regenerating the town. A 'Creative Quarter' has materialized amongst the old lanes, and brightly coloured materials are now layered on top of the fascias of old buildings,

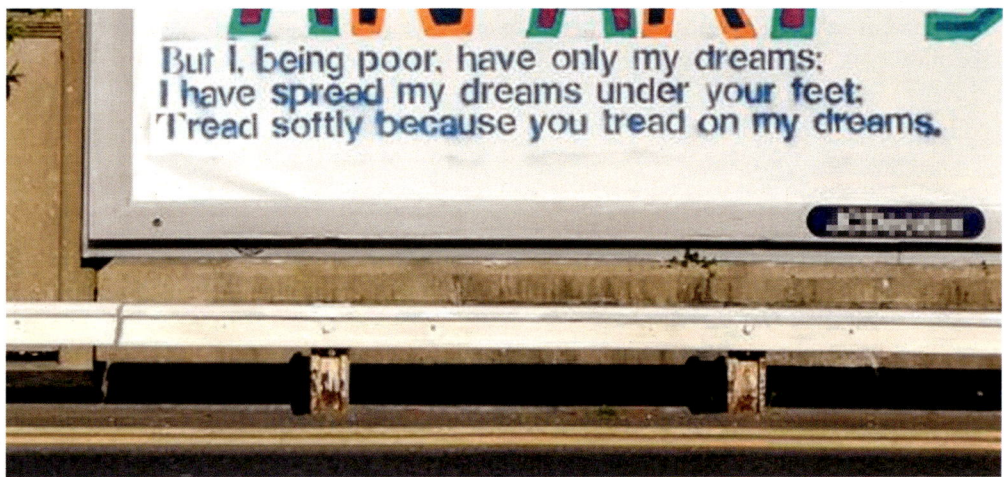

*Figure 17.2 A graffitied poster from Folkestone's Triennial Arts Festival
(Photograph by Lesley Hardy. Copyright reserved)*

like new clothes. This latest development has left its own distinctive mark, as yet another reinvention of the town and its communities. Whilst many are embracing this change, there are complex social challenges that bring into question its impact on community cohesion, and people's sense of place and belonging. These are inextricably linked to well-being, and heritage could play an important role in addressing such issues (DCMS 2016; HE 2017; HLF 2015; Reilly *et al.* 2018). This graffitied poster from Folkestone's recent Triennial Arts Festival bears the words from a poem by Yeats (Figure 17.2), expressing some of the feelings of anguish arguably linked to these changes.

Sitting within all of this, St Mary and St Eanswythe's churchyard is a place of liminality, of transition, where you can quite literally step between the old and new parts of the town. It is also a place with a residual sense of the past, marked in the historic building fabric of the church and its boundary walls. Even the town cross, re-built on the original medieval steps, is still a regular meeting place for people from all walks of life. It was only through spending time there that we began to appreciate the various ways in which people draw meaning and benefit from this place.

The 'People Before Us': A graveyard survey

When 'The People Before Us' was first conceived of, we had what was, in some respects, a traditional agenda. Graveyard surveys have been used as a tool by individuals and local and family history societies for many years. Fundamentally they are an exercise in recording and conserving, for which numerous guides and handbooks have been produced (e.g. HE 2011; Mytum 2000). They are an excellent and relatively low cost means of engaging community members in exploring and understanding local heritage, for highlighting conservation issues, and for producing a permanent record of social data for future research. At the outset, our project aimed to build on this. We also saw it as an opportunity to bring people together from different communities, and more broadly, to start conversations about the heritage of the town and its significance.

A formal call for participants was met with a reasonable response, and over the ten day period, groups and individuals joined us who were as diverse as local historical societies, military veterans, church members and primary school children, as well as a broad range of people from Folkestone and beyond. Some took part for the whole duration and others participated when they could. Numbers ebbed and flowed, but generally ranged from between seven to 15 at any given time. Our formal, structured activities included updating plans of gravestone and memorial positions across the six churchyard zones, and capturing a basic written (e.g. gravestone inscription, material, sculpture/symbols, damage etc.) and photographic record. Towards the end of the second day, however, it was apparent that progress was slow. This was for a range of reasons including the time needed to set up each day, clear litter, and train new people. The complexity of the heritage itself was also a key factor; many gravestones were poorly preserved and difficult to decipher. The rate of deterioration and change also became clear; reference to earlier surveys indicated that many stones had been moved, removed or crumbled away in recent years. Our experience of battling this inexorable decline and loss, combined with anxiety about completing our target to record the whole churchyard, seemed to create a particularly difficult dynamic. For whatever reason there was a discernible apprehension amongst some participants. In essence, this stemmed from a growing sense of unease and confusion over the project's expectations — and of those taking part — which we all shared. This changed one afternoon when we paused long enough to ask 'What are our priorities here?' It became apparent that we had not been approaching the project in the most effective way, missing the point in terms of participant and wider community engagement and enjoyment, but also in terms of our central purposes, and potential of the project.

Firstly, setting the distinct — and on reflection, unrealistic — targets, had placed unreasonable expectations on ourselves and the participants. The project began as task-focused, centred on achieving a distinct end-goal, rather than being about the process and experience of taking part. Such tensions surrounding 'obtainable goals' in community archaeology projects have been recognized elsewhere (Simpson 2009); there are underlying issues here relating to the strictures of funding and time that often characterize such heritage initiatives. Secondly, we erroneously assumed that people joined us to learn how to survey gravestones/memorials; we had not been explicit enough in asking what they wanted to do, were comfortable doing, and were hoping to gain from the experience. Thirdly, whilst engaging some members of the community (including those new to heritage projects) we quickly came to realize that others were being alienated. In response it seemed important to rethink the whole nature of participation; the boundaries between those inside and outside the project were much more porous than previously considered.

What emerged was that our sole focus on the formal participants, and the survey, had distracted us from the many others who have taken ownership over the site: the church-goers and wardens; the rough sleepers we would meet in the morning; the teenagers who congregate to socialize; the parents taking their children to school; those who 'pop in' to read, eat or even nap; and the passers-by and dog-walkers for whom the site is a staple within their daily routine. We had imposed ourselves on the place without really understanding how it functioned or how it was used. For some, our sudden presence was a source of resistance, perhaps stemming from a sense of temporary displacement — an unfortunate mirroring of some of the wider dynamics within the town. From others, however, we found attention and engagement that we had not anticipated. The importance of the site to these, and all the people who visited it, became one central question. As we relaxed and became less task orientated, less instrumental in our approach, we began to notice the many ways in which people were responding to being in the churchyard.

As we will discuss, reflecting on our aims and approaches early on, and responding to them, dramatically changed the direction and dynamic of the project. It became positive and inclusive, encouraged interaction with the wider churchyard communities, broke down social barriers, opened up dialogue, and enabled us and others to see this historic place — and its value — in new ways.

Doing things differently

Our activities

Over the following days, the project developed more organically. For those who actively took part, we aimed to respond to individual interests and rhythms, rather than imposing set activities. Initially we had reacted to 'What would you like me to do?' by taking the participant to a section of the churchyard and showing them how to record; we now let them direct us, asking 'What do **you** want to do?' making it clear that we had no agenda beyond encouraging people to join us in whatever way — and for whatever length of time — they wished. Importantly, we did not attempt to impose any rigid daily structure and no minimum participatory commitment was set; some people even joined us from the office in their lunch breaks. This fluidity allowed the project to mirror the natural daily rhythm — the ebb and flow — of activity

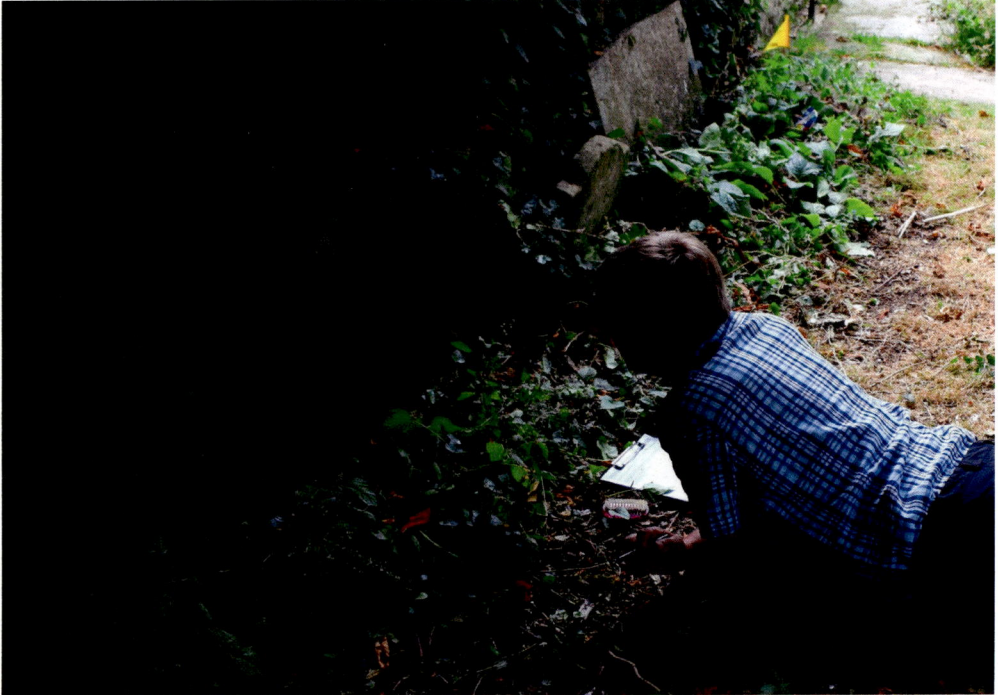

Figure 17.3 Participant Simon recording gravestones (Photograph by Eleanor Williams. Copyright reserved)

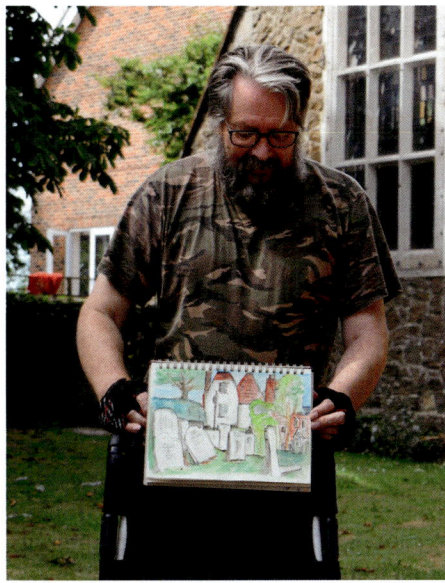
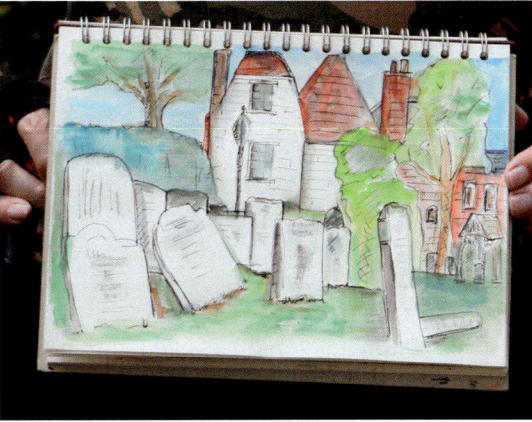

Figure 17.4 Artwork created during the project by Folkestone resident Steve McCarthy. (Photograph by Eleanor Williams. Copyright reserved)

in the churchyard. The project then became about 'making a start on the graveyard recording'; the overall dynamic became relaxed and people set their own, individual goals (Figure 17.3). There was a particularly memorable moment when we finally completed mapping a complex zone of the cemetery. Although one visitor commented 'Why don't you just use a GPS? It would be much quicker', speed and 'getting the job done' were not the point; we worked together, taught each other skills, and there was a collective feeling of accomplishment.

It was interesting how creative responses developed out of this approach. Hearing about the project through word of mouth, an artist joined us to sketch gravestones. Our daybook, in which people reflected on their experiences, included artistic interpretations of the place and our activities. Local resident Steve joined us most days, not to survey graves, but to pursue his hobbies: local history, photography, and painting. He drew our surroundings and activities, commenting that sketching allows him to not simply capture a specific moment, but also the place over time, and its mood (Figure 17.4). Importantly, for Steve and others, this was just as much about experiencing the place he was in and spending time with people, as it was about the activities themselves.

We observed that the project was valuable to people in various ways. Whilst at the beginning most found their own space, often working alone, this pattern changed to become more collaborative. One of our participants began the project mostly in isolation, photographing gravestones; it was the activity with which he was most comfortable. His confidence however grew; by the end, he was taking on a whole range of responsibilities and happily supporting others on how to record. One local resident who did prefer to survey independently, commented 'I've been feeling so blue lately, you can really lose yourself in this'. For some the project therefore offered an opportunity where they 'made friends', 'had a laugh' (as two comments recorded), and could socialize with a new — albeit temporary — community. For others, it was a chance to step out of a busy social context and become immersed in a particular task within a very different, yet familiar and safe, setting.

These aspects of the project appeared congruous with the nature of the churchyard; it is a space apart, clearly delineated from the busy urban environment surrounding it through its combination of heritage and green spaces, yet also open, permeable, and familiar. It was precisely these qualities that, despite some of its more 'risky' aspects, seemed to make the churchyard somewhere that people wanted to inhabit. For those keen to engage in a community heritage project but perhaps facing barriers (e.g. social anxiety, a lack of confidence in participating, accessibility issues, or time constraints) it offered the ideal setting; people felt that they could come and go on their own terms. We also argue that it is precisely this relative simplicity and flexibility that helped to encourage involvement from a broader range of people, allowing individual expressions and interests to evolve. Motivated by our common fascination with the site, and unprompted, certain community members started to bring along pieces of historical research that they had undertaken in tandem with the project; a 'sense of pride' for their unique local heritage — at times newly found — was arguably detectable amongst certain individuals. Fundamentally, our main role was in being a presence, and people felt able to respond to that in a number of different ways.

Our presence

A further observation was that, at the outset, our presence was having an altering effect on the wider community's use of the space. A project of this kind had never been conducted within this churchyard before, and whilst some people were clearly intrigued, others were suspicious. Perhaps some saw us as representative of authority or the civic world beyond the boundaries of the churchyard. Certainly we became aware of the sensitivities and convergences between the delineation of boundaries and authority, as discussed by Massey and Jess (1995). On our first day we positioned banners at the main entrances to the churchyard, and handed out flyers. Our intention was to simply raise awareness of the project, hoping that people would stop to talk, share their own experiences and possibly take part. We noticed that on the contrary, many avoided us. One individual, assuming that we were in some way related to the council and there to monitor behaviour, verbally challenged us. We had demarcated the churchyard as an official — and in some respects specialist — university project space, whereas for many it was theirs, a part of their everyday rhythms and routines. We had transposed a particular model of community heritage project onto the churchyard, treating it as a heritage 'site', one that was effectively 'ours' for the duration.

With some community excavation projects, a temporary delineation is created where people enter a specialist zone and adhere to defined roles and codes of conduct; this graveyard was not amenable to such a structure. Once aware of this, we endeavoured not to occupy the space, but rather to cohabit it, whilst observing and trying to understand, how the churchyard was used. We stopped unwanted flyering, removed the signage, and widened our attention. We met and talked with the different churchyard communities, as well as working with our own participants. This possibly altered the way in which we were seen. People in turn started to approach us, and a number of interested individuals stopped to participate on an ad hoc basis. By acting as a focus of attraction, the project created opportunities that brought together a diverse mix of people of different ages, backgrounds, and walks of life. We should not underestimate the value that people place on social connection and friendship networks that can arise from such projects (Power and Smyth 2016), but also how the coming together of individuals, including of different generations (Brady and Dolan 2009; Power and Smyth 2016), can have positive impacts. In some ways this churchyard can be seen as a microcosm of some of Folkestone's wider social tensions and divisions. For example, various people voiced opinions about the 'disrespectful kids' who use the site, but the interactions that developed over the project arguably helped to break down some of these barriers. Common ground existed in the mutual use of, and interest in, the site; this provided a platform to connect and to start conversations, including between particular groups of teenagers in the churchyard and some of the older community members. Heritage in this respect can provide an effective medium in which to bring communities together, potentially even contributing to greater levels of tolerance (EH 2014; HE 2017).

Seeing things differently

Through the process of actively seeking to break down the barriers inadvertently created at the beginning of the project, we instigated important dialogues. In this section, we provide examples and consider what these might mean for various groups and individuals who constitute the broad churchyard community. Our point here is that the internal and shared perceptions of the churchyard that became apparent to us during the project, revealed the depth and complexity of people's feelings about the significance of this site and its value for them.

On the fourth morning, two men who had been sleeping in the churchyard approached us. We introduced the project and in turn they shared their own understanding of the history of the site. One discussed a particularly emotive story on one of the gravestones — the drowning of a sailor — and asked 'What is the oldest grave here?' Interestingly, this was by far the most common question over the ten days; the site's antiquity, and the timespan of use by previous generations and individuals associated with the place, appeared at the forefront of many people's minds. On another day, one of our team went to investigate a commotion; a small group of rough sleepers who would meet at the town cross, had thrown out some teenagers. Asked what had transpired, one of the women replied 'We don't mind them coming here to smoke, but they shouldn't swear, it's a sacred, a special place'. Our initial assumptions surrounding why certain groups were using the place were challenged; instead of judgements about misuse and antisocial behaviour, we found that issues of ownership, concern, protection, connection and deep respect, were in evidence among the various churchyard communities. That is not to deny the community tensions which existed between different groups, but rather to reflect that these were more complex than originally assumed, and deserving of careful listening and observation.

Irrespective of people's age, background, or walk of life, common concerns were detectable in the responses to the place. On two days, children from three local primary schools joined us. This included St Eanswythe's Primary School, located adjacent to the churchyard. At the beginning, the children were asked to give one key word that came to mind when they considered their surroundings:

> '…gigantic church; Jesus; shiny stained glass; churchyard scary; delicate; safe in church; lots of history and old; calm; life and death; bodies; holy; spooky and dark.'

In small groups they then took part in a range of activities including exploring features of the church and churchyard, and finding named individuals and aspects of their life stories on gravestones. At the end of the two-hour session, we again asked for one keyword:

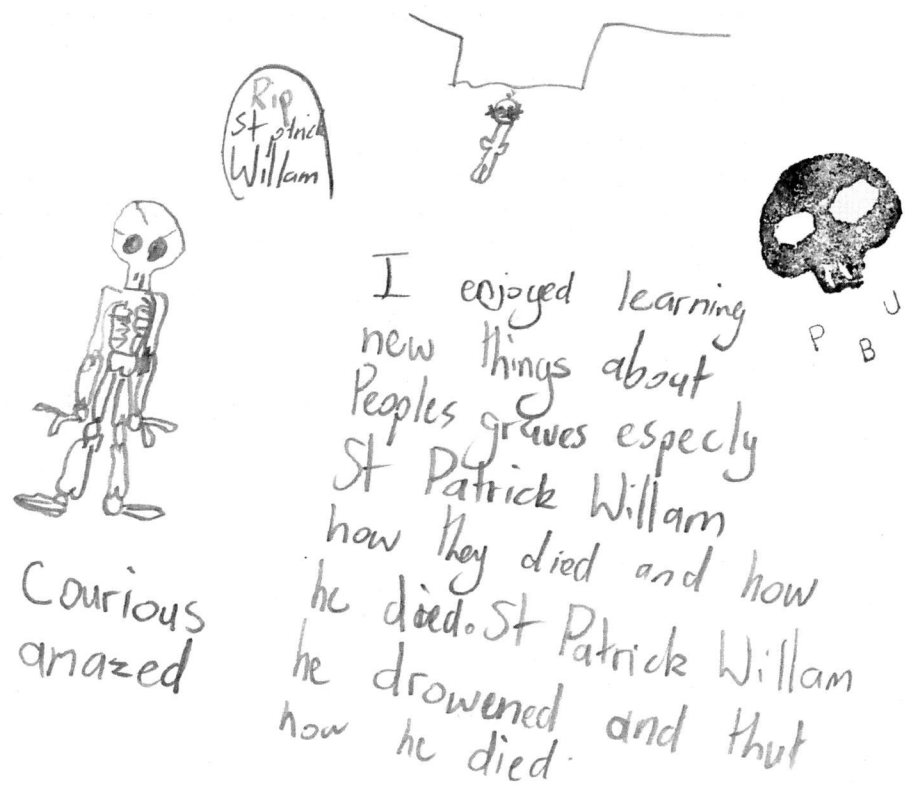

Figure 17.5 A drawing in response to the churchyard visit by a pupil at St Eanswythe's Primary School, Folkestone. (Drawing by a participant in school open day on July 3rd 2017. Copyright reserved)

'...peace; sacred; special; fragile; historical; careful; incredible; fascinating; delicate graveyard; calm; eye-catching; gentle; mouth-watering.'

There had been a detectable shift in the way that some viewed the place; no negative words were forthcoming. Instead, ideas of delicacy, gentleness, and peace were proffered. During the activities certain children from St Eanswythe's told us that their parents prefer to avoid the churchyard, and their own perceptions were of dark, unfriendly and even dangerous places. One child described it as being full of 'creepy dead people' and did not want to go near the gravestones. Attitudes noticeable shifted during the session and everyone actively explored the place. On the following days, some of the children brought their parents to meet us. Perspectives seemed to alter within a short period of time, arguably suggesting that feelings about one's locality, heritage, or landscape, can be challenged and reshaped, even by small-scale work such as ours. Figure 17.5 epitomizes many of the children's written/drawn responses. Overall they not only evidenced imagination and creativity, a connection with the past, and past people, but also a willingness to confront issues surrounding life and death. Many also chose to focus on aspects of nature within the churchyard.

Places such as churchyards have been recognized for their potential to improve health and well-being as they offer the ideal combination of heritage and nature, and provide much needed community green spaces in densely-populated areas (HLF 2018). Their significance, however, runs deeper. One aspect of this could be considered in terms of the place of the churchyard within its parish. As Rumsey (2017) suggests, the idea of the parish is deeply rooted and persistent, and although often invisible, its boundaries can still be felt. Whereas historic parish boundaries are now often unrecognized, their role as 'a fundamental agent of local welfare' (Rumsey 2017: 123) persists. The churchyard as a more visibly 'enclosed' and recognizable place, central to the parish, may maintain and concentrate some of these qualities; somewhere that people identify with as having special significance, a place of gathering and belonging, of the 'sacred', and an enduring locus of community identity. These places also have a particular symbolic and tangible power in that they contain the past, quite literally, within their boundaries; the dead share the space of the living, and through their memorialization offer an on-going and concrete connection to the past. As Power and Smyth (2016: 163–164) note, anxiety about the present can lead to an interest in one's heritage, where looking into the past can contribute to feelings of security and stability.

Reflections and conclusion

> 'Churchyards can be liminal places, peaceful and serene; places in which to wander or sit and think, and perhaps muse upon one's own mortality among the monuments to past lives' (Elders 2011: 29).

Over the course of the project, our goals were redirected; the individuals and communities we sought to engage joined us but with their own particular agendas and goals, which we absorbed and learned from. Our carefully planned activities evolved into opportunities for people to express their own interests, views and understanding of the site; this fostered a positive, inclusive and supportive environment. Early on we decided that what mattered was simply to be a presence, but also to observe and receive the many ways in which people found meaning here. At a basic level we offered a platform for dialogue. Through immersing ourselves in the site we came to understand that far from being overlooked, the churchyard was a place of constant activity. Although not expressed in a conventional way, much of this was about responding to the unique identity, history and meanings that this, like many other such places, contain. 'The People Before Us' showed us that small-scale projects like this could work at a deep level; they can address the association between people's well-being and the landscape as part of an understanding of our need for a sense of place and time, belonging, and security.

This chapter has aimed to show how such sites are therefore important to recognize, protect, and work with. For one reason, they can be integral, often in small personal ways, to individual well-being. Change can be emotionally and socially destabilizing, but the nature of such places – their permanency, and visible antiquity – can offer familiarity and stability amidst a rapidly shifting landscape. This is particularly relevant for a complex town such as Folkestone, where its physical landscape and identity continue to be reinvented, giving rise to profound uncertainty. These issues are possibly being expressed through the antisocial behaviour evident at the site, which is also having a negative effect on well-being by impacting upon some people's experience and enjoyment of the place. A sense of 'non-identity' can be linked to crime (Snell 2003: 99) or a lack of a sense of place can result in environmental degradation (Reilly *et al.* 2018). In addressing issues of well-being within a community, such places — these microcosms of wider social dynamics — are thus fundamental to acknowledge and work with. This should not be by imposition and occupation, but rather through immersion and cohabitation.

Projects working in these places need, if possible, to reflect these complexities. As others have already highlighted (e.g. HLF 2015; Simpson 2009), sustainability is important, as is finding practical ways to embed access to heritage within people's known landscapes. This inevitably raises questions about the short term nature of small-scale projects. Within the first days of 'The People Before Us,' individuals were already anticipating the end of the project and asking 'When will you be back?' The challenge is to work towards projects that are less short-term, more open and flexible, and situated in sites, practices, and places that are integral, and responsive, to **their** local environment, not simply created as a by-project of social or economic strategies that come and go. The question is how to evolve a practice which is compatible with the way that many community heritage projects — situated within current funding and resourcing models — must be set up, with rigidly defined budgets, timescales, objectives, and targets.

Lastly, we want to recognize that places such as the churchyard of St Mary and St Eanswythe can act in a profound way; they are everyday, but also extraordinary. They are redolent with the residual signs of the past; they speak of past lives, past experience, and for some, they exude a sense of immanence. They bring together the present, the recent and distant past; hundreds of years of named people visibly marked around you with dates, stories, and individual histories. In this respect, they stand as a witness to a collective, cultural recognition of the past and in that sense, can also seem to validate ourselves. Perhaps there is something comforting and reassuring about being able to place yourself on this timeline; you are a part of a long chain of events, and the knowledge that it is still going to be there in the future, a constant in the landscape.

Acknowledgements

This chapter is in memory of Father David Adlington, to whom we are extremely grateful for his support and enthusiasm. We would also like to thank Ian Gordon at the Church of St Mary and St Eanswythe, Dr Andrew Richardson and Canterbury Archaeological Trust, Francesca Clark (Kent County Council), Matt Rowe (Club Shepway), Nicholas Harrison (Soldier On!), Diarmaid Walshe, Keith Hingle, Paul Bingham, Tina Kilnan, and to everyone who joined us. We would also like to thank Canterbury Christ Church University and the HLF for the project funding.

Bibliography

Arnold, M. 2013. *Disease class and social change: Tuberculosis in Folkestone and Sandgate 1880-1930*. Newcastle: Cambridge Scholars Publishing.
Brady, B. and P. Dolan 2009. Youth mentoring as a tool for community and civic engagement: Reflections on findings of an Irish research study. *Community Development* 40(4): 359-366.
Camden, W. (trans. P. Holland) 1607. *Britannia*. London: George Bishop and John Norton.
Coulson, I. (ed.) 2013. *Folkestone to 1500: A town unearthed*. Canterbury: Canterbury Archaeological Trust.
DCMS 2016. *The culture white paper* [Online document]. London: HMG. Viewed 19 October 2018, <https://assets.publishing.service.gov.uk/government/uploads/system/uploads/attachment_data/file/510798/DCMS_The_Culture_White_Paper__3_.pdf>.

EH 2014. *Heritage counts 2014: The value and impact of heritage* [Online document]. Swindon: English Heritage. Viewed 24 October 2018, <https://content.historicengland.org.uk/content/heritage-counts/pub/2190644/value-impact-chapter.pdf>.

Elders, J. 2011. England's parish churchyards: A national treasure. *English Heritage Conservation Bulletin* 66 (The Heritage of Death): 29-30.

Hardy, L. 2013. A morsel too hard for time to chew, in I. Coulson (ed.) *Folkestone to 1500: A town unearthed*: 121-161. Canterbury: Canterbury Archaeological Trust.

HE 2011. *Caring for historic graveyard and cemetery monuments* [Online document]. Swindon: Historic England. Viewed 19 October 2018, <https://content.historicengland.org.uk/images-books/publications/caring-historic-graveyard-cemetery-monuments/caring-historic-graveyard-cemetery-mon.pdf/>.

HE 2017. *Heritage counts 2017: Heritage and the economy* [Online document]. Swindon: Historic England. Viewed 28 November 2018, <https://content.historicengland.org.uk/content/heritage-counts/pub/2017/heritage-and-the-economy-2017.pdf>.

HLF 2015. 20 years in 12 places: Improving heritage, improving places, improving lives [Webpage]. Viewed 28 November 2018, <https://www.hlf.org.uk/about-us/research-evaluation/20-years-heritage>.

HLF 2018. Walk among graves to improve health and wellbeing [Webpage]. Viewed 28 November 2018, <https://www.hlf.org.uk/about-us/news-features/walk-among-graves-improve-health-and-wellbeing>.

KCC 2015. *The English Index of Multiple Deprivation (IMD 2015): Headline findings for Kent. Business Intelligence Statistical Bulletin* [Online document]. Maidstone: KCC. Viewed 19 October 2018, <https://www.kent.gov.uk/__data/assets/pdf_file/0006/7953/Indices-of-Deprivation-headline-findings.pdf>.

Mackie, S.J. 1856. *A descriptive and historical account of Folkestone and its neighbourhood*. London: Simpkin and Marshall.

Massey, D. and P. Jess (eds.) 1995. *A place in the world? Places, cultures and globalization*. Oxford: Oxford University Press.

Mytum, H. 2002. *Recording and analysing graveyards (Practical Handbooks in Archaeology)*. York: CBA.

Philipot, T. 1659. *Villare Cantianum*. London: William Godbid.

Power, A. and K. Smyth. 2016. Heritage, health and place: The legacies of local community-based heritage conservation on social wellbeing. *Health and Place* 39: 160-167.

Reilly, S., C. Nolan and L. Monckton 2018. *Wellbeing and the historic environment* [Online document]. Swindon: Historic England. Viewed 19 October 2018, <https://historicengland.org.uk/images-books/publications/wellbeing-and-the-historic-environment/wellbeing-and-historic-environment/>.

Richardson, A. 2013. Late Roman and Anglo-Saxon Folkestone, in I. Coulson (ed.) *Folkestone to 1500: A town unearthed*: 55-76. Canterbury: Canterbury Archaeological Trust.

Rumsey, A. 2017. *Parish: An Anglican theology of place*. London: SCM Press.

Simpson, F. 2009. Evaluating the value of community archaeology: The XArch Project. *Treballs d'Arqueologia* 15: 51-62.

Snell, K.D.M. 2003. Gravestones, belonging and local attachment in England. *Past and Present* 179(1): 94-134.

Wells, H.G. 1905. *Kipps: The story of a simple soul*. London: Macmillan.

Chapter 18

Landscapes of mental health: The archaeology of St Wulstan's Local Nature Reserve, Malvern, England

Andrew Hoaen, Bob Ruffle, and Helen Loney

Abstract

The St Wulstan's Local Nature Reserve was developed in 1997, on the site of a former military hospital built for US military casualties of the Second World War D-Day landings and subsequent actions. After the war, the hospital was absorbed by the NHS, closing in 1986, with subsequent site redevelopment including the nature reserve. The planting of the reserve partly aimed to preserve something of the hospital's heritage, through the use of trees and shrubs from the former hospital grounds. This paper presents part of a four year research project at the University of Worcester, investigating the archaeology of nature reserves and landscapes in Worcestershire and the elsewhere in the UK. The paper explores the ways in which the environment has been used to enhance and improve mental well-being. It then describes the history of both the original St Wulstan's Hospital and the more recent nature reserve, going on to describe the present research project and present interim results from its first year. The discussion explores the ways in which the St Wulstan's Local Nature Reserve may be considered a healing environment, and how such studies can assist with the understanding of post-war environmental changes.

Keywords: Contemporary archaeology; Hospital sites; Mental health; St Wulstan's; Trees

Introduction

This study forms part of a wider investigation into the archaeology of nature reserves and landscapes within Worcestershire and elsewhere in the UK (Hoaen in press a; b). The former hospital site at St Wulstan's was part of a series of five US military hospitals built during the Second World War (WWII) in Malvern Wells, Worcestershire to receive casualties from the D-Day landings in Normandy from June 1944. After the war it was taken over by the NHS and used first as a tuberculosis (TB) hospital and then as a psychiatric hospital before closing in 1986. The site was redeveloped for housing, and the hospital buildings were subsequently demolished in 1994–1996 with the eastern half of the site declared a Local Nature Reserve in 1997 (Figure 18.1). Part of the reasoning behind the declaration was to maintain the planting of specimen trees and shrubs from the grounds and thereby maintain the heritage of the hospital.

The research was developed and conducted following the *Archaeology of the West Midlands: A Framework for Research* (Watt 2011). Our focus has been on understanding and enhancing our archaeological knowledge of the following themes identified by Belford: Capitalism, Globalization, and Consumption (2011: 229), as well as sub-themes of Conflict, Death and Disease, and the Home (2011: 237–238). Hickman has noted a gap in our knowledge around the landscapes of mental health after the 1930s (2013). At the time of writing, the project has just completed its first year and it is intended to run for a further three years, forming part of the archaeological and heritage training provided for first year archaeology students at the University of Worcester.

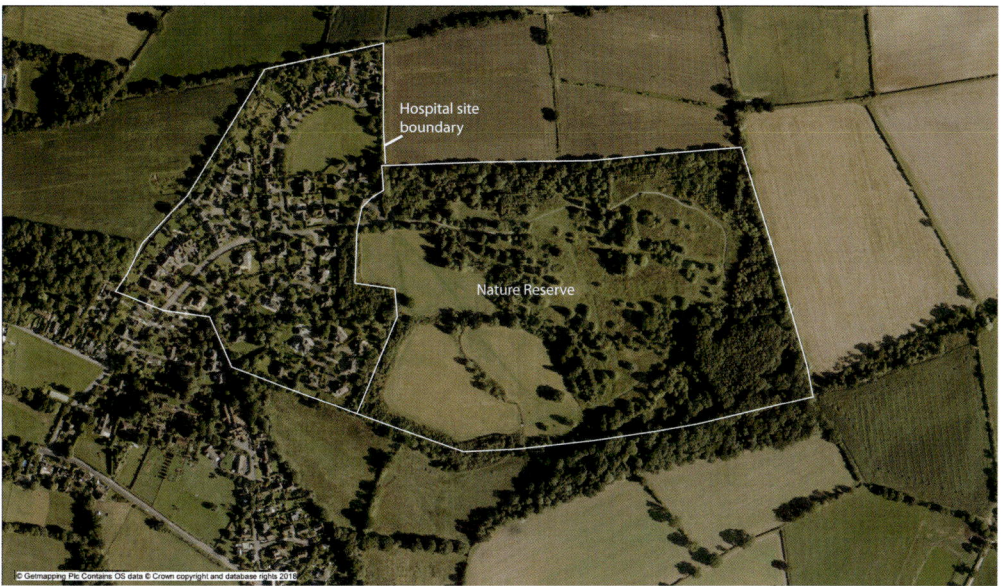

Figure 18.1 St Wulstan's Local Nature Reserve in 2009 showing boundaries of the former hospital and new buildings. (Based on Digimap 2018a, used under license)

Environment, and what we might call the 'environmental *sensorium*', has long been considered an important part of medical practice, although the weight given to this factor has varied through time (Hickman 2013). The concept of gardening and other outdoor and physical work as a helpful practice for the traumatized, can be seen in Voltaire's satire Candide (Voltaire 1759) and was also pioneered in America by physicians such as Benjamin Rush in the late eighteenth century (Plankinton 1973). Since the 1990s it has been recognized that work such as gardening together with structured outdoor activities has a role to play in therapeutic practice, and contributes to the mental well-being of the general public (c.f. Bragg *et al.* 2015; Bragg and Atkins 2016; Sempik and Aldridge 2006). On a personal note, one of the authors (Hoaen) discovered in 2012 that he had been suffering from a long-standing complex post-traumatic stress disorder. One of the therapeutic outcomes of the recovery process was the suggestion to return to writing and delivering conference papers, but also to work out of doors in natural surroundings. Consequently, all of his subsequent research has been into the archaeology of contemporary environments, particularly nature reserves and ancient woodlands. He finds these environments much less stressful to work in than other archaeological contexts, and overall better for his mental well-being whilst conducting fieldwork.

Approaches for the environmental analysis of contemporary archaeological landscapes

The hospital grounds at St Wulstan's present a challenge to archaeological practice with regard to how and what to record in order to capture the environment both as it exists today and in the recent past. We are investigating a number of interlinked questions: how has the environment of the hospital changed through time; did the gardens play a therapeutic role in the life of the hospital, either overtly or subconsciously; to what extent can we consider the other organisms at the site to have possessed agency; what can we determine about the environmental *sensorium* of the location.

Whilst environmental historians (e.g. Crumley 1994) are quite used to investigating recent landscape change, the analysis of recent and contemporary landscapes from the perspective of environmental archaeology is relatively new (Richer and Geary 2017). The concept that environment might have a determining role in human society and on the individual, is one that has been overlooked within archaeology in recent years. Environment, we will argue, has a critical role to play in understanding people's sensory world, both in the past and in the present. As Ingold (2000: 47) has said, environment is central in hunter gatherer societies to individuals' understanding of themselves: 'In their account there are not two worlds of nature and society but just one....'. We would agree with Ingold that if we are to understand the environment, we need to move away from these binary divisions between mind and body, and culture and nature.

To do this we will structure our investigation of the environment around the concepts of use and delight as outlined by Smout in *Nature contested* (Smout 2000: 7) and which ultimately derive from Horace and Georgian poetry (*sensu* Hardie 2001). The fields of ecocriticism (Garrard 2004) and the environmental humanities (Bate 1991) draw on literary and philosophical approaches to investigate concepts such as the 'pastoral' and the 'wild', both rather undertheorized in archaeology.

Archaeologies of the senses have been a developing area within archaeology for some time (Tilley 1994; MacGregor 1999), and a sensory approach appears suited to interpreting the archaeology of former hospitals and the subsequent nature reserve at St Wulstan's. In order to document the sense of 'delight' and the sensual world at specific sites, it is important to be able to understand the plantings and the buildings that constitute and constituted the environmental *sensorium*. Delight is both abstract and yet concrete; we know when we are delighted, but what constitutes delight is very much an individual experience. As a qualitative variable of experience it is a difficult concept to pursue archaeologically.

Two useful theoretical approaches to delight are the concepts of affordances as suggested by Gibson and subsequently developed by Ingold (2011), and that of charisma (Lorimer 2015). Here we might consider what role the gardens had in creating a pleasant experience for the staff, patients, and visitors to the site, and what this may have contributed to their well-being. The idea of charisma was first developed by the biologist Uexküll, who considered the qualities of organisms that either brought them to the attention of other organisms or led them to being ignored. Lorimer has used this to analyse the way in which certain animals (e.g. elephants) are charismatic for people and act as a focus around which a whole series of conservation measures may be built (2015). In a similar way, certain plants also have charisma and may be deliberately selected for their affordances as well as their charisma. Apple trees, for example, provide flowers in the spring and apples in the autumn so have a dual purpose when seen in this way. Some trees such as conifers are charismatic because of their sensory qualities at different seasons of the year. Lorimer points out that the vast majority of life forms are not ecologically charismatic and consequently are rarely considered when planning gardens. To be selected, a plant has to be both noted and notable. Lorimer also observes that organisms have an aesthetic charisma that will be culturally contingent. Insects, for example, provoke both loathing and likeability (Hillman 1988). By combining these concepts of affordances, charisma, and delight, we may also begin to detect where plants and animals have developed agency within human decision-making. The concept of the environment having agency is a relatively new one (Bennett 2009), but an examination of the St Wulstan's Local Nature Reserve and hospital site suggests that some elements within that environment have their own agency and are capable of influencing human decisions.

The roles of the environment and the senses appear to have been recognized relatively early in recuperation. For example, Hickman quotes Florence Nightingale on the beneficial effects of a view from a window or a vase of flowers (2013: 206). The role of the environment in therapy, and in particular the use of gardens and horticultural work, appears to have declined after the 1930s (Sempik and Aldridge 2006) and was noted by Monty Don on *Gardener's World* on the BBC (SweetTree Farming for All 2015). This has been attributed to a lack of funds and labour after both the Great Depression and WWII, coupled with a new medical focus on interior spaces and drug-based therapies.

History of St Wulstan's Hospital and Local Nature Reserve

The site at St Wulstan's was originally known as the Long Meadow and was recorded by the Land Utilization Survey of Britain as poor-quality grazing land in the 1930s (Stamp 1937). Analysis of Ordnance Survey mapping, post 1945 aerial photographs, and building plans enables us to reconstruct developments at the site with a reasonable degree of accuracy. To these we can add information derived from oral history and documentary archives (Unaccessioned materials deposited in Worcester City Council Archives, 2009). Unfortunately, the documentary archive from the St Wulstan's history archive project has yet to be accessioned. Consequently, documents used from that archive will be referred to by name rather than document number.

Malvern has been regarded as a place of well-being since the middle of the eighteenth century. The long-term consequences of that specialization have included the marketing of the area for tourism, as people sought peace and quiet. With the start of WWII, Malvern and the county of Worcestershire became an important location for a variety of government and military institutions, both technological and respite in nature. When America joined the conflict in 1942, a series of five hospitals was established in the vicinity of Malvern. One of these, the site at Brickbarns (St. Wulstan's) was the home of US 96th General Hospital (Turley and Turley 2000). Originally planned as a surgical unit, the hospital subsequently became a psychiatric hospital for shell shock cases from D-Day June 1944 onwards.

The original layout of the main buildings was to a standard pattern on all the Malvern sites: parallel lines of long, single-storey ward buildings, grouped end to end in pairs of lines, with an access path between them. There were two such pairs of lines in the eastern half of the site, in the area that is now the Nature Reserve. The other buildings, including staff accommodation, were in the western half. The hospital incorporated the mature trees and most of the hedging from the pre-existing agricultural landscape (Figure 18.2), which meant in some cases that wards were sited between these trees.

The military hospital closed in 1945, and after a short period of use as a refugee camp for displaced persons, the site was given to the NHS and developed as a TB hospital that opened in 1950. It was during this phase that thought was given to refurbishing the buildings and developing the gardens. The *Malvern Gazette* notes that 'Outside the blank dreary wastes of land are blossoming into gardens, avenues of silver birches, poplars and flowering trees' (1950).

Historic Landscapes and Mental Well-being

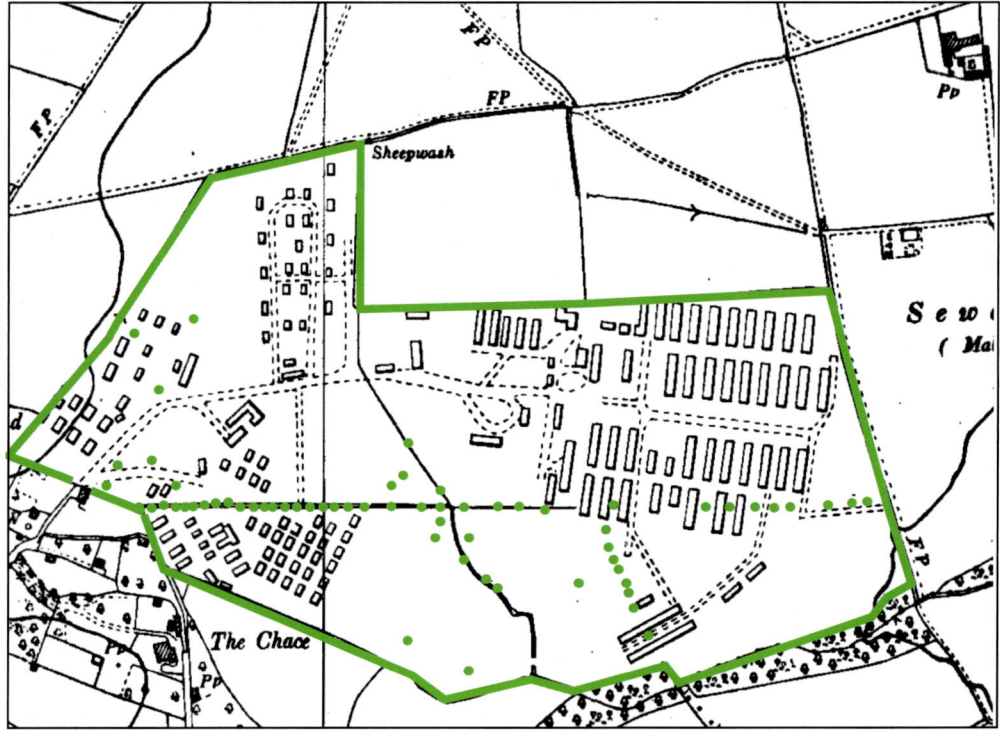

- Tree from pre hospital landscape
- Pre hospital hedge lines

Figure 18.2 St Wulstan's hospital site at 1955, with pre-hospital landscape trees and hedgerows shown. (Based on Digimap 2018b, used under license)

With the discovery of a cure for TB, the hospital was closed in 1960. By this point however, the investment of the staff and health board, together with the charitable activities of the local community, had produced a valuable asset with its well laid out grounds. The health authority therefore looked for alternative uses for the site.

It was decided to reopen the site as a psychiatric hospital, specializing in the rehabilitation and return to the community of long stay patients from across the West Midlands, under the medical superintendent Dr Roger Morgan. Dr Morgan adapted the hospital to use a form of industrial therapy in order to help people move from long term hospital living to the community. Industrial therapy was a development of the post-war period, that aimed to train patients in a variety of tasks within their region (Long 2013; Morgan 1970). Records from this period include several accounts by the medical superintendents of the ways in which this therapy was used at the site (e.g. Morgan, Cushing and Manton 1965). As this type of therapy became popular and the site attracted both national and international interest, a visiting American psychiatrist, T. Query, provided a further useful account (1968).

Most work took place indoors in approximations of the type of industrial metal working workshops that could be found throughout the West Midlands at that time. The 'business' proved successful; patients were paid, and through work, were found jobs and homes both in the Malvern area and further afield. Gardening and other outdoor work was seen as secondary, and used for male patients who were considered unsuitable for the workshops. Women were trained in secretarial, cooking and cleaning work.

The hospital remained open until 1986, during which time the western half was redeveloped extensively (Figure 18.3). Gardens and ornamental plantings were laid out along with allotments and orchards. Subdivisions using ornamental hedges were created along with tree lined avenues. An oblique photo taken in 1992, shows the hospital grounds a few years after abandonment (Figure 18.4). Woodland regeneration can be seen in various places, but the main tree and shrub plantings amongst the wards and around the administrative buildings can be clearly seen. It is noticeable that hedges have been used to screen the living accommodation of the staff from the site.

The site was used for various purposes after closure, but eventually, in the early 1990s, plans were brought forward by Bovis to redevelop the old staff quarters in the Crescent and to build new houses on the remainder of the site. A successful campaign by the council and local residents led to the site being split; the western half would be used for housing, whilst the eastern half would be cleared and landscaped to form a nature reserve (Figure 18.1).

University of Worcester research project methodology

The project was divided into two parts. The first part consisted of documentary research at the Worcestershire archives in 'The Hive', together with online sources such as Digimap and

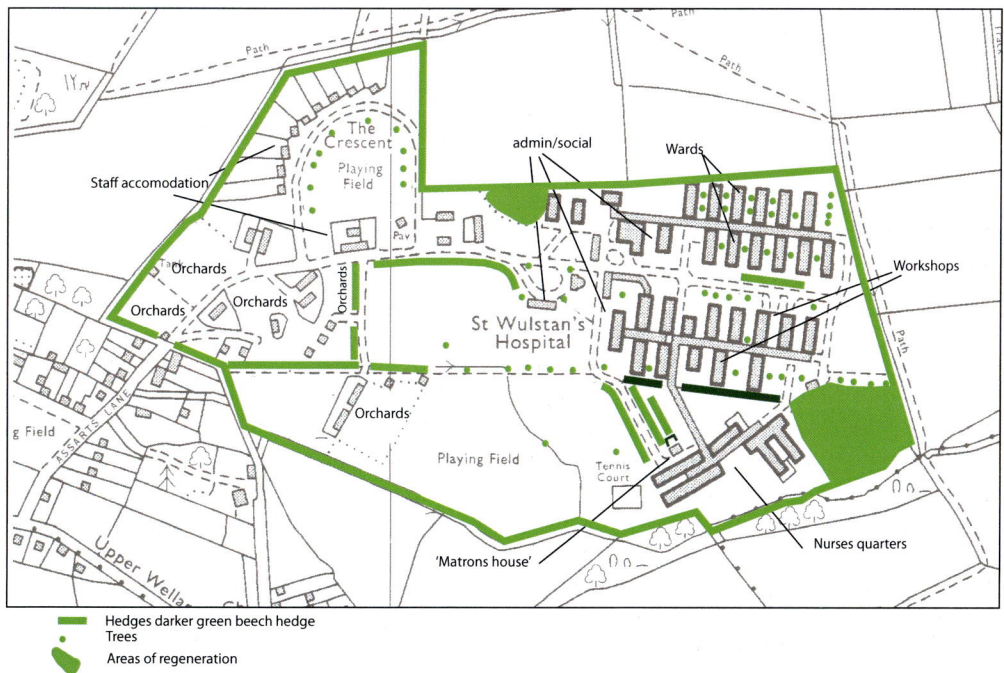

Figure 18.3 St Wulstan's hospital site in 1971 showing main areas of 1960s planting including orchards and hedges. (Based on Digimap 2018c, used under license)

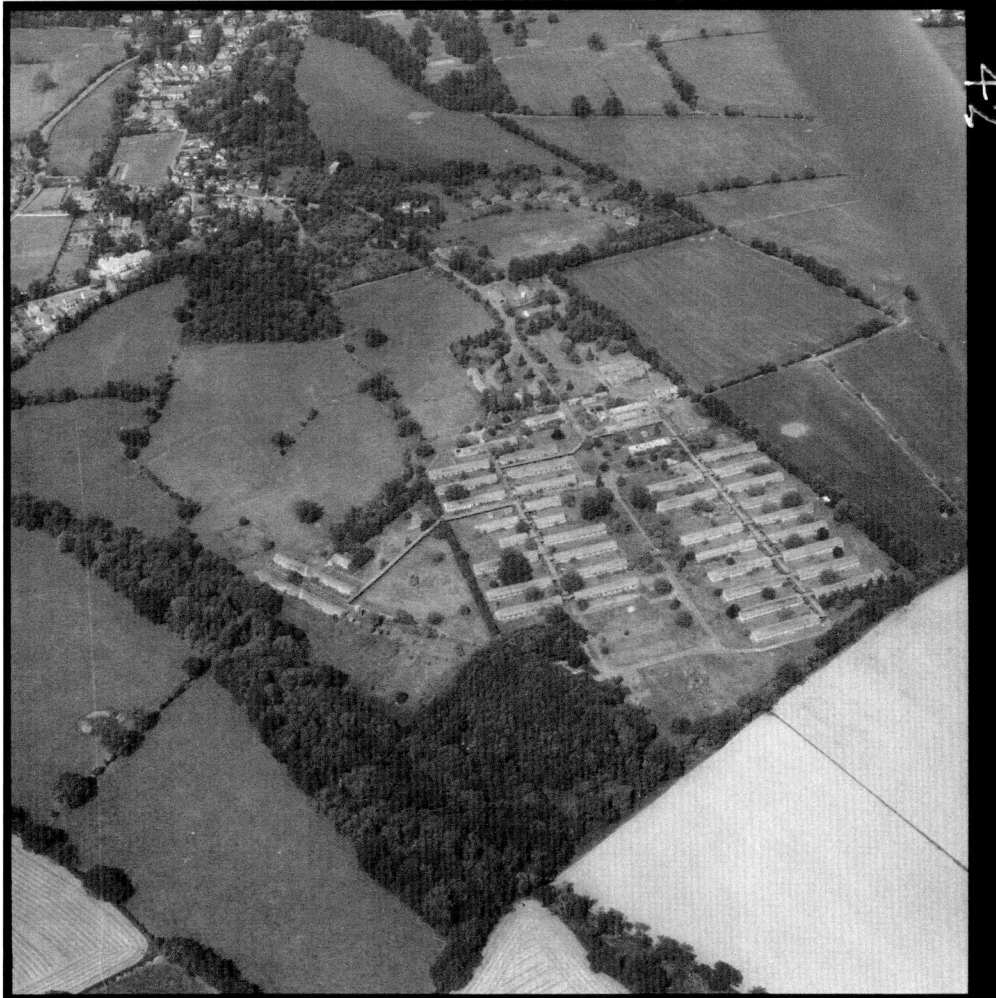

Figure 18.4 Aerial photograph showing the site after closure in 1992. (Courtesy of the Historic England Archive MNR SU 7481/7. Crown copyright reserved)

Google Earth. The second part comprised fieldwork conducted by first year students for the University of Worcester Archaeology and Heritage degree program, as part of their fieldwork requirement. We conducted geophysical survey of an earlier monument at the site, off set survey of parts of the hospital gardens, and a pick-up survey of pottery disturbed by pond digging. This section will focus on the documentary research, the tree survey (Handley and Rotherham 2013), the finds and a well-being survey.

The well-being survey consisted of an anonymized, self-administered questionnaire, sent out on 12 March 2018 (Denscombe 2017; Oppenheim 1992). The questions were based on established well-being and mental health self-assessments such as those on the Good Medicine website (Hawkins 2018). Participants were asked to provide basic personal information, including frequency of visits to the Nature Reserve. Participants were then asked to provide ranked responses to questions about their knowledge of the site, and their emotional engagement with their visits.

University of Worcester research project results

Maps plans and documents

The results of the St Wulstan's history archive project are held by Worcestershire County Council (Ward 2009). Whilst these are invaluable social records of the site, they are missing the official records of the hospital including the daybook, the location of which is not currently known. Few of the records in the archive deal directly with the hospital gardens and grounds. Where they do, they contain interesting insights into the work of the hospital but shed little light on the species that were planted. There are, however, documents that enable us to understand how the staff and residents felt about the hospital and its gardens, and to understand the role they played in softening the utilitarian aspects of the buildings.

The temporary nature of the original US army hospital suggests that the grounds were managed largely by mowing, with little thought as to how they might be improved as the setting for a hospital. An aerial photograph (US/31GR/LOC20 frame 9) from 1945 suggests that sport and recreation were important elements of the use of the ground; a baseball diamond can be clearly seen, along with an oval running track. Oral history recounts that local boys were not allowed to play baseball but had to make do with softball.

The first major attempts at improving the grounds are recorded in the *Malvern Gazette* (1950), during preparation for the conversion to a TB hospital. Evidence for the planting of cherries, birch and poplars can be seen in an aerial photograph dating to between 1945 and 1969 A series of young trees and shrubs can be seen, along with surviving mature trees and hedgerows of the pre-existing landscape. The plantings are concentrated away from the wards and instead are focussed around the entrance and administrative buildings.

An aerial photograph taken in 1969 (Williams pers. comm.) shows that an area of woodland has developed in the southeast corner of the site by that time. At the present day, this part of the site is considered to be dangerous due to the earlier dumping of hazardous waste, which may be why woodland was allowed to grow up here. Elsewhere, orchards have replaced housing in the west of the site and planting has continued around the site. It is noticeable that trees and shrubs were planted between the ward blocks, and that the ends of ward blocks have flower beds. Also, by 1969, formal flower beds are present, with formal hedges and lawns completing the gardens. It appears that hedges and blocks of woodland were used to screen the living accommodation of the staff from the patients (Figure 18.3).

The grounds were also used for fetes and festivals, not only by the staff and patients, but also by the local community. As the site was not enclosed, patients were able to leave and members of the public were welcome to use the facilities. As well as the gardens, the hospital also had a cricket pitch and tennis courts, and later, football pitches. After 1969, the main change to the grounds is the addition of conifers to the administrative areas around the 'flagpole', and along major walkways.

From the documentary records, we can see that the gardens and the general setting of the hospital played an important but possibly subconscious role in the life of the patients, staff and local residents. The superintendent Dr Morgan makes it clear in his writings that gardening was mostly carried out by professional staff, and that only suitable patients were employed in

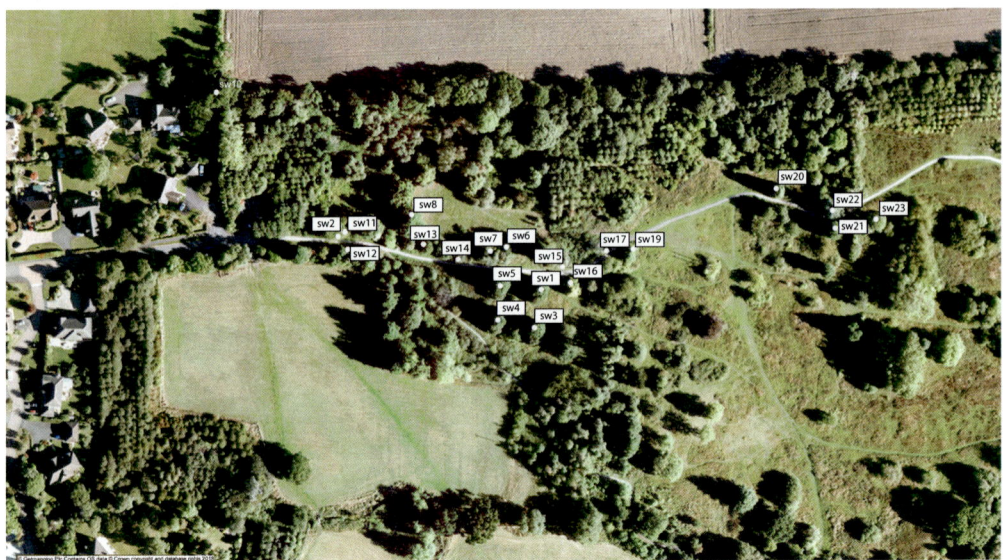

*Figure 18.5 Plan of the 2018 tree survey on the 2009 Digimap aerial photo.
(Based on Digimap 2018d, used under license)*

this activity. Nonetheless, according to Query, the hospital took a holistic approach based on gestalt theory, wherein the patient's environment, both psycho-social and sensual, is crucial to their recovery. The pleasant environment created by the gardens is frequently commented on in the hospital's newsletter. For example, the editor often comments on the gardens with statements such as:

'I consider myself lucky to work in such a setting of peace and tranquillity'
(*St. Wulstan's Newsletter* June 1981).

Similarly, patients write in poems and notes about how the environment is one of peace and beauty. For example, in *Our surroundings* by Anne Forrest, she praises the tranquillity that she finds whilst wandering around the grounds. However, the grounds and pleasant surroundings of the hospital could occasionally interfere with a patient's rehabilitation. Query relates that one woman was helped to retrain as a secretary so that she could return to work, and she was then found a position in a factory. She soon returned to the hospital, commenting:

'How can you expect us to give up the green tranquillity of the rehabilitation hospital for the hell of a factory' (Forrest 1967: 53).

Tree survey

The initial woodland survey in 2018 was carried out along the northern margins of the site (Figure 18.5; Table 18.A). An additional reconnaissance walk-over survey subsequently identified the remains of a garden enclosed by a beech hedge next to the 'Matrons House', a second beech hedge to shield the nurses' quarters from the workshops, and the remains of the pre-1945 hedges (Figure 18.3). The species identified by the survey are mainly conifers, but also include decorative trees such as maples and walnuts.

Table 18.A *Tree species identified by survey undertaken in 2018.*

Tree Species	ID Number
Leyland Cypress	SW1–5, SW10, SW12, SW16, SW20, SW22, SW23
Scots Pine	SW6
Unidentified	SW7, SW13, SW15, SW17,
Lebanon Cedar	SW8
Oak	SW9
Walnut	SW11
Western Red Cedar	SW18, SW19, SW21, SW22
Maple	SW14

Finds

An area of disturbed ground was field-walked, resulting in the collection of early to mid-twentieth century pottery and glass. The marked glass includes a Badoit mineral water bottle base, a Pond's cold cream container, and several fragments of what may be medicine or poison bottles. A total of 67 pottery sherds were collected. As might be expected, these comprised a mixture of stoneware and earthenwares, with a few pieces of porcelain/bone china. The identifiable pieces of porcelain and/or bone china included a likely late nineteenth century Limoges fragment, as well as wares from a number of British manufacturers such as T.G. Booth of Tunstall. There was also a well-preserved Lovatt & Lovatt ink bottle, and a complete Virol bone-marrow paste pot. This sample may predate the main phase of the NHS hospital. It possibly dates to the period of the American hospital or earlier. Other finds include an NHS plastic tea mug and bowl and a surgical steel implement, all collected by the reserve warden, Martin Barnett.

Well-being survey

A total of 21 questionnaires were completed and submitted for analysis, and the following information summarizes the results. About 57 per cent of respondents were over 65 years of age, and 71 per cent were female. The age demographic is a reasonable reflection of the time and day of the week in which this survey was conducted. This was mid-day during the working week, and so would favour both retirees, approximately 51 per cent, and women of working age who maintain a household. There were three respondents between the ages of 18 and 24 who were students.

Overall, 50 per cent of participants reported that they visited the site more than once a week, with 19 per cent reporting that they visited the site daily. Some 86 per cent of participants reported they were here to walk a dog, but when asked what prompted visits more than once a week, 67 per cent responded for 'regular exercise', 29 per cent suggested an interest in plants and animals, 19 per cent bird watching, and 14 per cent 'to clear their head'.

Question Ten asked participants to rank their feelings regarding visits to St Wulstan's on a scale from 1 to 5, with 1 'Strongly disagree' and 5 'Strongly agree'. The highest score possible is 105. The question 'Do you think your visits help you relax?' received an agreement score of

90 per cent, with 'Do you think your visits help you to be cheerful?' receiving an agreement score of 74 per cent. The question 'Do you think your visits help you solve problems?' scored 51 per cent. Finally, Question 11 asked participants about their awareness of the history of the site as a WWII hospital for service men with shell shock, as a TB hospital and as a psychiatric hospital. Responses were incomplete, so the absence of an answer was taken as a 'No' response. Nonetheless, the bulk of respondents, 81 per cent, were aware of the site's history as a WWII hospital, 72 per cent also knew that it had been a psychiatric hospital, and 62 per cent knew of its time as a TB hospital.

Discussion

From its early beginnings as a temporary site for casualties from the D-Day landings of June 1944 to the present day, St Wulstan's has been subject to constant and rapid change. From fields to hospital buildings, back to fields, and then back to fields and houses. If nothing else, the site tells us about the frenetic state of human activity in the post-WWII medical landscape. It suggests that doing something new is almost as important an activity as the provision of care. Gardens and horticulture therapy were not considered significant elements of mental health rehabilitation services in the early post-war period. Despite this, the site at St Wulstan's suggests that the quality of one's surroundings — the environment in which patients and staff lived — was also considered significant; it was just no longer the role of patients to provide that service.

Within the hospital site, significant living elements of the historic environment have survived despite, or because of, the constantly changing landscape. The most obvious of these are the hedges and the trees incorporated in them. Along the central hedge line that runs directly through the site, many trees survived the hospital's construction, despite it being a time of war and the hedge apparently being very much in the way. Elsewhere on the site, parkland trees also survived this initial phase of construction and became incorporated into the life of the hospital. Whilst there may have been many different reasons for this, it could be that the aesthetic charisma of isolated trees in a park setting gave certain trees agency that favoured their survival. It may also be that as large mature trees, they were simply too much trouble to remove, again suggesting the agency of this element of the environment.

After the conversion to a TB hospital, both the NHS and the local community contributed to the creation of attractive landscaped grounds. The environmental setting within the Malverns, with the visible presence of the hills and the fresh air, helped create a suitable *sensorium* for a sanatorium treating TB. The wards were redesigned to allow the patients access to fresh air, with photographic records showing rows of patients in beds outside the hospital buildings, enjoying the view and the air. This idea of an open-air hospital for the treatment of TB can dated back to the mid nineteenth century (Hickman 2013). Interestingly the early plantings in the TB hospital grounds were based around seasonal deciduous plants. The planting was carried out by professional staff, with materials to improve the life of the patients donated by the local community (Ward 2009).

This collaboration between the NHS and the local community appears to have continued with its conversion to a psychiatric hospital. It is during this phase, after around 1960, that many of the trees and plantings occurred that give the site its unique character. These gardens, as we have discussed above, were not considered a primary part of therapy at the site. They were the creation of the management of the hospital, working with mainly professional gardeners and a small number of patients. However, the gardens, trees and shrubs all connected with the inhabitants, and it is clear from the documents that the environment they created contributed to the overall well-being of the people at the site. By inviting the community into the site for fetes, sports and recreation, Dr Morgan created a facility that was not only for the benefit of his patients, but was also greatly admired and respected in the local area. Consequently, despite changing patterns in the health service and the costs associated with maintaining the buildings, the hospital was able to survive repeated plans to close it.

When closure did finally occur, the site held a great deal of importance for the local community. The trees and the 'natural' feel of the gardens encouraged a campaign to save all or most of the site as a nature reserve. This campaign was very successful; the developers constructed houses on one half of the site, but also paid for the demolition of the hospital buildings and landscaping of the other half.

Conclusion

As an environment for healing, St Wulstan's appears ideal. There was a long history of care and therapy in the Malvern community into which the hospital was inserted. The location is one in which there is an abundance of space, quiet, and fresh air, with excellent views towards the Malvern Hills. Whether these factors contributed to the initial selection of the site, or whether there were more prosaic factors such as the cost of the land, proximity to railway stations and distance from hostile forces, we cannot know. Once the site became established as a place of healing, these and other factors had a role to play as contingent elements in the choices made around the changes of use of the site.

St. Wulstan's is now a mature nature reserve, but the remains of the hospital plantings are still present; together with the earlier field systems, they still structure the layout of the site. Long Meadow is still a meadow. The Matron's Residence is now a buried concrete pad, but the beech hedge of her garden is still present in the landscape. Our small survey suggests that aside from the utilitarian need to 'walk the dog', users of the nature reserve find it a place helpful for peace and reflection. They also are very aware of its history as a hospital. We would argue that in part, this is due to its aesthetic charisma, firstly as a well-appointed hospital garden and secondly because of the way in which the design of the nature reserve has preserved elements of the former hospital. In this short paper it has not been possible to fully explore the history of this important post-war hospital. Instead, we have attempted to show that an understanding of the environmental settings of such places can contribute to our overall interpretation of change in the post-war period.

Acknowledgements

We are grateful to the staff of the Worcestershire County Council archives, for their assistance in consulting the St Wulstan's records. We wish to thank Countryside Site Officer, Martin Barnett of St Wulstan's Nature reserve for his help.

Bibliography

Bate, J. 1991. *Roman ecology*. London: Routledge.
Belford, P. 2011. The archaeology of everything — grappling with post-medieval, industrial and contemporary archaeology, in S. Watt (ed.) *The West Midlands research framework*: 211-236. Birmingham: University of Birmingham.
Bennett, J. 2009. *Vibrant matter: A political ecology of things*. Durham, NC: Duke University Press.
Bragg, R. and G. Atkins 2016. *A review of nature-based interventions for mental health care, Natural England Commissioned Reports, Number 204*. York: Natural England.
Bragg, R., C. Wood, J. Barton and J. Pretty 2015. *Wellbeing benefits from natural environments rich in wildlife* [Online document]. Colchester and Newark, Notts: University of Essex and The Wildlife Trusts. Viewed 30 November 2018, <https://www.wildlifetrusts.org/sites/default/files/2018-05/r1_literature_review_wellbeing_benefits_of_wild_places_lres.pdf>.
Crumley, C.L. 1994. *Historical ecology*. Santa Fe: School of American Research Press.
Denscombe, M. 2017. *The good research guide for small-scale social research projects* (Sixth edition). London: The Open University Press.
Digimap 2018a. St Wulstan's Nature Reserve in 2009 showing boundary of former hospital and new buildings, Malvern Wells, [AP], Scale 1:5000, Aerial Roam Series [Online map]. Viewed 27 August 2018, <http://digimap.edina.ac.uk/>.
Digimap 2018b. Hospital site at 1955, with pre-hospital landscape trees and hedgerows shown, Scale 1:10560, Ordnance Survey National Grid 1:10560, 1st Revision 1949–1981 [Online map]. Viewed 28 September 2018, <http://digimap.edina.ac.uk/>.
Digimap 2018c. Hospital site in 1971 showing main areas of 1960s planting including orchards and hedges, Scale 1:2500, Ordnance Survey National Grid 1:2500, 3rd Revisions 1960–1992 [Online map]. Viewed 28 September 2018, <http://digimap.edina.ac.uk/>.
Digimap 2018d. Plan of tree survey on 2009 aerial view of St Wulstan's Nature Reserve, Malvern Wells, [AP], Scale, Aerial Roam Series [Online map]. Viewed 5 October 2018, <http://digimap.edina.ac.uk/>.
Forrest, A. 1967. *Our surroundings*. Worcester City Council archive document
Garrard, G. 2004. *Ecocriticism*. Abingdon: Routledge.
Handley, C. and I.D. Rotherham 2013. *Shadow woods and ghosts: A survey guide*. Sheffield: Wildtrack Publishing.
Hardie, P.R. 2001. Virgil, in J.A. Palmer, D.E. Cooper and D. Cooper (eds.) *Fifty key thinkers on the environment*: 17-22. London: Routledge.
Hawkins, J. 2018. Good medicine [Website]. Viewed 30 November 2018, <http://goodmedicine.org.uk/about>.
Hickman, C. 2013. *Therapeutic landscapes: A history of English hospital gardens since 1800*. Manchester: Manchester University Press.
Hillman, J. 1988. Going bugs. *A Journal of Archetype and Culture* 48: 40–72.
Hoaen, A. in press a. Conceptualising the wild in contemporary environmental archaeology. *Internet Archaeology*.
Hoaen, A. in press b. Fragments of the wild: Yew trees, Wordsworth and contemporary archaeology. *International Review of Environmental History*.
Ingold, T. 2000. *The perception of the environment: Essays on livelihood, dwelling and skill*. London: Routledge.
Ingold, T. 2011. *The perception of the environment: Essays on livelihood, dwelling and skill* (Second edition). London: Routledge.

Long, V. 2013. Rethinking post-war mental health care: Industrial therapy and the chronic mental health patient in Britain. *Social History of Medicine* 26(4): 738–758.

Lorimer, J. 2015. *Wildlife in the anthropocene.* Minneapolis: University of Minnesota Press.

MacGregor, G. 1999. Making sense of the past in the present: a sensory analysis of carved stone balls. *World Archaeology* 31(2): 258–271.

Malvern Gazette 1950. St Wulstan's a Miniature Village of Healing. *Malvern Gazette* June 30 1950.

Morgan, R. 1970. The industrial rehabilitation of long-stay psychiatric patients in hospital. *Proceedings of the Royal Society of Medicine* 63(12): 1332–1335.

Morgan, R., D. Cushing and N.S. Manton 1965. A regional psychiatric rehabilitation hospital. *British Journal of Psychiatry* 111(479): 955–963.

Oppenheim, A.N. 1992. *Questionnaire design, interviewing and attitude measurement.* London: Pinters Publishers.

Plankinton, H. 1973. Horticulture as a work program for therapy. Unpublished PhD thesis, University of Delaware.

Query, T. 1968. *Illness, work and poverty: The hospital / factory in rehabilitation.* San Francisco (CA): Jossey Bass.

Richer, S. and B.R. Gearey 2017. From Rackham to REVEALS: Reflections on palaeoecological approaches to woodland and trees. *Environmental Archaeology* 23(3): 286–297.

Sempik, J. and J. Aldridge 2006. Care farms and care gardens: Horticulture as therapy in the UK, in J. Hassink and M. van Dijk (eds.) *Farming for health: Green-care farming across Europe and the United States of America*: 147161. New York: Springer Publishing.

Smout, T.C. 2000. *Nature contested: Environmental history in Scotland and northern England since 1600.* Edinburgh: Edinburgh University Press.

Stamp, L.D.1937. *The land of Britain: The Report of the Land Utilization Survey of Britain.* London: Geographical Publications.

SweetTree Farming for All 2015. BBC's Monty Don: Gardening as mental health therapy [Webpage]. Viewed 30 November 2018, <http://www.sweetreefarmingforall.org.uk/sweettree-farming-for-all/bbcs-monty-don-gardening-as-mental-health-therapy/>.

Tilley, C. 1994. *A phenomenology of landscape: Places, paths, and monuments.* Oxford: Berg.

Turley, A. and N. Turley 2000. *The US Army at Camp Bewdley and locations in the Wyre Forest area 1943-1945.* Worcester: Adrian and Neil Turley.

Voltaire 1759 [Trans. T. Cuffe 2007]. *Candide, or optimism.* London: Penguin Classics.

Ward, P. (ed.) 2009. *Nature to nurture: A history of the St Wulstan's Hospital site.* Worcester: Worcestershire County Council.

Watt, S. (ed.) 2011. *The archaeology of the West Midlands: A framework for research.* Oxford: Oxbow Books.

# Chapter 19

Archaeology and mental health: War memorials survey in Ceredigion

William Rathouse

Abstract

Inspired by projects including Operation Nightingale and The Past in Mind project, Mind Aberystwyth has been offering its members the opportunity to participate in archaeological digs since 2014. In 2016 they began planning a service-user led project to survey war memorials in Ceredigion. The purpose of the project was twofold: the memorials were photographed and their details recorded, so that their condition would be on record and, should any of them be damaged or destroyed, they could be reconstructed. It was also intended that participation would benefit mental health service users by enhancing self-confidence, promoting well-being, and supporting recovery. This chapter details the conduct of the project from planning through field research and onwards to data recording and presentation. It also examines data indicating the effectiveness of the project in achieving its mental health outcomes.

Keywords: Archaeology; Ceredigion; Mental health; Mind; War memorials

Introduction

This chapter reports on a project that the author designed and undertook with members of Mind Aberystwyth, focusing on War Memorials in Ceredigion. Following on from Mind Herefordshire's Past in Mind (Past In Mind 2014; Lack 2014) and the Ministry of Defence's Defence Archaeology Group (DAG) Operation Nightingale (DAG 2018; MOD and DIO 2019), this project was intended to create records of the monuments and to support the mental well-being of the participants.

From an early stage in the organization's history, Mind Aberystwyth has run group activities. Art and craft activities have long played a significant role, and a woodland ecotherapy group has been run since around 2010. Attendees can try their hand at woodland management work and greenwood crafts, or simply enjoy being out of doors in a wooded setting. In 2013, after reading about the Past in Mind project (Lack 2014), Fiona Aldred (then Chief Executive of Mind Aberystwyth) suggested that members might be provided with an experience of archaeological fieldwork as an activity to support their mental health. Thus in 2014 and 2015 the author involved service users from Mind Aberystwyth in digs at the Cistercian sites of Llanllyr and Strata Florida. These were run by Dyfed Archaeology and the University of Wales Trinity Saint David (Mind Aberystwyth 2015). The feedback from participants in all these projects was very positive and led on to the Archaeology for Mental Health War Memorials Survey.

Aims

The Archaeology for Mental Health War Memorials Survey addressed two areas: archaeology and mental health. The archaeological aims of the project were to:

1. Produce photographs and detailed records of war memorials in and around Ceredigion, so that in the event of serious damage, they could be repaired or replaced.
2. Provide data for online databases including War Memorials Online (2018) and the Imperial War Museum (IWM) War Memorials Register (2018).
3. Produce a written report to be disseminated to local and national stakeholders.

The mental health aim can be summed up as: To provide participants with an experience of archaeological survey work, and by so-doing to improve their self-esteem, assist with the formation of coping strategies and develop skills transferrable to paid employment.

The Project

Preparation

Having established these aims and drawn up an outline plan for the conduct of the project, Mind Aberystwyth staff approached the Heritage Lottery Fund (HLF) for a grant under their 'First World War: Then and now' scheme (HLF 2018a). The funding was agreed by November 2016, and training began on Saturday 28 January 2017, running from 10am to 4pm. It included an initial briefing by the author and a presentation from Dr Lester Mason (University of Wales Trinity Saint David) on the history of war memorials. The process to monitor well-being outcomes was explained, and informed consent sought for data collection. A second training day ran on Monday 6 February from 10am to 4pm. Menna Bell from Dyfed Archaeology Trust instructed volunteers in how to photograph, measure and record the appearance, condition and design of war memorials. Project members also met with a BBC radio journalist, who interviewed participants (BBC 2017).

Survey techniques were practiced on the Aberystwyth Allegory Memorial at Aberystwyth Castle and the Aberystwyth War Memorial plaque at St Michael's Church. A planning session was run on Monday 13 February. This followed the example provided by The Past in Mind project to involve participants in planning, giving them a greater sense of ownership of the programme. A list of known sites recorded by War Memorials Online, the Imperial War Museum's list, and West Wales War Memorial Project (WWWMP 2018) was drawn up, and memorials known by participants were added. A tentative schedule for visiting the listed memorials was then agreed. Transport hire was available, but in the event, private cars of project staff were sufficient. Participants seemed less than enthusiastic about this planning element of the project.

Fieldwork

On Saturday 18 February the first fieldwork without an external trainer was undertaken in Aberystwyth town centre. The Aberystwyth Boat Club's clubhouse was visited, but it transpired that this did not contain a memorial as initially supposed. Other memorials visited were: Ardwyn School Memorials at Aberystwyth Library (Figure 19.2); the Hermann Ethé memorial; Penparcau Memorial Hall; Penparcau Cross; Llanbadarn Cross; Burma Star Window; Plaques to Capt. & Lt. Powell. The second fieldwork day was Wednesday 22 February (12:30pm to 3:30pm) and involved visits to Llandysul Memorial Field and St Tysul's church. On Thursday 23 February (1:45pm to 2:30pm) the Aberystwyth University Memorial was surveyed. On Saturday 25 February (1pm to 5pm) there were visits to Goginan (Figure 19.1), Ystumtuen, Devil's Bridge, and Hafod Estate. Ystumtuen Chapel and Hafod Church were locked and keyholders not available, so these sites were not surveyed. On Monday 27 February (1pm to 5pm) the Allegory Memorial at a new housing development was surveyed, on the site of the old Tabernacle Chapel. The day continued with visits to St Michael's Church at Llandre and Rhydypennau Hall in Bow Street, finishing with Capel Y Garn, also in Bow Street. On Saturday 4 March the weather was sufficiently inclement that field survey work was postponed and writing up commenced at the Mind Drop-In Centre. The next session ran on Monday 6 March (1pm to 4pm) and involved field survey work at Bow Street's Noddfa Chapel. Plaques at Talybont Memorial Hall were also visited. On Wednesday 15 March (12:30pm to 3:30pm), Llanybydder Obelisk (located in Carmathenshire but close to a client's home) was surveyed. On Monday 20 March (1pm to 5pm) the plaques at the NatWest Bank and Post Office were recorded, and additional information gathered at Penparcau Memorial Hall. On Monday 27 March the author visited Bronant Chapel alone in the morning and then, in the afternoon, visits were made at Llanfarian Pentre Bont, Llanilar Church, and the memorial at Ysbyty Ystwyth (Figure 19.3). Saturday 1 April (1pm to 5pm) saw visits to Llanafan, Pontrhydfendigeid, and Ystrad Meurig. In the latter case, participants were unable to enter the church, but examined monuments in the churchyard. Monday 3 April involved surveys at Borth and Taliesin. On Wednesday 5 April memorials at the University of Wales Trinity Saint David's Lampeter campus were surveyed. The final field research day took place on Monday 10 April (1pm to 5pm) and involved the monuments at Penuwch, Llangeitho, Llanddewi Brefi, Ystrad Meurig.

By the end of the project we were confident in our ability to quickly prepare scale photographs and to record inscriptions (Figure 19.4). One task involved the production of scale drawings of a surveyed memorial that featured an allegory of peace or victory (Figure 19.5). This was created using software intended for controlling lathes for machining metal. Copies of this and other images produced were shared with an archaeologist specializing in building recording who forwarded

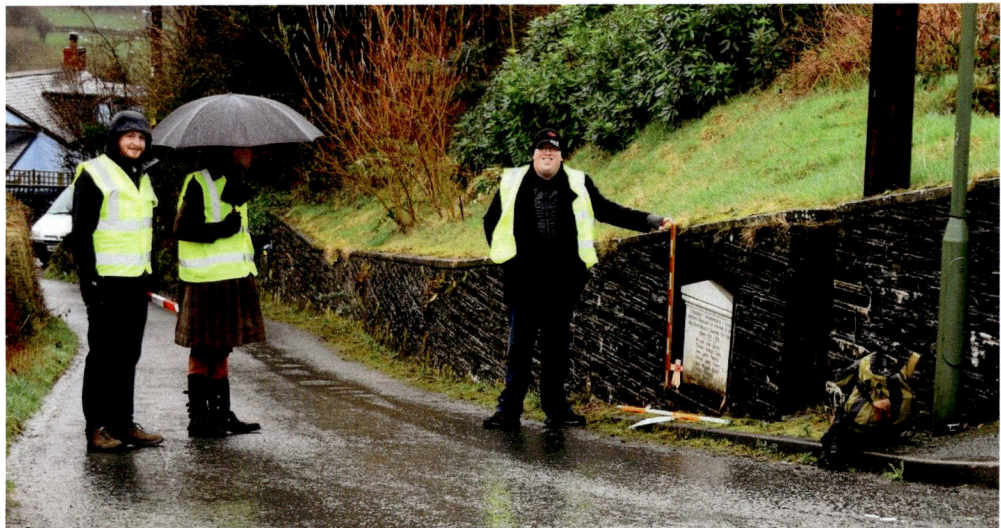

Figure 19.1 Team members pose next to the memorial in the village of Goginan, west of Aberystwyth. (Photograph by William Rathouse. Copyright reserved)

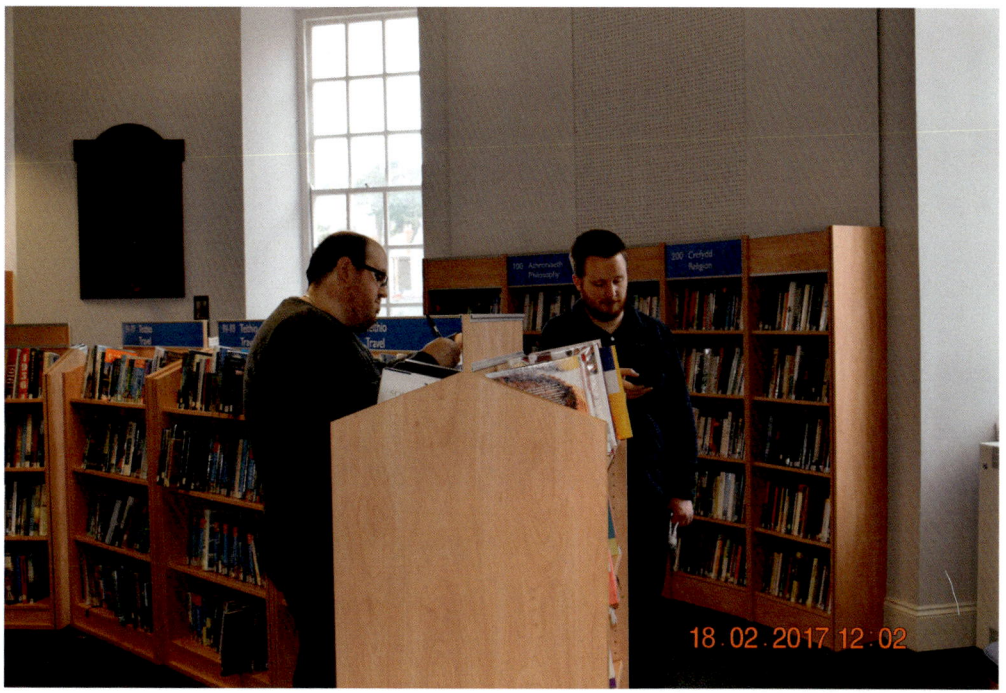

Figure 19.2 War memorial plaques re-erected in Aberystwyth library are surveyed. (Photograph by William Rathouse. Copyright reserved)

congratulations to the participant who produced them on a highly professional job. This praise appears to have provided a much needed boost to this person's self-esteem and self-confidence.

There followed nine days of data entry between 15 April and 14 October, during which results were uploaded to War Memorials Online and the written report prepared. A full report on the archaeological work of the project is available from the Royal Commission on the Ancient and Historical Monuments of Wales, Dyfed Archaeological Trust, The National Library of Wales, and can be downloaded from the internet as online document (Rathouse 2018).

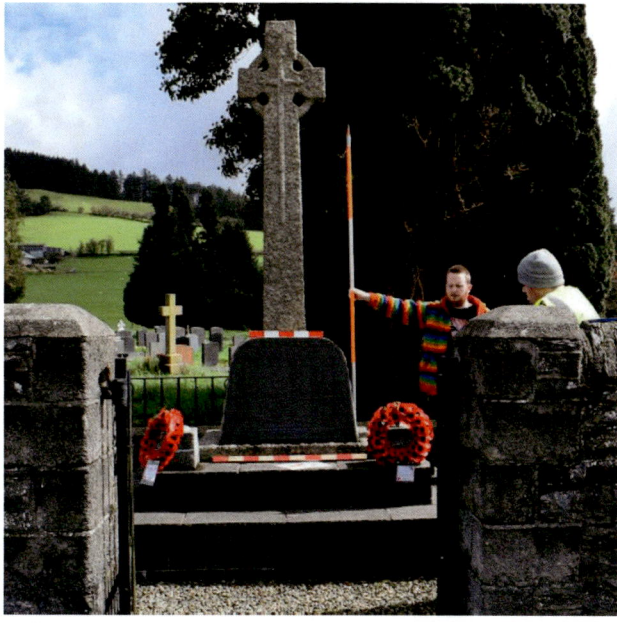

Figure 19.3 Staff volunteer and service user measure and prepare scale photographs of Ysbyty Ystwyth War Memorial. (Photograph by William Rathouse. Copyright reserved)

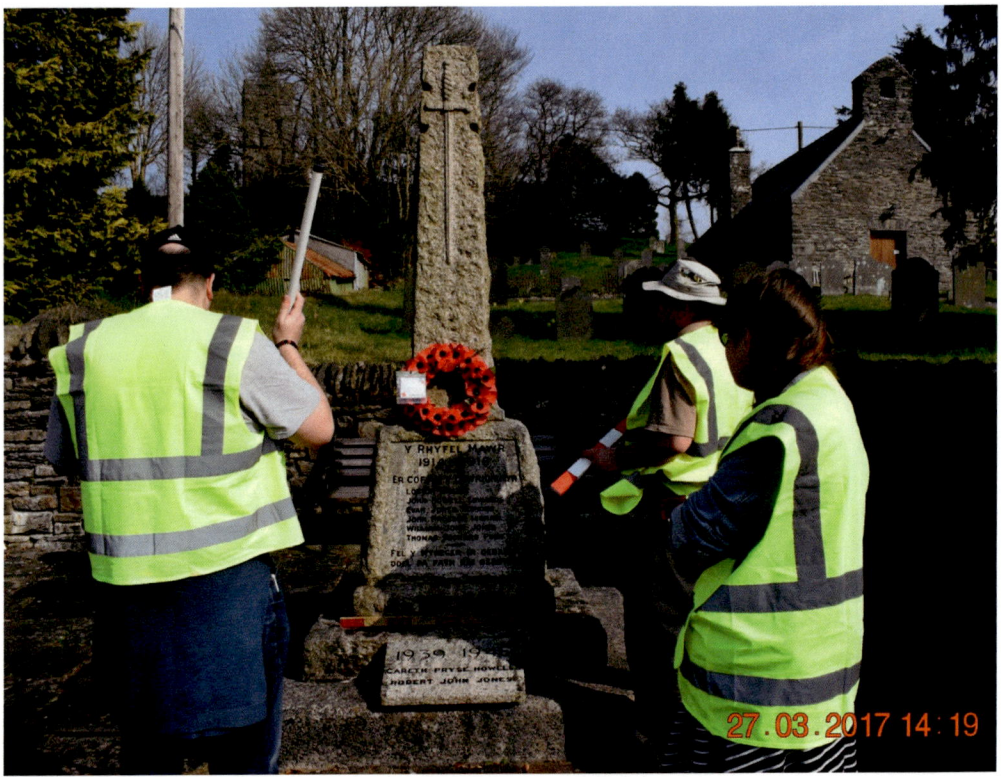

Figure 19.4 Preparing scale photographs and recording inscriptions.
(Photograph by William Rathouse. Copyright reserved)

Results

As a relatively novel concept, data on the effectiveness of archaeological fieldwork in promoting good mental health has been limited until recently. However, as other papers in this volume demonstrate, this area of research is gaining momentum. Whilst anecdotal evidence cannot be taken as proof of a general rule, can be a valuable form of qualitative data indicating possible outcomes.

Monitoring and analysis of mental health outcomes was therefore built into the Archaeology for Mental Health War Memorials Survey. Both quantitative and qualitative data were gathered. The quantitative data was generated at the start and end of each session by asking participants to complete a Warwick-Edinburgh Mental Wellbeing Scale form. This tool presents participants with 14 statements about their feelings and asks them to ascribe a number to each describing if they have experienced that feeling: (1) none of the time; (2) rarely; (3) some of the time; (4) often; or (5) all of the time. The feeling statements were as follows: I've been feeling optimistic about the future; I've been feeling useful; I've been feeling relaxed; I've been feeling interested in other people; I've had energy to spare, I've been dealing with problems well; I've been thinking clearly; I've been feeling good about myself; I've been feeling close to other people; I've been feeling confident; I've been able to make up my own mind about things; I've been feeling loved; I've been interested in new things; and, I've been feeling cheerful.

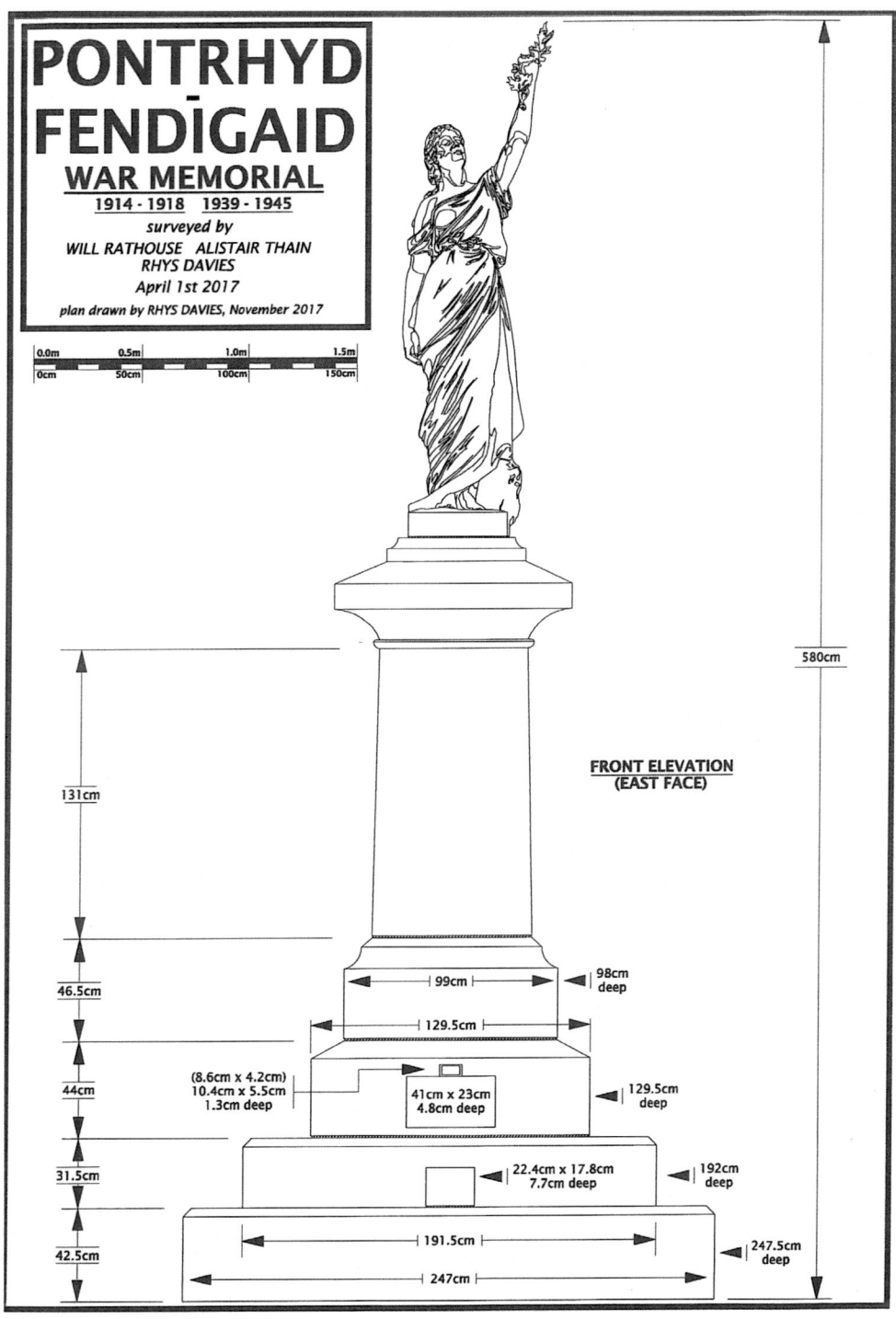

Figure 19.5 A scale drawing of a memorial we surveyed featuring an allegory of peace or victory. (Drawing by Rhys Davies. Copyright reserved)

Qualitative data was gathered in the form of photographs and short reports by participants, describing the experience of the project and its impact on their mental health. When writing these reports, the participants were urged to include criticisms and highlight areas where such projects could be improved. Records were also kept of who attended each session and the tasks undertaken therein.

The quantitative results were based on surveying at 43 sites. This work involved three staff members, one volunteer, and eight participants. Nine of the sessions had recorded outcomes. Average scores were noted for each participant, from the beginning to the end of the recorded sessions.

Outcomes

Qualitative

To the author, the most revealing evidence of the success or failure of this kind of project was critical review from participants. They were asked to write a short account of the project and its effects, being as critical as possible and highlighting areas where future projects might improve.

A participant diagnosed with psychotic depression, who attended one fieldwork session and two write up sessions, described her experiences thus:

> 'In the beginning I was nervous got worked up before coming to the sessions, now I am more relaxed about it and being with everyone, my mixing skills still need improvement, but it's been good to be around other people. I have also enjoyed taking part in the typing up of the couple of records I have done, but frustrated at my speed and general computer skills, as these are declined badly now, to what I use to be able to do and know., but in spite of this, I have enjoyed coming along to has been nice to feel a little useful. I hope there is another project along these lines again that I could maybe participate and contribute to in the future.'

> 'Before going on these projects I'd never done anything like this or ever known much about archaeology but, I have discovered it does fascinate me a bit, how much history can be found or discovered, from a chip of stoneware or just a stone or a little plaque, age of things etc.'

Another participant diagnosed with an autistic spectrum condition, social anxiety, and depression, who attended 15 sessions, described his experiences as follows:

> 'I found that the project really helped me in giving me a weekly goal to work towards, which has really helped anchor me during a time of unemployment, anxiety and depression. I found my mood elevated after each session, spending time in the open air in good company being a very positive experience.

> In terms of how the project could be improved I feel further outreaching to prospective participants would help. Many of those who joined us towards the end of the project

expressed regret at having not come aboard sooner, and I feel that there are others among Mind Aberystwyth's clients who would feel the same way. Further funding to extend the number of field trips we could take would also be beneficial.'

Quantitative

The quantitative data suggested some positive impact on the well-being of participants across each session, but failed to demonstrate a significant positive outcome from the beginning to the end of the project. Seven improvements were found, with five lower scores and one with no change. Only one participant had a higher average score at the end of the project than at its beginning. However, qualitative data, especially the written reports, show significant positive value to participants.

It is important to consider that quantitative results across the project as a whole may be skewed by feelings associated with it ending. It also fails to account for the effect of other life experiences during the period of the study that may have affected the mental well-being of participants. Another issue is that not all of the feelings described in the Warwick-Edinburgh Mental Wellbeing Scale were expected to be addressed by the activities undertaken in the project. It was anticipated that participants might feel more useful, relaxed, interested in others, able to deal with problems, capable of thinking clearly, feel good about themselves and close to others, more confident and interested in new things. However, it was not anticipated that the project was particularly likely to help participants feel optimistic about the future, loved, or (immediately) more energetic. It should also be borne in mind that, when applying figures to feelings (quantitative data), it is hard to demonstrate consistency of measure. It can also be argued that quantitative data is more useful in showing numbers of people experiencing simple distinctions of (for example) a good or bad experience. However, the breadth and depth of that impact may be better revealed by qualitative description. Furthermore, the significance of this data is restricted by the small sample size.

Future Projects

Recommendations

There are areas for improvement suggested by the Archaeology for Mental Health War Memorials Survey. In addressing these, better outcomes might be provided for more participants, and more robust data can be gathered on the efficacy of such projects. The following improvements are proposed.

A larger number of participants should be engaged in similar projects, with robust data capture implemented. Not only does this ensure that more people benefit, but it also provides a larger participant sample, and hence, more representative data for analysing outcomes. In the project to which this chapter refers, the small sample number is probably the most significant weakness.

There is some concern that participants in such projects who experience improvements, may simply fall back into their original situation or condition, after the end of their project. Ongoing, open-ended, funding and running of mental health archaeology schemes would therefore be desirable. Currently this appears rare, with most projects being of fixed duration. Notable exceptions Operation Nightingale (DAG 2018; MOD and DIO 2019) and the Thames Discovery Programme (TDP) based at the Museum of London Archaeology unit (TDP 2018). It is important, and funders such as the Heritage Lottery Fund are wise to stipulate, that the projects they fund should demonstrate benefits for individuals and communities as well as heritage (HLF 2018b). Alternatively projects might be integrated with housing, monetary and psychological interventions and/or job placements.

Improvements in outcome monitoring might be achieved by standardizing a quantitative analysis tool. The full Warwick-Edinburgh Mental Wellbeing Scale may not be the most appropriate tool; as discussed above, it sometimes includes the measurement of feelings that projects do not expect, or intend, to influence. The Museums Association (MA) suggests a range of techniques for measuring well-being outcomes within museums (MA 2018), particularly the UCL Museum Wellbeing Measures Toolkit (UCL 2018) and The Happy Museum Project 'Happy Tracker' (The Happy Museum 2018). However, a proliferation of measurement tools and techniques around the use of archaeology and heritage to improve well-being, may lead to discrete datasets that cannot be directly compared either within specialisms or with other sectors.

Archaeology in the the future for Mind Aberystwyth

With these experiences and recommendations, and following the feedback from participants in the projects thus far undertaken, Mind Aberystwyth is planning future work in this area. In order to ensure greater numbers of participants, the build-up phase of future projects will be longer. This will allow for liaison with, and visits to, other mental health support organizations, in order to solicit the involvement of their clientele. Mind Aberystwyth has already approached other local Mind branches in the wider Carmarthenshire and Pembrokeshire areas, as well as other local service providers in Lampeter and Aberystwyth. They are seeking funding of extended duration, that will allow future projects to run longer - a year or more - and permit more fieldwork.

Specific projects under consideration include extending and expanding on the war memorial survey already completed, by undertaking this research in Carmarthenshire and Pembrokeshire. It has also been suggested that Mind Aberystwyth could take on part of a larger project, recording vanishing rural infrastructure, in particular, the stone and concrete platforms built to facilitate collection of milk churns by the Milk Marketing Board. They are also keen to undertake excavation fieldwork. One landowner, who has hosted the woodland ecotherapy group at the site of an old lead mine, has expressed an interest in finding out where the workers cottages were on their land.

Mind Aberystwyth are also keen to run heritage walks in historic landscapes in Ceredigion, inspired by the Restoration Trust's Human Henge project. As a trial of this idea they have looked at the area around Strata Florida Abbey, that includes Bronze Age cairns, post-medieval metal mines, and the abbey buildings and environs. Another area under consideration is in North Pembrokeshire near the Nyfer estuary. This landscape includes a Mesolithic settlement on the North bank, Neolithic cromlechs at Newport and Pentre Ifan, a hengiform monument at Castell Mawr, early medieval stonework at Nevern Church, and the reconstructed Iron Age settlement at Castell Henllys. Another element that could be added to future projects, is an arrangement for participants to take up work placements in the heritage sector (K Gibbons pers. comms.). Assistance could also be provided in helping participants to access university courses in history, archaeology, heritage and related disciplines, as demonstrated by Breaking Ground Heritage (BGH 2018) and Operation Nightingale (DAG 2018; MOD and DIO 2019).

Conclusion

The evidence collected in Mind Aberystwyth's 2017 Archaeology for Mental Health War Memorials Survey, has demonstrated some support for the idea that archaeology is effective in developing recovery or coping strategies, for people affected by poor mental health. However, the positive effects were but not as strong as had been anticipated. It is believed that the quantitative data is less representative of the efficacy of the project, than the qualitative descriptions. The author remains convinced that archaeology is unusually well placed to support mental health, because it provides a 'purposeful activity and meaningful occupation' Creek (2002:75): concentration and focus that mirror distraction and mindfulness techniques; physical exercise; sunlight and fresh air; teamwork and positive social interactions; and a sense of cultural connection. The author is therefore keen to run more projects in order to further test this hypothesis.

Bibliography

BBC News 2017. Aberystwyth WW1 archaeology projects for mental health [Webpage]. Viewed 23 November 2018, <https://www.bbc.co.uk/news/uk-wales-mid-wales-38706017>.

BGH 2018. Breaking Ground Heritage [Webpage]. Viewed 23 November 2018, <http://www.breakinggroundheritage.org.uk/>.

Creek, J. 2002. Treatment, planning and implementation, in J. Creek (ed.) *Occupational therapy and mental health* (Third edition): 119-139. Edinburgh and London: Churchill Livingstone.

DAG 2018. Defence Archaeology Group: About [Webpage]. Viewed 23 November 2018, <http://www.dag.org.uk/page18.html>.

HLF 2018a. First World War: Then and now [Webpage]. Viewed 23 November 2018, <https://www.hlf.org.uk/looking-funding/our-grant-programmes/first-world-war-then-and-now>.

HLF 2018b. HLF: The difference we want your project to make [Webpage]. Viewed 23 November 2018, <https://www.hlf.org.uk/looking-funding/difference-we-want-your-project-make>.

IWM 2018. Imperial War Museum: War Memorials Register [Webpage]. Viewed 23 November 2018, <https://www.iwm.org.uk/memorials>.

Lack, K. 2014. *Past in mind: A heritage project and mental health recovery.* Bromyard: Privately published.

MA 2018. Measuring socially engaged practice [Webpage]. Viewed 23 November 2018, <https://www.museumsassociation.org/museums-change-lives/measuring-socially-engaged-practice/19032018-methods-for-measuring-social-impact>.

Mind Aberystwyth 2015. Therapeutic archaeology dig @ Mind Aberystwyth [Webpage]. Viewed 23 November 2018, <http://mindaberystwyth.org/therapeutic-archeology-dig-mind-aberystwyth/>.

MOD and DIO 2019. Operation Nightingale [Webpage]. Viewed 6 February 2019, <https://www.gov.uk/guidance/operation-nightingale>.

Past in Mind 2014. Blog from the bog: The official blog for the Herefordshire Past in Mind project [Blog]. Viewed 6 November 2018, <https://pastinmindproject.wordpress.com/>.

Rathouse, W. 2018. *Archaeology for mental health war memorial survey* [Online document]. Viewed 1 June 2019, <https://www.academia.edu/36525041/Archaeology_For_Mental_Health_War_Memorials_Survey_Dedication>.

TDP 2018. Thames Discovery Programme [Webpage]. Viewed 23 November 2018, <http://www.thamesdiscovery.org/>.

The Happy Museum Project 2018. 'Happy Tracker' wellbeing measurement tool [Webpage]. Viewed 23 November 2018, <http://happymuseumproject.org/happy-tracker/>.

UCL 2018. UCL Museum Wellbeing Measures [Webpage]. Viewed 23 November 2018, <https://www.ucl.ac.uk/culture/projects/ucl-museum-wellbeing-measures>.

War Memorials Online 2018. War Memorials Online [Webpage]. Viewed 23 November 2018, <https://www.warmemorialsonline.org.uk/>.

WWWMP 2018. West Wales War Memorial Project [Website]. Viewed 23 November 2018, <https://www.wwwmp.co.uk/>.

Chapter 20

Waterloo Uncovered: From discoveries in conflict archaeology to military veteran collaboration and recovery on one of the world's most famous battlefields

Mark Evans, Stuart Eve, Vicki Haverkate-Emmerson, Tony Pollard, Eleonora Steinberg, and David Ulke

Abstract

Waterloo Uncovered is a ground-breaking conflict archaeology project focused on the Waterloo battlefield in Belgium. Established in 2015 (the battle's bicentenary year) to learn more about the battle that shaped modern Europe, it supports serving personnel and veterans (SPV) in their well-being, recovery (from mental and physical injury), education, vocation and transition into civilian life. The project brings together professional archaeologists, students, SPVs, and volunteers in a mutually beneficial collaboration. It has five founding partner organizations: SPW (Service Public de Wallonie); The Centre for Battlefield Archaeology (University of Glasgow); L-P: Archaeology; ORBit team, Department of Soil Management (Ghent University); and University College Roosevelt (Utrecht University). The charity is also dedicated to educating the general public about its findings. These are changing the way we understand both the Battle of Waterloo and how we support our armed forces. This paper discusses the project so far, and outlines our future research goals.

Keywords: Archaeology; Collaboration; Recovery; Transition; Veteran

Introduction

Archaeology is emerging as an exciting and promising tool in supporting the recovery of serving military personnel and veterans (SPV) who have experienced physical and/or psychological trauma (Finnegan 2016; Osgood and Andrews 2015; Ulke 2018). Equally, SPV have numerous skills applicable to archaeology and they can be great assets for public engagement. In this paper, we present findings from our project, Waterloo Uncovered. This combines world-class archaeology on the site of one of the greatest battles in European history, with SPV support, education, and transition into civilian life. SPV support is at the forefront of the project's mission, together with expanding our knowledge of the battle. A commitment to professional standards of archaeology underpins this charitable project, alongside multinational collaboration and public engagement. In this paper we will focus on how we select and support SPV participants, the outcomes we have recorded so far, and the potential wider benefits and future direction of this project.

It bears explanation that 'SPV' is standard military terminology; both project co-ordinators and the serving and veteran military personnel themselves, use the term to identify this community. For the purposes of this paper, serving personnel (SP) are defined as and including those currently employed by the Army, Navy, and Air Force in a regular (full-time), reservist (part-time), or training capacity (including the Officers Training Corps (OTC) and Cadet Force. Veterans (V) are defined as those who have served in the British Armed Forces for at least one day (which would include as little as a single day in training).

Waterloo Uncovered

The Battle of Waterloo can, with some justification, lay claim to being the single most significant day (18 June 1815) of fighting in European history. Other battles were longer, fought over larger areas, or involved more combatants. However, few can be said to have settled a war in a single afternoon, and to have produced, in their conclusion, the peace that characterized the continent for so long after 1815. It may be one of the best-documented battles in history, but over the last 200 years there has been very limited archaeological work carried out on the site. In that time, wear-and-tear, and illicit metal detecting and looting, have depleted the available archaeological evidence. Our project began on the bicentenary of this battle and, despite the depletions, has made significant archaeological discoveries (the details of which will be presented in forthcoming publications).

Fittingly, the project was founded by two SPV with archaeology backgrounds and a significant link to the Battle of Waterloo. Waterloo Uncovered founders Mark Evans and Charlie Foinette studied archaeology together at the Institute of Archaeology, University College London. Completing their MAs in Museum Studies and Public Archaeology respectively, they both changed tack and joined the British Army as officers in the Coldstream Guards; a regiment that made an important contribution to, and suffered significant losses at, Waterloo. Early in their military careers they both spotted the potential for archaeology to benefit the military, not only by uncovering new and important finds about regiments and battles, but as a means of educating serving personnel about their military history. Both saw the potential in archaeology for meaningful engagement with soldiers; its physical, outdoor process and direct involvement could improve on book- and lecture-based learning and build on the soldiers' skillsets. For injured veterans, other physical, outdoor programmes that built confidence, skills, and social connections, were showing positive outcomes; archaeology offered an obvious parallel. This programme therefore combines support for SPV recovery and transition into civilian life with public archaeology, giving a structure where non-professional archaeologists make a meaningful contribution to the field. Waterloo Uncovered additionally has five founding partner organizations: SPW (Service Public de Wallonie); The Centre for Battlefield Archaeology (University of Glasgow); L-P: Archaeology; ORBit team, Department of Soil Management (Ghent University); and University College Roosevelt (Utrecht University). The mutual benefits of this socially-engaged, community-based archaeology, will be discussed in more detail below.

In the UK, both SPV support and archaeology have unmet needs, to which Waterloo Uncovered contributes. The Ministry of Defence (MOD) recently reported that among the military personnel that served between 1991–2014, approximately 66,000 will need physical or mental health support. For these, the greatest need is for mental health provision (MOD 2017). Support is available from clinical, welfare, and psychological programmes. However, the need continues to outweigh provision, and a significant number of veterans experience varying degrees of difficulty in adjusting to civilian life and recovery from their injuries (Duvall and Kaplan 2014). Veteran populations have historically had negative perceptions about mental health treatment (Caddick *et al.* 2015; Hoge *et al.* 2004). For example, compared to other civilians, veterans with post-traumatic stress disorder (PTSD) are less likely to engage in help-seeking behaviours (Murphy *et al.* 2015). Meanwhile, the All Party Parliamentary Group on Archaeology (APPAG) concluded that despite considerable and growing public interest in archaeology, funding and staffing for archaeology projects are still falling short of needs. This leaves professional archaeologists overworked, whilst commendable community archaeology projects lack proper liaison with professional groups (Aitchison 2017; APPAG 2004). The last decade or so has seen the appearance of a number of diverse community archaeology projects, including those that involve SPV; the most notable of these is Operation Nightingale (Finnegan 2016). At its inception in 2014, Waterloo Uncovered looked to some of these initiatives for guidance on best practice in the integration of SPVs into archaeological projects. Since then, it has developed, and continues to refine, its own holistic approach (Ulke 2018). This approach has benefited greatly from encouraging partnerships and collaborations with leading practitioners from fields such as veteran care, clinical psychology, professional archaeology, and the world of academia. Underpinning all of this, though, is the integration of community (most notably SPV), professional, and student archaeology. In achieving this, Waterloo Uncovered aims to achieve benefit for (and from) all its participants; our evaluations suggest that volunteers and staff gain as much as the SPV from the experience.

Mutual benefits

For SPV participants, some of the factors promoting well-being through archaeology align with those inherent to other successful SPV support projects. These include outdoor activity, social interaction, and learning new skills (Duvall and Kaplan 2014; MOD 2012). Additional benefits from archaeology include its 'meditative' quality (complete concentration on detailed practical tasks to the exclusion or more disruptive thoughts), and the fact that the work is purposeful in ways that contribute to tangible and lasting outcomes. Both are common features of projects that are successful in supporting mental and physical recovery (Carless *et al.* 2013; Finnegan 2016; Ulke 2018).

Beyond this, there are features of our archaeology project, we believe, that may have unique mutual benefits for SPV and archaeologists alike. Firstly, we and other assisted-archaeology projects have seen how the military skillset overlaps with the skills needed for professional archaeology (Finnegan 2016; Osgood and Andrews 2015). Both groups are hardened to (and even enjoy) outdoor work in varying weather conditions. They develop skills in mapping, scanning, and surveying the ground, are proficient in teamwork and team leadership, are accustomed to meticulous reporting, and are experienced in group living. This makes SPV involvement a genuine asset on the excavation (a term here which is taken to encompass a wide variety of field activities); they contribute effectively from the outset, with moderate additional training, due to their existing skillset and hardiness. Indeed, exposure to the 'camaraderie' of a dig can in itself be the benefit that SPV seek, as the environment and interaction is reminiscent of military living.

Secondly, archaeology provides a connection to heritage, history and identity for the SPV, in the same way that heritage contributes meaning to people's lives across the UK (MORI 2000). For some of the participants Waterloo Uncovered provides a direct link between soldiers who have served, or are still serving, to the contribution of their own regiment at the Battle of Waterloo. For others, the archaeology links them more broadly to past soldiers. Again, this link is also an asset to battlefield archaeologists. Waterloo Uncovered recognizes that SPV have crucial insight into the human experience of being in battle. They have an inherent understanding of how this affects decision-making, and that this can add considerable value to archaeologists' interpretation of conflict sites. Additionally, despite changes in modern warfare, SPV have applicable knowledge involving the ballistics of fired weapons, military tactics and their application, the terrain of a battlefield and how to exploit it, and military injuries and losses. As such, SPV are perhaps uniquely placed to provide meaningful insights into the interpretation of new and existing knowledge about the Battle of Waterloo.

Methods

As our programme and the research within it is ongoing, we will detail our programme structure for all our participants (SPV, archaeologists, students, and volunteers), together with the common research framework and data collection on well-being for all our cohort. Omitted are our methods for archaeology conducted on the programme. A more comprehensive account of our methods can be downloaded from our website (WU 2018), and a discussion of archaeological methodologies adopted and the results of this research is in preparation.

The Waterloo Uncovered team

Around a quarter to one-third of the Waterloo Uncovered excavation team are recruited as 'beneficiaries', whom we refer to as SPV. The remainder of the programme team consists of staff members, volunteers (including welfare officers, archaeological and research directors, archaeological supervisors, technical specialists, etc.), and students. Notably, a number of these team members are also serving or ex-military, so around half the team are actually SPV. Since our programme started, past beneficiaries have returned as volunteers or staff. In this report, although we acknowledge that this additional military background may be an important factor in the Waterloo Uncovered programme, we refer only to 'beneficiaries' as SPV.

Participant selection

When we recruit SPV, archaeologists, students, and volunteers for the Waterloo Uncovered programme, we consider it important to have a diverse group; in gender, nationality, ethnicity, military background and, type and degree of injury. Our process for recruiting non-SPV involves an interview and briefing about the nature of the project and a general discussion of the benefits and challenges of taking part. Optionally, students, volunteers, and archaeologists are given the opportunity to take mental health first aid courses.

SPV selection follows an established protocol. Each year, we estimate how many SPV we can support on the excavation, and recruit until we have an excess of applicants to allow for withdrawals and (rarely) exclusions. SPV recruitment begins in February when we review application forms. To recruit veterans, we work with other organizations including Combat Stress, Help for Heroes, and Walking With The Wounded amongst others to identify individuals who would most benefit from taking part. Injured serving personnel are recommended to us by Personnel Recovery Units or by their units. Additionally, throughout the project, a proportion of SPV have 'self-referred', that is they applied to us directly rather than through an organization. These self-referred SPV are important to us; the issues they face, such as social isolation, are not necessarily addressed by other organizations. A recent report published by Forces in Mind (Rafferty *et al.* 2017), interviewed 62 military veterans about barriers to accessing support. A key finding was that, as well there being recognized stigma for military and ex-military needing support (for detailed discussion of stigma, see Caddick *et al.* 2015; Sharp *et al.* 2015), veterans often feel that they are not entitled to, or eligible for, support programmes (Rafferty *et al.* 2017: 23). For example, SPV can feel that they have already had 'their portion' of care but are somehow not yet 'fixed', as opposed to viewing their recovery as a transition towards self-regulation (Rafferty *et al.* 2017: 9). We recognize that approaching Waterloo Uncovered, whether as a first point of contact or as a referral from another organization, sometimes requires SPV to overcome significant barriers.

In March, applicants undergo a 30–40 minute interview. During this, a staff member and welfare officer verify the SPV's background, discuss their motivations and aims for their time on their excavation, and how best to manage their welfare. We aim to be as inclusive as we can; we have a 'can-do' attitude towards supporting people with injuries. Exclusion criteria apply only when there is a serious risk of harm for the participant in taking part, a significant risk to others from the participant, or if the SPV's specialist care requirement exceeds available resources (although we are happy to host carers on the dig). Aiming to have the most diverse team possible, we select participants from a wide range of ages, genders, background and injuries. Selection is complete by April, and we take care to inform unsuccessful candidates in an appropriate and considered fashion. They are encouraged and provided with information to apply to other (UK-based) archaeological excavations that cater for SPV. Where appropriate, they are offered contact details and encouraged to contact other charities and services that might be able to address their needs. Some of the unsuccessful applicants are also given the option of a place on the Waterloo Uncovered reserve list and, if selected candidates withdraw, these reserve applicants are invited in their place.

The Waterloo Uncovered programme

For the SPV, the programme begins once they accept the invitation. We aim to build our relationship with each SPV through regular email and phone contact. For some of our applicants, attending a project like this is physically and/or mentally challenging, so we spend three months making individual preparations and building trust and confidence in our participants. Negative experiences or preconceptions can block a veteran's decision to engage or continue with support programmes (Rafferty *et al.* 2017). We aim to keep communication open so that candidates can voice concerns about coming on the programme, and, where possible, we manage stress and anxiety to keep them engaged. We collaborate with case workers, clinical teams and more general support networks (including family) where necessary.

Our two-week excavations have so far centred on Hougoumont Farm, a key site on the battlefield of Waterloo in Belgium. UK-based SPV, staff, students, archaeologists, and volunteers travel together from London, meeting other international participants on arrival. To cater for the full range of medical needs on the team, everyone is housed at a 3* hotel near the excavation site that offers self-contained catering and has proved extremely accommodating to the varying needs of our groups. To support group cohesion and social interaction, we aim to house team members in twin rooms with exceptions only for special requirements.

Days on the excavation have consistent structure and routine. Socialization is encouraged, with morning briefings and evening debriefings, shared mealtimes and evening activities. Although our approach to support is holistic, our plan for each SPV is founded on a detailed risk assessment for physical and mental health (using a Casualty, Evacuation / Repatriation Plan) and a duty welfare and administrative team is available around the clock.

The first two days of the programme are dedicated to orientation and training. We introduce SPV to the principles of archaeology and the events of the Battle of Waterloo, with a day of briefings and a battlefield tour. On the second day, SPV are trained in site safety and basic archaeology skills in small teams of five or six, in a 'round-robin' system commonly used in the military. This initial orientation is a chance for team leaders, SPV and the welfare team to see how best to include and support all participants. The working groups, supervised by an archaeologist, remain the same throughout the dig and, from day three until the end. The groups work at a flexible pace, tailored to the injuries and limitations of each team-member. We provide the SPV alternatives to trench archaeology that include surveying, finds processing, and photography — and there are opportunities to alternate between these four. All our SPV are given the option of having their progress in archaeology validated in an accredited 'skills passport'. The skills passport is backed by major employers and the Chartered Institute for Archaeologists (BAJR 2019) and supports a transition towards professional archaeology for those who want it, by documenting formal experience and training. In addition to archaeology, the programme offers optional creative activities to all team members, such as art, photography, model painting and creative writing. Purposeful and creative activities such as these have a known stress-relieving effect and can enhance health and well-being (Gutman and Schindler 2007).

At the conclusion of the dig, the UK elements return to London together before dispersing, and Waterloo Uncovered continues email and phone contact with SPV for roughly two more months. During this time we perform a handover to their referral organizations, support network, or caregivers. We also supply all our SPV with information on other welfare services that they may find useful, and guidance on how to continue developing any interest in heritage and archaeology. After the two month point, Waterloo Uncovered remains available to those wanting information or advice regarding archaeology and heritage, and regularly invites SPV to take part in public engagement and events organized by the charity (in early 2019 this included a residential conflict archaeology and heritage weekend in Scotland, hosted by the University of Glasgow — a project partner — and Northlight Heritage). We also facilitate ongoing social contact through social media and reunion events, maintaining an 'alumni' network that many participants find helpful.

Assessment

We assess the effect of the programme on both 'non-military' (archaeologists, students, volunteers, and staff) and SPV. To track well-being, SPV complete self-reporting questionnaires on the first and last day of the excavation, plus three months post-excavation. Within the questionnaire, we include the Warwick-Edinburgh Mental Well-being Scale (WEMWBS; Warwick Medical School 2016) and ICEpop CAPability measure for Adults (Al-Janabi *et al.* 2012) to obtain quantitative scores and track changes in well-being. We also rely on qualitative feedback from the participants in a debrief interview in the last few days of the dig and a feedback survey sent after their return home. Since 2017, we have also held focus groups and collected qualitative feedback from the archaeologists, students, volunteers, and staff. For everyone who takes part in the Waterloo Uncovered programme, the questionnaires assess the impact of taking part in the excavation on well-being, motivation, and education.

Outcomes

Participation, age, rank, nationality, and gender

We have aimed to host a diverse range of people, with as little hierarchy as possible and in a structure that encourages social mixing. Since its start in 2015, 77 SPV beneficiaries have come through the Waterloo Uncovered programme. Another 106 participants have taken part as archaeologists, staff, volunteers, and students. SPV ages ranged from 18 to 78, while other participants' ages ranged from 17 to 68. The gender split across the excavations was 28 per cent female and 72 per cent male. Notably, this gender split was more uneven among SPV, with a 13 per cent female / 87 per cent male split. However, the female component exceeds the most recent figures for gender representation in the Armed Forces. In 2018, 10 per cent of the Armed Forces were female, and this number has been far lower historically and is reflected in veteran populations — for example, in 1990, less than 6 per cent of the Armed Forces were women (Dempsey 2018). During the programme, SPV were treated equally, regardless of previous or serving rank in the military. The mix of SPV on the programme represented 21.7 per cent commissioned officers and 78.3 per cent non-commissioned officers. Overall, our participants over three years represented 14 nationalities; SPV hosted so far have been 87 per cent British, 9 per cent Dutch, and the remainder from USA, South Africa, and Switzerland.

SPV well-being

We have seen our participants' well-being improve during and after the Waterloo Uncovered programme. Good well-being, according to the UK mental health charity Mind (2013), allows you to do the following:

- Feel relatively confident in yourself and have positive self-esteem
- Feel and express a range of emotions
- Build and maintain good relationships with others
- Feel engaged with the world around you
- Live and work productively
- Cope with the stresses of daily life
- Adapt and manage in times of change and uncertainty

We have seen a number of the above parameters improve for our SPV beneficiaries. Over the last three years, we have been collecting quantitative data on well-being using the WEMWBS and ICECAP-A scoring systems. Both are showing a trend towards improvement in scores in paired comparisons before and after the excavation part of the programme (Ulke 2018). We are now aiming to accumulate enough data for a well-powered large-scale paired analysis.

Qualitative feedback from SPV has identified a number of factors that contribute to their improved recovery. It is worth noting that not all factors were beneficial to all people, while some showed more improvement than others (Ulke 2018). Our feedback supports the recommendation that the type of SPV support needed, depends on the individual (British Legion 2018).

However, interaction with other SPV, with a diverse group of civilians, and engagement with archaeology, were often cited as beneficial, as the following testimonial extracts demonstrate:

'Really, what made my experience on the project was not only learning about the battle and how it was fought compared to modern warfare, but uncovering the truth, whilst remembering all those who fought for something greater than themselves. The project also brought new life to me as it was somewhere where other soldiers and veterans could be together; we all have that same like-minded mentality and humour. I have since made amazing friends and seen how the project has helped others in ways that could not be put into words.'

'My whole social network other than family, are all military, even my wife. Meeting the archaeologists and students was an unexpected benefit to me.'

'The overall programme was a great experience and has increased my confidence in myself and other areas. I really enjoyed the interaction with the non-service personnel which I found a great help in my case. (We were all part of the same team). Meeting people of different nationalities and cultures was a good experience as well. I learnt that that there can be a life after the service (if you look for it)'

SPV transition, life skills, and vocation

While some of our SPV may have had a pre-existing interest in archaeology, it is our observation that taking part in the Waterloo Uncovered programme provides a significant proportion of our cohort with new skills, interests and sometimes a full new career path. Of the 77 SPV we have hosted so far, six have gone on to study archaeology at university (three undergraduate degrees and three masters degrees). A further 15 SPV have continued onto other heritage of archaeology projects, for example: volunteering in a museum; metal detecting; or joining other programmes such as Breaking Ground Heritage or Operation Nightingale. Our public engagement programme to disseminate findings from the archaeological dig has benefited from the involvement of ten SPV, and we have had 12 people return as staff or volunteers for the Waterloo Uncovered team. One SPV described his transition in the following way:

'I learnt a lot about myself, I felt like I had truly found myself and a purpose again. I now know I have a keen interest in archaeology and I will be carrying it on. I haven't felt this happy in a long time and everyone comments on how happy I look when I'm digging therefore, it's really helped me learn who I am, who I want to be and what I want to do. Following the dig I've done another dig with OP WALBEA and I'm doing another dig with Op Nightingale. Next year I'm hoping to return and do more archaeology with both of these projects.'

Archaeologist feedback

Over the last three years archaeologists and students have reported that they too had a positive experience of taking part in the programme. A common theme has been the benefit of coming into contact with people from different backgrounds and life experiences, despite the challenges of having differing humour or political views. In 2017, we began recording this feedback through focus groups. In a discussion with 12 returning staff and students, although some had previous interaction with SPV, there was unanimous agreement that taking part in the programme changed their perspective and encouraged them to share a new respect for military veterans with friends, family and colleagues (Haverkate, preliminary data). For example, one focus group member remarked that prior to the programme, they could not understand why anyone would join the army and that they had a 'very naive understanding of the military'. After the programme, this changed to 'an understanding of [sic] they are people who are attempting to do something so much braver than I could ever attempt'. There was an observation that academics studying military history have a reluctance to engage with veterans, but that our programme helped change that outlook for the participating academic staff and students.

Social mixing progressed in our programme but was by no means complete. In the focus groups and in feedback, archaeologists have commented on the distinct military culture but welcome its integration into archaeology:

> 'As an archaeologist the opportunity to excavate and produce archaeological results at the site of one of the most important events of the nineteenth century is a privilege. To do this with military personnel, who have infinitely more combat experience than I shall ever acquire, and to provide them with some respite, recovery and change adds to that satisfaction. In many ways I remain an outsider, a lifetime archaeologist among a group of professional military personnel, people who share experience, humour and camaraderie. It is truly humbling to think that something that has been so important to me, archaeology, can also provide some help to those who need it.'

Discussion

Waterloo Uncovered is changing our understanding of the history of the battle and, at the same time, transforming the lives of many people involved in the project. A central tenet is collaboration and sharing of information, including open-source research materials and public engagement. It is a model for conflict archaeology and social change that will continue to develop; a model that we feel could contribute effectively to research on well-being, archaeology practice, recovery and military history.

In its own right, Waterloo Uncovered does not have any specific recovery or clinical output. However, the holistic nature of the process, from application to completion of a trip, provides an environment, challenge and experience that can be used to support the recovery pathway for SPV. Both goal-setting (Doig *et al.* 2009), and a participatory structure like ours (Nutbeam 2000) have proven associations with better health outcomes. By including participants in the programme from the outset and conducting extensive interviews beforehand, the SPV engage in meaningful participant-centred goal-setting, that reflect how they would like to be involved and what they would like to gain from the experience. The programme structure also has parallels with graded return to work and progressive goal attainment practices, which have shown to significantly improve recovery and workplace participation (NICE 2009, Appendix C). In particular, it introduces structure and timekeeping (for travel, the working day and the application itself). It exposes SPV to a flexible workplace environment, provides the opportunity to progressively repeat experiences that may have previously caused anxiety (e.g. travel, eating in public, socializing), allows SPV with disabilities to practice mobility in a non-familiar, non-clinical environment, and builds confidence through challenging and purposeful activity. Our tracking of SPV recovery and transition trajectories is still on-going, and thus it remains to be determined whether participation in Waterloo Uncovered has significant effects on health outcomes and work participation.

Social connectedness has a long-standing positive association with emotional, physical and psychological well-being. More recently, it has been recognized that well-being interventions, such as ours, need to provide meaningful social roles outside the formal mental health system. For long-term mental health recovery, individuals need to believe that their social contribution is valued, and they also need to broaden their connections in order to enhance the diversity of their social group (Webber and Fendt-Newlin 2017). Our programme is characterized by group work, group socializing, shared accommodation and, contrary to the military culture that SPV may be used to, a flattened hierarchy. A key outcome is the interaction of civilians, military and veteran communities as they collaborate to gain deeper understanding of one of the most important battles in the history of Europe. This interaction fosters an improved integration of veterans into civilian life, both in their transition and in their acceptance and recognition by other civilians. This integration is, we believe, a significant factor in the improvement of well-being that we have observed. SPV come from the civilian population and returning to it is part of their life cycle. However, veteran and military communities can often become isolated from the rest of the civilian population through their choice of subsequent profession, their social circle and their belief system (Finnegan 2016; Murphy *et al.* 2016). Despite a common value system, serving personnel and veterans also have limited interaction (Hatch *et al.* 2013; British Legion 2018) and even veterans socially interact within their peer group, branch and rank, as opposed to across the full veteran population. Although fragmented, all these groups share a distinct military and veteran culture, with which members of our staff, our founders and welfare officers are familiar. Whilst our programme is not clinical, participants have commented on how their well-being is improved by feeling at ease and being amongst understanding peers. As the project has evolved, including SPV as returning staff and volunteers has also seen us benefit from their lived experience of injury and recovery, affecting the ways in which we support participants (WHO 2017). Overall, our findings support the proposal that cultural sensitivity —in this case to SPV values and identity — in the provision of welfare support, promotes better well-being outcomes (Heaslip 2015).

We have seen that the ultimate benefit of our programme comes from shifting perspectives and social mixing, from which we have measured benefit to both civilians and SPV. An extensive survey conducted by the British Legion (2018) found that, in addition to injury, Armed Forces culture is a contributor to the risk of social isolation and loneliness faced by veterans. Within this culture, there was a perception that civilians misunderstand or even show disdain for SPV (Demers 2011) and, simultaneously, veterans were reluctant to transition back to civilian life for fear of losing their identity (British Legion 2018). We saw noticeable improvements in self-esteem and positive views on civilian life after SPV were included in a mixed-gender, multinational group that combined civilians, military personnel and veterans, during both work and leisure. Previous studies have also reported that reduced social integration and loss of old military friendships among veterans carries an increased risk for PTSD and other mental health conditions (Hatch *et al.* 2013). Here we show, perhaps unsurprisingly, that the reverse — social integration and reconnecting with other SPV — has a positive effect on well-being. The British Legion (2018) recently identified as an important gap in evidence: the 'effectiveness of interventions with the [Armed Forces], including those that specifically target military identity'. Because Waterloo Uncovered deals with the full breadth of military identity — historical identity through archaeology and SPV identities — we are uniquely placed to fill this gap in evidence, and thus to develop best practice models for SPV recovery and full transition into civilian life. Further research is needed and some of our future direction is outlined below.

Future direction

Waterloo Uncovered initially aimed to support a few veterans and perform some exploratory archaeology, but it has since evolved into a much larger project. We now aim to use archaeology as a lens through which to view the Battle of Waterloo and understand the impact of war on people. We want to benefit all participants on our programme — SPV, archaeologists, volunteers and students — and to gain deeper insight into the benefits of collaboration and discovery.

Our project models several forward-looking recommendations for both archaeology and health support (Heaslip 2005; Thomas 2004; WHO 2017). By including SPV in our battlefield excavation, we work with a distinct social group that has a meaningful connection and interest in conflict history, and engage them in dialogue rather than didactic teaching. Further still, we give them tools to continue their exploration of their own heritage (Thomas 2004). We have not encountered any insurmountable challenges in training or supervision by performing archaeology in this way, so it serves as an ongoing proof-of-concept that community archaeology can combine with social engagement. From 2019, we plan to expand our archaeology beyond the Hougoumont Farm site and to increase our inclusion of international veterans. Additionally, we aim to use the lived experience of our SPV to inform both how we support their welfare (WHO 2017) and the ways in which we collaborate on conflict archaeology. By recording well-being scores and vocational outcomes for our SPV beneficiaries, we also have an increasing dataset with which to research the impact of our programme on SPV transition and recovery. For further study, we aim to introduce an Impact of Events Scale assessment to our SPV questionnaire and to expand and continue our qualitative analysis. Currently, we are in the process of developing a research framework that will allow us to make the best use of our data and to collaborate with other research groups.

Bibliography

Aitchison, K. 2017. *Archaeological market survey 2016-17* [Online document]. Sheffield: Landward Research Ltd. Viewed 17 January 2019, <https://www.archaeologists.net/sites/default/files/Archaeologicalper cent20Marketper cent20Surveyper cent202016-17per cent20101117.pdf>.

Al-Janabi, H., T.N. Flynn and J. Coast 2012. Development of a self-report measure of capability well-being for adults: The ICECAP-A. *Quality of Life Research* 21(1): 167–176.

APPAG 2004. Revised summary of issues from submissions [Webpage]. Viewed 17 January 2019, <http://www.appag.org.uk/report/summary_issues.html>.

BAJR 2019. Learning: Education and courses [Webpage]. Viewed 17 October 2018, <http://www.bajr.org/BAJREducation/>.

British Legion 2018. Loneliness and social isolation in the armed forces community [Webpage]. Viewed 17 January 2019, <https://www.britishlegion.org.uk/get-involved/campaign/loneliness-and-social-isolation/>.

Caddick, N., B. Smith and C. Phoenix 2015. Male combat veterans' narratives of PTSD, masculinity, and health. *Sociology of Health and Illness* 37(1): 97–111.

Carless, D., S. Peacock, J. McKenna and C. Cooke 2013. Psychosocial outcomes of an inclusive adapted sport and adventurous training course for military personnel. *Disability and Rehabilitation* 35(24), 2081–2088.

Demers, A. 2011. When veterans return: The role of community in reintegration. *Journal of Loss and Trauma* 16(2): 160–179.

Dempsey, N. 2018. *UK defence personnel statistics* (House of Commons Library Briefing Paper CPB7930) [Online document]. London: HMG. Viewed 17 January 2019, <http://researchbriefings.files.parliament.uk/documents/CBP-7930/CBP-7930.pdf>.

Doig E., J. Fleming, P.L. Cornwell and P. Kuipers 2009. Qualitative exploration of a client-centred, goal-directed approach to community-based occupational therapy for adults with traumatic brain injury. *The American Journal of Occupational Therapy* 63(5): 559–568.

Duvall, J. and R.J. Kaplan 2014. Enhancing the well-being of veterans using extended group-based nature recreation experiences. *Journal of Rehabilitation Research and Development* 51(5), 685–696.

Finnegan, A. 2016. The biopsychosocial benefits and shortfalls for armed forces veterans engaged in archaeological activities. *Nurse Education Today* 47: 15–22.

Gutman, S.A. and V.P. Schindler 2012. The neurological basis of occupation. *Occupational Therapy International* 14(2): 71–85.

Hatch, S.L., S.B. Harvey, C. Dandeker, H. Burdett, N. Greenberg, N.T. Fear and S. Wessely 2013. Life in and after the armed forces: Social networks and mental health in the UK military. *Sociology of Health and Illness* 35(7): 1045–1064.

Heaslip, V. 2015. Experiences of vulnerability from a gypsy / travelling perspective: A Phenomenological Study. Unpublished PhD thesis. Faculty of Health and Social Sciences. Bournemouth University.

Hoge C.W., C.A. Castro, S.C. Messer, D. McGurk, D.I. Cotting and R.L. Koffman 2004. Combat duty in Iraq and Afghanistan, mental health problems, and barriers to care. *The New England Journal of Medicine* 351(1): 13–22.

Mind 2013. How to improve your mental wellbeing [Webpage]. Viewed 17 January 2019, <https://www.mind.org.uk/information-support/tips-for-everyday-living/wellbeing/>.

MOD 2012. The Battle Back Programme: Sport and training for wounded, injured and sick personnel from across the armed forces [Webpage]. Viewed 17 January 2019, <https://www.gov.uk/guidance/the-battle-back-programme>.

MOD 2017. *Defence people mental health and wellbeing strategy 2017-2022* [Online document]. London: HMG. Viewed 17 January 2019, <https://www.gov.uk/government/uploads/system/uploads/attachment_data/file/689978/20170713-MHW_Strategy_SCREEN.pdf>.

MORI 2000. What does 'heritage' mean to you? [Webpage]. Viewed 17 January 2019, <https://www.ipsos.com/ipsos-mori/en-uk/what-does-heritage-mean-you>.

Murphy, D., G. Hodgman, C. Carson, L. Spencer-Harper, M. Hinton, S. Wessely and W. Busuttil 2015. Mental health and functional impairment outcomes following a 6-week intensive treatment programme for UK military veterans with post-traumatic stress disorder (PTSD): A naturalistic study to explore dropout and health outcomes at follow-up. *BMJ Open* 5(3) [Online journal]. Viewed 17 January 2019, <http://dx.doi.org/10.1136/bmjopen-2014-007051>.

Murphy, D., L. Spencer-Harper, C. Carson, E. Palmer, K. Hill, N. Sorfleet, S. Wessely and W. Busuttil 2016. Long-term responses to treatment in UK veterans with military-related PTSD: An observational study. *BMJ Open* 6(9) [Online journal]. Viewed 17 January 2019, <http://dx.doi.org/10.1136/bmjopen-2016-011667>.

NICE 2009. Workplace health: Long-term sickness absence and incapacity to work. Public health guideline [PH19] [Webpage]. Viewed 17 January 2019, <https://www.nice.org.uk/guidance/ph19>.

Nutbeam, D. 2000. *Health promotion effectiveness — the questions to be answered. In. IUHPE A report for the European Commission by the International Union for Health Promotion and Education.*

The Evidence of Health Promotion Effectiveness: Shaping Public Health in a New Europe, Part 2 (Second edition) [Online document]. Saint-Maurice, France: International Union for Health Promotion and Education . Viewed 17 January 2019, <https://www.iuhpe.org/images/PUBLICATIONS/THEMATIC/EFFECTIVENESS/HPE_Evidence-2_EN.pdf.>.

Osgood, R. and P. Andrews 2015. Excavating Barrow Clump: Soldier archaeologists and warrior graves. *Current Archaeology* 306: 28–35.

Polusny, M.A., C.R. Erbes, P. Thuras, A. Moran, G.J. Lamberty, R.C. Collins, J.L. Rodman and K.O. Lim 2015. Mindfulness-based stress reduction for post-traumatic stress disorder among veterans: A randomized clinical trial. *Journal of the American Medical Association* 314(5): 456–465.

Rafferty, L., S. Stevelink, N. Greenberg and S. Wessely 2017. Stigma and barriers to care in service leavers with mental health problems [Webpage]. Viewed 17 January 2019, <https://www.kcl.ac.uk/kcmhr/publications/Reports/index.aspx>.

Sharp, M-L., N.T. Fear, R.J. Rona, S. Wessely, N. Greenberg, N. Jones and L. Goodwin 2015. Stigma as a barrier to seeking health care among military personnel with mental health problems. *Epidemiologic Reviews* 37(1), 144–162.

Thomas, R.M. 2004. Archaeology and authority in the twenty-first century, in N. Merriman (ed.) *Public archaeology*: 191–201. London: Routledge.

Ulke, D., 2018. The Legacy of Mars: The impact of participation in archaeology on the mental well-being of military personnel and veterans. Unpublished undergraduate dissertation, University of Leicester.

Warwick Medical School 2016. WEMWBS user guide [Webpage]. Viewed 17 January 2019, <https://warwick.ac.uk/fac/med/research/platform/wemwbs/researchers/userguide/>.

WHO 2017. Promoting recovery in mental health and related services — WHO quality rights training to act, unite and empower for mental health (pilot version) [Webpage]. Viewed 17 January 2019, <http://www.who.int/iris/handle/10665/254811>.

WU 2018. *Waterloo Uncovered. Project review volume 1* [Online document]. Viewed 1 June 2019, < http://www.waterloouncovered.com/learn/project-review-volume-1/>.

Chapter 21

Crafting, heritage and well-being: Lessons from two public engagement projects

Zena Kamash

Abstract

In this chapter I discuss the design and results of two public engagement projects: Remembering the Romans in the Middle East and North Africa (RetRo); and Rematerialising Mosul Museum. They brought together heritage with arts and crafts to promote both more positive narratives about the Middle East and North Africa (MENA) and the well-being of participants. I start with an overview of the existing research into heritage and well-being, and crafting and well-being, showing how pulling these strands together can be beneficial and might have therapeutic effects for people suffering from trauma. I then present a summary of my two projects before discussing the feedback from the participants to explore ways in which being part of the workshops contributed to well-being. In the final part I suggest potential ways forward for future work in this area.

Keywords: Crafting; Heritage; Iraq; Middle East and North Africa; Trauma

Introduction

Existing research into heritage, crafting, and well-being, indicates that a combination of these fields might be therapeutic for those suffering from trauma. Recent projects, Remembering the Romans in the Middle East and North Africa (RetRo) and Rematerialising Mosul Museum, both used these factors to engage groups of people of different backgrounds and abilities in order to explore the ways in which they experienced these benefits in the form of improved well-being.

Definition of well-being

For the purposes of my work, and for this chapter, I follow the What Works Centre for Wellbeing's definition using three dimensions of well-being (What Works Wellbeing 2018):

1. The personal dimension: confidence, self-esteem, meaning and purpose, increased optimism and reduced anxiety;
2. The cultural dimension: coping and resilience, capability and achievement, personal identity, creative skills and expression; and
3. The social dimension: belonging and identity, sociability and new connections, bonding, reciprocity and reducing social inequalities.

Crafting, museums and well-being: An overview

There is a burgeoning amount of evidence for links between heritage, well-being, and art and craft activities. For the UK context, a lot of this work has been helpfully synthesized by the All-Party Parliamentary Group on Arts, Health and Wellbeing Inquiry Report on creative health and the use of the arts for health and wellbeing (APPGAHW 2017; additional scoping work on crafting and well-being is also being carried out currently by the Yarnfulness Project: Yarnfulness 2018). In this overview, I will draw out salient points from this report as well as explore some of the more specific research into crafting and well-being, particularly in the treatment of trauma.

Having access to heritage, and the ability to take part in heritage activities, has been shown to increase life satisfaction (APPGAHW 2017: 65). The Heritage in Hospitals project, for example, which ran from 2008 to 2011, demonstrated that taking museum objects into care homes significantly increased wellness and happiness that could be measured quantitatively (Ander *et al.* 2013a; Ander *et al.* 2013b; Lanceley *et al.* 2011; Solway *et al.* 2015; Thomson *et al.* 2011; Thomson *et al.* 2012a; Thomson *et al.* 2012b. Also see Chatterjee and Noble 2013). The opening up of ways to take part was key here, as co-production and inclusion in decision-making are important for health (APPGAHW 2017: 66). There is, however, a continuing problem over access as demonstrated by the Taking Part Survey — a study undertaken for the Department for Digital, Culture, Media and Sport, Arts Council England, English Heritage, and Sport England — which showed that the majority of people both visiting museums and galleries and taking part in creative activities were well-educated professionals aged 55–74 who also had had access to such activities when young (Inglis and Williams 2010). Furthermore, museum visitors and creative activity participants are most likely to be white and unlikely to be black or Asian (Inglis and Williams 2010: 2). Clearly, then, there are significant barriers to access that still need to be overcome. In addition, given that access to heritage and co-production are so important for well-being and health, then what happens when that heritage is forcibly taken from you, for example through destruction? And how can we work to overcome the barriers that might further prevent the same people from having that access? These questions are discussed further below.

Similar to heritage, there is also increasing evidence that engaging in craft activities can have a positive influence on well-being. It promotes motivation, a positive sense of self, personal growth, and a sense of competence and achievement, as well as a sense of being in control and able to make choices (Bedding and Sadlo 2008; Hacking *et al.* 2006; Perruzza and Kinsella 2010; Riley 2008; Reynolds 2009; Tzanidaki and Reynolds 2011; for a useful overview, see Riley *et al.* 2013). Crafting with textiles and fibres seems to be particularly beneficial for well-being. Participants in the Stitchlinks Project (Stitchlinks 2018), for example, which surveyed 3545 people from 31 countries, reported that when they knitted they felt calmer and happier. The reasons cited for this benefit revolved around several themes. The rhythmic and repetitive nature of knitting was deemed to have therapeutic and meditative qualities that provide a 'mental break' and help to prevent negative thoughts creeping in (Riley *et al.* 2013: 52–53). Respondents also commented that knitting was a way of being socially active, including giving things to other people, and gave them a sense of accomplishment: 'a touchable feelable result' (Riley *et al.* 2013: 55). This tactility of the craft was reflected by 46 per cent of respondents commenting that they felt texture affected their mood. In addition, as well as opening up new skills, including other crafts, respondents felt that it gave them a connection to tradition. This was also found to be the case in the study by Boerema *et al.* (2010) of sewing and well-being amongst immigrant women in south Australia, for whom sewing also provided a link to cultural traditions. This perceived link between crafting and tradition opens up a space for heritage, crafting and well-being to come together in concert, as will be discussed further below.

Also of relevance in this context is current research into trauma, mindfulness and creativity. Trauma, in particular post-traumatic stress disorder (PTSD), manifests itself both as a strong desire to avoid thinking about the original trauma and as unbidden memories, often referred to as 'flashbacks', and nightmares (see Caruth 1995; Smelser 2004; van der Kolk and van der Hart 1995). Fear of triggering the trauma can lead to social isolation and avoidance of pastimes that were previously enjoyed. Traditional treatment for PTSD has focused on exposure-based therapies in which patients gradually confront their anxiety and trauma. More recently, there have been moves to supplement these traditional therapies, which treat the trauma-related psychopathology, with alternatives that may be gentler, help people feel safer and foster personal strength and growth (Smyth and Nobel n.d.; Southwick *et al.* 2015; Talkovsky and Lang 2017). These alternatives frequently draw on mindfulness as a technique to promote resilience, especially in adults. In bringing thoughts back to the present through mindfulness, life can be engaged more in the present rather than fixating on the past and future. Attention can be controlled in order to decrease negative biases, regulate emotions and improve threat appraisal (Smyth and Nobel n.d.: 4; Southwick *et al.* 2015: 3).

There is a similarity here with the rhythm and absorption of arts and craft practice that provides potential for these practices to be used as alternative treatments (APPGAHW 2017: 40). Where work has been done in this area, it has tended to focus on PTSD in military veterans (for a summary of projects, see APPGAHW 2017: 111), though the Mental Health Foundation's Amaan Project has been working with asylum-seeking women in Glasgow (Mental Health Foundation 2018; see also APPGAHW 2017: 113). As well as the mindfulness benefits of crafting, crafting as part of a group also has other positives for PTSD sufferers as it recognizes that individuals are part of wider social groupings and structures (on the need for this recognition, see Southwick *et al.* 2015: 1).

Group-based activities can both help increase social inclusion for people who have avoided social activities and aid in creating community cohesion between, for example, host communities and newly-arrived refugees (APPGAHW 2017: 113; Kidd *et al.* 2008; Smyth and Nobel n.d.: 3-4). Finally, taking a 'craftivist' approach — the gentle act of protest through crafting — may also be beneficial for people experiencing trauma. Often a contributing element to trauma is the lack of any sense of control over a situation (on health and a sense of control, see APPGAHW 2017: 20). If, through crafting and craftivism, a participant is able to regain a sense of control that could be potentially very powerful indeed.

Remembering the Romans in the Middle East and North Africa (RetRo) and Rematerialising Mosul Museum: Overview and design

In this section, I will present an overview of the two public engagement projects, before discussing how, and why, they were designed with the promotion of well-being in mind. It should be noted from the outset that neither project had a psychology professional on the team. This means that neither project can be deemed to constitute therapy, though individuals may have experienced therapeutic outcomes (see below). In addition, due to the possibility of triggering trauma in some of the participants, ethical consent was sought for both projects.

RetRo took place in the spring of 2016 and was funded by an AHRC Cultural Engagement Fund grant. The project saw two day-long workshops at the Petrie Museum in London and two

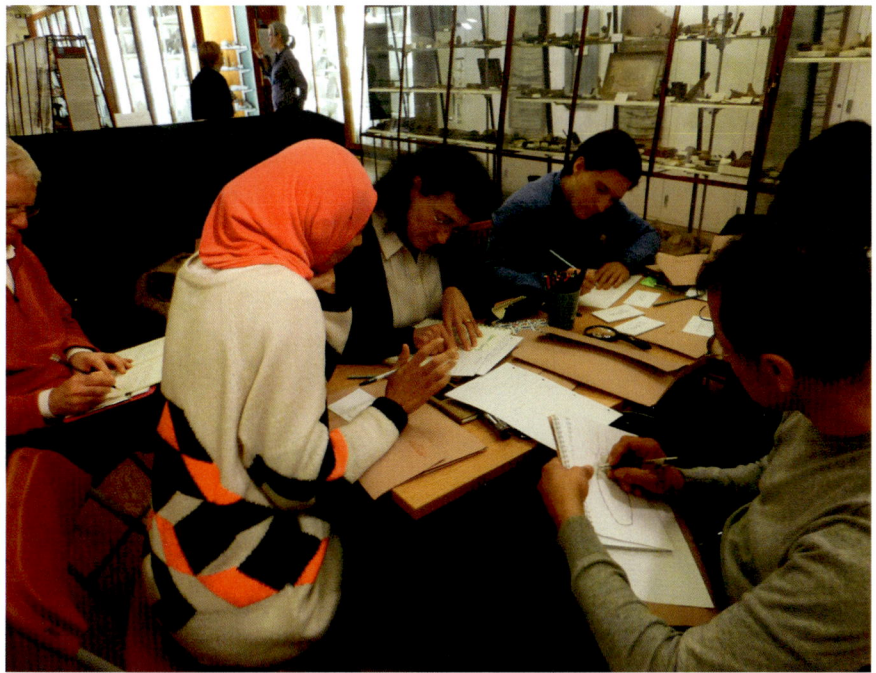

Figure 21.1 RetRo workshop in progress at the Petrie Museum, London: creative writing and drawing. (Photograph by Zena Kamash. Copyright reserved)

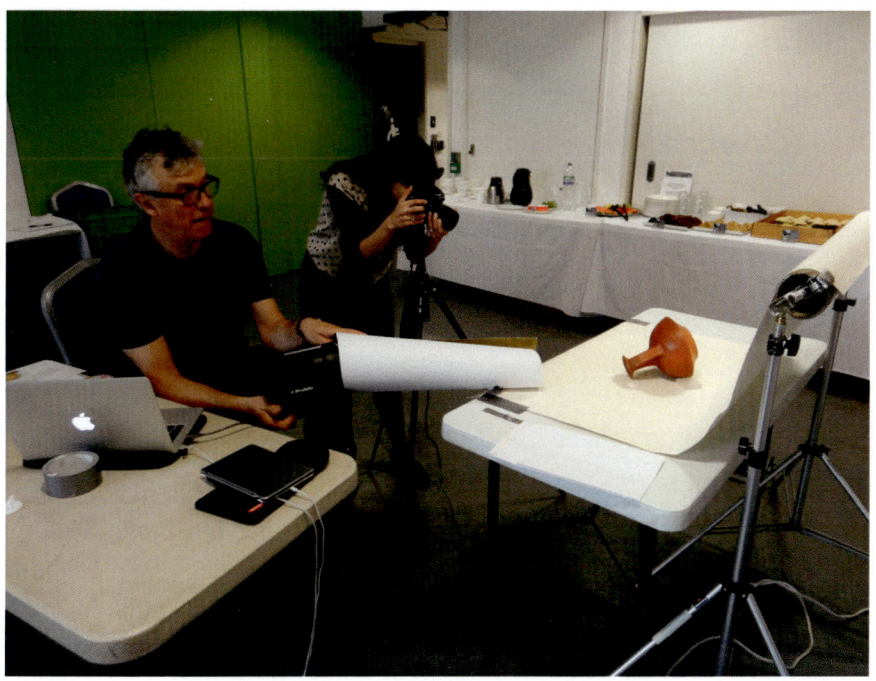

Figure 21.2 RetRo workshop in progress at the Great North Museum, Newcastle: photography. (Photograph by Zena Kamash. Copyright reserved)

day-long workshops at the Great North Museum in Newcastle, as well as a side project called Postcard to Palmyra, which is discussed in detail in elsewhere (Kamash 2017). The workshops were collaborations with the museums and with artist Miranda Creswell, photographer Rory Carnegie, and creative writing specialist Sarah Ekdawi. During the workshops, the museum curators gave a brief tour of their collections, then participants were invited to choose either an object or objects from either a pre-selected set of objects or any object on display, and to respond to it through drawing, photography, and/or creative writing with the guidance of Miranda, Rory and Sarah (Figures 21.1 and 21.2). Participants (32 across all workshops) included people with a Middle Eastern or North African background, and people with an interest in the archaeology of the region.

Rematerialising Mosul Museum grew out of the RetRo project and was funded by the British Institute for the Study of Iraq and the Institute of Classical Studies. The project took place in the summer of 2018 when two workshops were held at Cheney School, Oxford. These workshops were a collaboration with fibre artist Karin Celestine. Photographs of objects that had once been in Mosul Museum (from: Project Mosul 2017) were used as inspiration during the workshops, together with photographs of monuments in the city (from: Monuments of Mosul 2018), images of objects from the British Museum and the Ashmolean Museum, actual objects that I inherited or received as gifts from family members and, at the second workshop, postcards of various sites in Iraq brought by one of the participants. During each workshop,

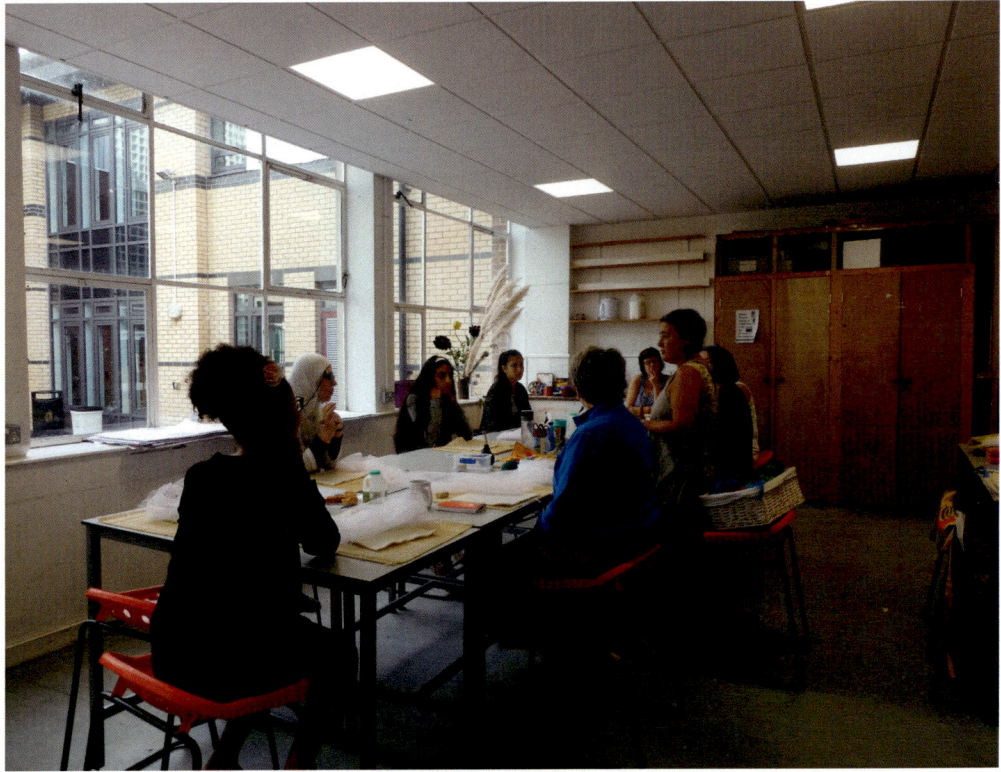

Figure 21.3 Felting workshop in progress at Cheney School, Oxford. Karin Celestine (standing) explains the wet felting technique to the participants. (Photograph by Zena Kamash. Copyright reserved)

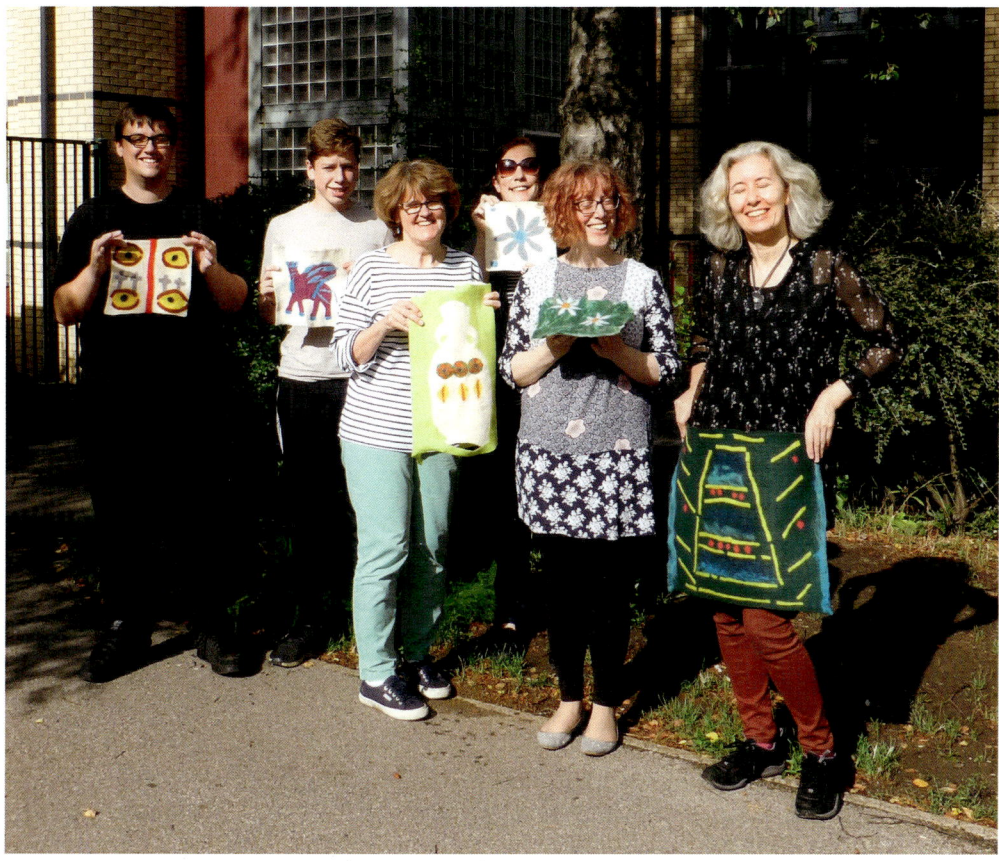

Figure 21.4 Participants of the first felting workshop with their final felted panels. (Photograph by Karin Celestine. Copyright reserved)

Karin demonstrated the wet felting technique so that participants could make a felted panel inspired by their chosen picture or object (Figures 21.3–5). Participants (14 across both workshops) included people with an Iraqi background, people learning Arabic who wanted to learn more about associated cultural aspects, and people who wanted to learn a new craft skill, as well as being interested in archaeology and Iraq.

Both workshops were motivated by a desire to shift the narrative towards the MENA region and its heritage. An important element in this was to make an effort to amplify voices of people from that region and, in so doing, try to break down some of the barriers to access outlined above. Adverts for the projects were bilingual (in English and Arabic), and flagged to cultural organizations working with MENA communities in the UK. There were two major hurdles encountered here. Firstly, in the RetRo project it seemed that using museum spaces for the workshops may have imposed a further barrier, being off-putting for people who were not already used to being in these spaces. As a consequence, the Rematerialising Mosul Museum felting workshops were held in a state secondary school which seems to have helped this problem, at least in part. The second hurdle, however, has been harder to overcome so far. This barrier came from cultural organizations themselves, especially refugee organizations,

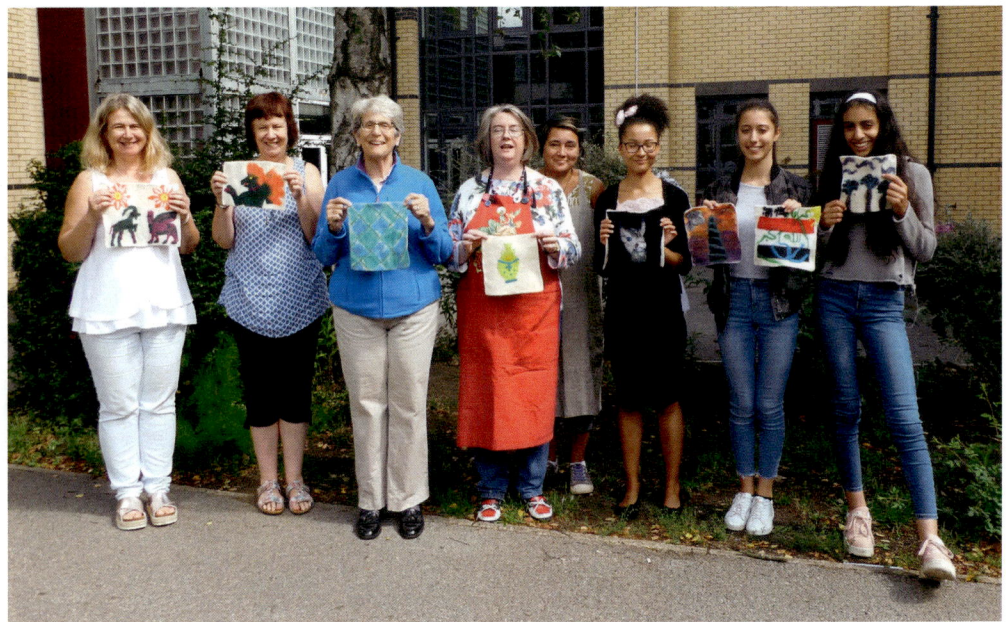

*Figure 21.5 Participants of the second felting workshop with their final felted panels.
(Photograph by Zena Kamash. Copyright reserved)*

who have been extremely reluctant to engage. There seem to be a couple of potential reasons for this reaction: first, a concern over the ethics of this kind of work (i.e. potentially provoking trauma in vulnerable individuals); and second, an under-appreciation of the potential value of this kind of work (for example one organization considered this not to be their type of 'helpful' work). The first is, of course, a legitimate concern and was considered by seeking ethical consent prior to each project. The second is more frustrating and indicates the need for more work to demonstrate this potential – this volume is, of course, one step, hopefully, in that direction.

As well as wanting to promote a more positive narrative around MENA heritage, these projects were also a reaction to the current trend for cultural heritage reconstruction projects, especially in Syria and Iraq. A key problem for me in many (though not all – see e.g. #NewPalmyra 2018) is the lack of consultation and participation, particularly of people connected to the region. Given the growing evidence for co-production for health in decision making outlined above, it seems likely that the same would be true of reconstruction projects. There is, therefore, not only a moral imperative to include people's thoughts and views, but also a healthcare imperative. These workshops represent a first step in exploring that imperative and in finding ways for people to re-establish connections with their heritage that have been forcibly removed through destruction.

As such, a key aim for both projects was that the space provided should be open, supportive and friendly in order to promote creativity and sharing. There were various ways in which this was achieved. Some were quite simple, such as providing Middle Eastern treats like baklawa and dates, as well as tea and coffee, for participants. In all workshops the focus was on 'gentle engagement' i.e. chatting informally to participants one-on-one or in small groups about what they were doing and the objects they had chosen. As part of this 'gentle engagement' process, opening talks were kept short and light in order to help break down any perceived barriers between 'experts' and 'participants'. In particular, I felt it important that I participate alongside everyone else at the workshops, and learn the new skills myself. This helped to make everyone feel at ease, especially people who may have felt nervous about their artistic abilities (see below) — I was a novice, learning just as much as everyone else. This meant that everyone participating could feel that they had their own kind of expertise and experience to share with the rest of the group and that these flows were multi-directional.

As a result of this 'gentle engagement', guest books were used instead of feedback forms, where people were welcome to share any thoughts about the workshop (and were equally welcome not to write anything at all). One consequence of this decision is that neither project has gathered quantitative data about how the participants felt during the workshops. In order to mitigate this, however, follow-ups were conducted for each project after the workshops. For the RetRo project, all participants (including museum curators and creative practitioners) were invited to reflect on their experiences and what they had learnt one year on from the workshops; these responses have been published as a co-authored journal article (Kamash *et al.* 2017). For Rematerialising Mosul Museum, an email survey was sent out two months after the workshops that asked explicitly for reflections on the three well-being dimensions outlined above.

Measuring well-being during and after the workshops

In this section, I will present the feedback from participants in order to analyze how the workshops measure against the What Works Centre for Wellbeing's well-being dimensions (see above). This feedback is taken from the guestbooks and from the co-authored *Epoiesen* article written one year after the RetRo workshops (Kamash *et al.* 2017), where participants were not asked explicitly to reflect on well-being. In the case of the Rematerialising Mosul Museum project, participants were asked to comment directly on these three dimensions, two months after the felting workshops had taken place; all participants, including fibre artist Karin, responded to the feedback request. All participants providing feedback have been asked whether they wish to be anonymous in this publication; where anonymity has been requested, names have been redacted, otherwise participants are referred to by their first name. The respondents who have requested anonymity are referred to here as 'Respondent 1' and 'Respondent 2' and so on. Several respondents self-identify as suffering from generalized anxiety, with at least two being unable to work at the time of the workshops due to anxiety-related issues. Phrasing in direct quotes from respondents has been kept as in the original.

Under the personal dimension, several themes recurred in the feedback around confidence, pride and anxiety, coping and resilience, and identity and self-esteem. This dimension sees significant overlap with the cultural dimension, so these factors are discussed together here. Some participants in the felting workshops commented on the process of felting itself being calming and therapeutic (Respondent 1) with Rana, Yasmin and Deema explicitly noting that the rhythmic nature of the process helped to reduce anxiety. This echoes some of the findings from Stitchlinks, as well as linking with the mindfulness aspects noted above. The task was also key to how Respondent 2 felt about the process as there was a 'defined outcome' (i.e. making a felted panel), but there was also 'room within the definition for me to have to make some decisions'. Respondent 2 goes on to say that making choices related to the crafting 'increased my confidence in making other, wider choices' and also that:

> 'Completing the felt piece and sharing pictures of it with friends was really positive. Look, I'm someone who can create something. I made this. I am not just someone who is incapable of doing... I didn't feel like a proper person for a while, and... doing this helped.'

This ability to make creative choices within the task was also identified as a positive aspect by Lucia. This seems to demonstrate that a feeling of control and self-determination is an important element in activities that aim to promote well-being; this may be even more important for people who have lost a sense of control over their lives during conflict.

A sense of achievement and pride was also noted by Karen, Christina, and Alec. Some respondents also highlighted that the positive effects on their confidence had continued after the workshops. In relation to the RetRo workshops, for example, Jayne (in Kamash *et al.* 2017) stated that participating had given her more confidence in her studies. Commenting on the felting workshop, Respondent 1 said:

> 'The workshop most definitely had a tremendous "feel good" effect on me. I had a sense of pride in my achievement, both whilst at the workshop and afterwards.'

One of the most interesting aspects of this kind of developing confidence came from several respondents for whom participating was in some way anxiety-inducing in the first place. Thinking about the RetRo workshop, Muna commented that she had felt 'terrified' about being in a room with artistic people, but that choosing to photograph an object she felt she could identify (i.e. a ceramic jug) meant that she was 'freed up from the worry' about her 'lack of creative ability' (Kamash *et al.* 2017). Having built her confidence at RetRo, Muna also came to a felting workshop. In addition, Florence who was very nervous at the start of the RetRo workshop, flourished with some gentle encouragement. Her daughter, Thandi, who accompanied her to the workshops, wrote: 'Archaeology is now a passion of hers.... she [Florence] has gained such confidence in herself and her ability to relate to history' (email communication 20.10.17; quoted with permission).

Worrying about a lack of creative skill was also raised as an issue for Karen at the felting workshop, because 'it is something that at an early age I was identified as not being very good at'. By being able to prove that anxiety wrong Karen says that:

> 'it has taught me to have more regard for what I can do and in that respect helped to increase my confidence in stepping outside what I know and my self-esteem in relation to what I can achieve if I try.'

Furthermore for some people even the act of getting to a workshop can be anxiety-inducing; both Karen and Christina commented on how nervous they were about journeying to the felting workshops. Again, for both, feeling that they had overcome that anxiety was a source of pride and a reason to feel increased confidence: 'It has given me [Christina] confidence in knowing that I can overcome my fears and anxieties'. These instances remind us that not everyone feels immediately comfortable about participating in these kinds of activities, so creating a space and an atmosphere in which people can gently be encouraged is key, as noted above.

An additional and vital layer within this, of course, has to be that these workshops were intended to tackle and open up a range of challenging issues, some of which related very directly to difficult elements of some participants' identities. Muna, for example, explained:

'I was very keen to attend [the felting workshop] as I am of Iraqi origin and have found it extremely challenging to remain optimistic in relation to long running turmoil there. There is also an all pervasive negative narrative that can come from being of Arab origin... It was also extremely important to me that my teenage son has the experience of being around positive Arabic role models and learns about Iraqi culture as a counter balance to some of the stereotypes that he will have to be able to navigate. He hides his identity all the time, even from his friends, so things like this help to ensure that he has self-esteem.'

In relation to this, the nature of the activity was highlighted as an important element. For example, Heba reflected that taking a creative approach in the RetRo workshops helped her to 'feel more empowered to write my own story freely.' Similarly, Rana, Yasmin, and Deema said 'it [the felting] provided people with the means to portray their personal identity through a media other than words — this was refreshing for our Iraqi identity.' The importance of non-verbal expression — especially for people who may have experienced trauma, and so find 'putting it into words' difficult — cannot be underestimated. It may be aspects such as this that make these activities effective supplements to traditional therapies. In addition, the use of the 'gentle engagement' method was key to creating the right kind of atmosphere during the workshops. Thandi commented:

'You and Karin created an ambiance for peaceful reflective thought about identity, memories, politics and academic value which is often rather tricky to tackle in conversation alone without getting super-heated.'

Within this, time and space to reflect were identified as some of the most important aspects of the workshops, in an anonymous comment in the felting workshop guestbook and by Muna:

'It is not really possible to over emphasis how important I feel it is to allow people time and space to explore this culture... There are many layers of anxiety associated with being connected to this area that have often spanned a lifetime and continue to stretch in front of you into the future. There is often not time for your mind to process as it is not a one off traumatic event that you can "move forward" from. It is rather a way of being that you learn to live alongside. The time to spend in this workshop in a positive way surrounded by Arabic culture was fantastic and left me feeling elated.'

Moving into the cultural dimension of well-being, where this did not overlap with issues of resilience, achievement, personal identity etc. discussed above, the majority of respondents commented on creative skills and expression. Numerous respondents commented on the value of learning or enhancing a skill for their well-being, and the value of having help, especially from Karin, to build on their creative skills and expression. For Lucia, Sarah, and Respondent

2, this was also a reminder of the importance of creativity in their lives, and it provided a focus for wanting to introduce more creativity into their lives in the future. One anonymous person in the felting workshop guestbook commented that it was fun to experiment with ways of being artistic that are not provided for in schools. Muna also noted that linking with a creative side 'allowed the workshop to appeal to all ages' and to include people who had differing levels of archaeological knowledge.

As well as learning skills, participants also commented on other kinds of learning that fit into the social dimension of well-being. Two respondents discussed how being at the felting workshops meant they knew more about Iraq and Iraqis afterwards. Karen talked about hearing stories from Iraqis at the workshop that:

> '…made me realize that this was something that although seemingly a part of daily life through the news media, that I knew nothing about beyond what I am told in the news… [The experience] made Iraq to me feel like more than just a place I hear of on the news (sort of 3D rather than 2D if you know what I mean).'

This has culminated in Karen reading a book about Iraq and its politics that she had been given some time ago 'but had put… aside'. Similarly, Respondent 2 described how creating their piece led them to following up news articles and blog posts to learn more about Iraq:

> 'I have much more of an appreciation of it [Iraq] as a real place with a long history, a complex and varied culture, a diverse geography, life, people, hope; and not just a place of destruction. This survival, rebuilding, adapting, flourishing, shines a light on how strong people are… it adds to my understanding of the world, and my place in it… Having a focus outside yourself helps change your perspective too.'

These kinds of reciprocity and broadening out of understandings are what Muna, above, was hoping could be achieved. They are amongst the values of having mixed groups at such events, though it should be noted that Respondent 2 participated from home, rather than coming to a workshop. Respondent 1 observed that they felt such interactions benefited and developed their own cultural identity and knowledge. Indeed, Lucia, Muna, Christina and Alec all commented on the value of being with people from other backgrounds, with Lucia particularly valuing the opportunity to share the workshop with Iraqis, whom she described as being 'survivors of their culture so to speak'. Furthermore, for Rana, Yasmin, and Deema, being part of a large group gave them 'a sense of overall understanding and ultimately belonging'. Herein, then, lies the value of continuing to break down the barriers to access discussed above.

People also commented on how having 'shared, yet individual, goals' make workshops socially inclusive, with people helping each other out. Karen also commented that having this 'common reason' meant there were 'no barriers to communication', even though people may come from very different backgrounds; she felt this was one of the biggest contributing factors to her well-being as it helped her through the anxiety of making new connections with people. Linked to this, it was interesting to observe at both the RetRo and the felting workshops that numerous people came with friends or family; only one or two came alone. This may also be connected to the anxieties around participating that were noted above. As a consequence, several people commented on how the workshops gave them an opportunity not only to create new bonds, but also to enhance existing friendships, including, in the case of Sarah, those with Iraqi people who were not at the workshop she attended. Overall, it appeared that seeing the range of responses, and witnessing other people's enjoyment, was a source of well-being for many of the participants. Karin encapsulated these observations neatly in her reflection on her experience of running workshops, including these ones:

> 'The crafts give a focus of attention and the rhythm of working means that often conversation flows more easily than when just sat together with nothing to do... The sense of community is increased, not just in the meetings of new people, but how we work together. People naturally help each other out, offer to roll the wool, or get hot water. They work together and in that sharing, new bonds and ideas are opened up. In this workshop in particular, having people of different races, religions, backgrounds made this even more great an experience... Sharing a creative experience gives us a way in to someone else's life and culture. The smell of a soap, triggers a conversation and a memory and an understanding that would not happen in normal interaction. That is a golden opportunity.'

Conclusions and recommendations for the future

These workshops demonstrate that there is significant potential for these kinds of engagement, involving heritage and crafting, to have a beneficial impact on well-being, and even to be therapeutic for those suffering from anxiety and trauma. In addition, this work shows that continuing the efforts to break down the barriers to accessing to heritage and crafting activities is worthwhile. For people from a range of backgrounds and traditions, participating in these workshops provided opportunities to explore potentially difficult parts of their identities and their link with their heritage, in some cases non-verbally, and to feel part of a wider community. Bringing people together who might not ordinarily mix, created a space for reflection about our interactions in the wider world and seems to have encouraged deeper empathy with those different to ourselves. These workshops also demonstrate the value in continuing the survey work of other projects such as Stitchlinks, and of expanding that research to include a broader range of people who may not come to crafting by themselves.

Clearly, this work has been on a very small scale so far. Further research on a larger scale, potentially including a longitudinal study, will be key to providing more robust evidence of its efficacy. In this, working with psychologists will be vital to unpicking the various strands of evidence and gaining a deeper understanding of what works and why. This may help to overcome the gate-keeping issues encountered with, for example, refugee charities. I hope that such opportunities to increase well-being, which draw on the therapeutic benefits of heritage and crafting, become more routinely offered in future.

Bibliography

#NewPalmyra 2018. The #NewPalmyra digital reconstruction project [Website]. Viewed 28 November 2018, <https://www.newpalmyra.org>.
Ander, E., L. Thomson, A. Lanceley, U. Menon, and K. Blair 2013a. Using museum objects to improve wellbeing in psychiatric and rehabilitation patients. *British Journal of Occupational Therapy* 76(5): 208–216.

Ander, E., L. Thomson, A. Lanceley, U. Menon, and G. Noble 2013b. Heritage, health and well-being: assessing the impact of a heritage focused intervention on health and well-being. *International Journal of Heritage Studies* 19(3): 229–242.

APPGAHW 2017. *Creative health: The arts for health and wellbeing. Inquiry report* (Second edition). London: APPGAHW.

Bedding S. and G. Sadlo 2008. Retired people's experience of participation in art classes. *British Journal of Occupational Therapy* 71(9): 371–378.

Boerema C., M. Russell and A. Aguilar 2010. Sewing in the lives of immigrant women. *Journal of Occupational Science* 17(2): 78–84.

Caruth, C. 1995. Introduction: Trauma and experience, in C. Caruth (ed.) *Trauma: Explorations in memory*: 3–12. Baltimore: John Hopkins University Press.

Chatterjee, H. and G. Noble 2013. *Museums, health and well-being*. Farnham: Ashgate.

Hacking S., J. Secker, L. Kent, J. Shenton and H. Spandler 2006. Mental health and arts participation: The state of the art in England. *Journal of the Royal Society for the Promotion of Health* 126(3): 121–127.

Inglis, G. and J. Williams 2010. *Models of sporting and cultural activity: Analysis of the Taking Part Survey*. London: Department for Culture, Media and Sport.

Kamash, Z. 2017. 'Postcard to Palmyra': Bringing the public into debates over post-conflict reconstruction in the Middle East. *World Archaeology* 49(5): 608–622.

Kamash, Z. with H. Abd el Gawad, P. Banks, A. Bell, F. Charteris, S. Ekdawi, Z. Glen, J. Howe, A. Laidlaw, M. Mitchell, A. Nafde, A. Parkin, F. Wilson, L.T. Wilson, and A. Wood 2017. Remembering the Romans in the Middle East and North Africa: Memories and reflections from a museum-based public engagement project. *Epoiesen* 1: 69–89 [On-line document]. Viewed 28 November 2018, <dx.doi.org/10.22215/epoiesen/2017.9>.

Kidd, B., S. Zahir and S. Khan 2008. *Arts and refugees: History, impact and future*. London: Arts Council England, The Baring Foundation and Paul Hamlyn Foundation.

Lanceley, A., G. Noble, M. Johnson, N. Balogun and H. Chatterjee 2011. Investigating the therapeutic potential of a heritage-object focused intervention: A qualitative study. *Journal of Health Psychology* 17(6): 809–820.

Mental Health Foundation 2018. The Amaan project [Webpage]. Viewed 28 January 2019, <https://www.mentalhealth.org.uk/scotland/improving-mental-wellbeing-asylum-seekers-and-refugees>.

Monuments of Mosul 2018. Monuments of Mosul in Danger project [Website]. Viewed 28 November 2018, <http://www.monumentsofmosul.com>.

Perruzza N. and E.A. Kinsella 2010. Creative arts occupations in therapeutic practice: A review of the literature. *British Journal of Occupational Therapy* 73(6): 261–268.

Project Mosul 2017. Project Mosul/Rekrei [Website]. Viewed 28 November 2018, <https://projectmosul.org>.

Reynolds, F. 2009. Taking up arts and crafts in later life: A qualitative study of the experiential factors that encourage participation in creative activities. *British Journal of Occupational Therapy* 72(9): 393–400.

Riley, J. 2008. Weaving an enhanced sense of self and a collective sense of self through creative textile-making. *Journal of Occupational Science* 15(2): 63–73.

Riley, J., B. Corkhill, C. Morris 2013. The benefits of knitting for personal and social wellbeing in adulthood: finds from an international survey. *British Journal of Occupational Therapy* 76(2): 50–57.

Smelser, N.J. 2004. Psychological trauma and cultural trauma, in J.C. Alexander, R. Eyerman, B. Giesen, N.J. Smelser and P. Sztompka (eds.) *Cultural trauma and collective identity*: 31–59. Berkeley (CA): University of California Press.

Smyth, J. and J. Nobel n.d. Creative, artistic, and expressive therapies for PTSD. White paper for the Arts and Healing Foundation. Unpublished report, Arts and Healing Foundation.

Solway, R., L.J. Thomson, P.M. Camic and H.J. Chatterjee 2015. Museum object handling in older adult mental health inpatient care. *International Journal of Mental Health Promotion* 17(4): 201–214.

Southwick, S.M., R.H. Pietrzak, J. Tsai, J.H. Krystal and D. Charney 2015. Resilience: An update. *PTSD Research Quarterly* 25(4): 1–10.

Stitchlinks 2018. Stitchlinks [Website]. Viewed 28 November 2018, <http://www.stitchlinks.com>.

Talkovsky, A.M. and A.J. Lang 2017. Meditation-based approaches in the treatment of PTSD. *PTSD Research Quarterly* 28(2): 1–10.

Thomson, L., E. Ander, U. Menon, A. Lanceley and H.J. Chatterjee 2011. Evaluating the therapeutic effects of museum object handling with hospital patients: A review and initial trial of wellbeing measures. *Journal of Applied Arts and Health* 2(1): 37–56.

Thomson, L., E. Ander, A. Lanceley, U. Menon and G. Noble 2012a. Enhancing cancer patient well-being with a non-pharmacological, heritage-focused intervention. *Journal of Pain and Symptom Management* 44(5): 731–740.

Thomson, L., E. Ander, A. Lanceley, U. Menon and G. Noble 2012b. Quantitative evidence for wellbeing benefits from a heritage-in-health intervention with hospital patients. *International Journal of Art Therapy* 17(2): 63–79.

Tzanidaki, D. and F. Reynolds 2011. Exploring the meanings of making traditional arts and crafts among older women in Crete, using interpretative phenomenological analysis. *British Journal of Occupational Therapy* 74(8): 375–382.

Van der Kolk, B.A. and O. van der Hart 1995. The intrusive past: The flexibility of memory and the engraving of trauma, in C. Caruth (ed.) *Trauma: Explorations in Memory*: 158–182. Baltimore: John Hopkins University Press.

What Works Wellbeing, 2018. What Works Centre for Wellbeing [Website]. Viewed 28 November 2018, <https://whatworkswellbeing.org>.

Yarnfulness 2018. The Yarnfulness Project [Website]. Viewed 27 October 2018, <https://yarnfulnessproject.org>.

Afterword

Alex Coulter

When I was invited to speak at the 2018 conference *Historic Landscapes and Mental Well-being* at Bournemouth University I knew a little about the Human Henge project, but had no idea that the conference would be so varied, rich, and dynamic. With many new ideas swirling around in my head, I was very daunted by my task, which was to draw the threads together at the end. There were many deeply felt and thoughtful presentations, and interesting exchanges on the power of heritage and the past to engage us emotionally, intellectually, and spiritually, in body and in soul. This afterword is a reflection on that day, as well as on the papers in this volume.

My experience is firmly centred in the world of arts and health. I have a background in the visual arts, worked in a hospital arts programme for 15 years, and now run a regional network known as Arts & Health South West. However, over the last 20-odd years I have seen the field grow exponentially. My recent role, project managing the All-Party Parliamentary Group on Arts, Health and Wellbeing's two-year inquiry, and the publication of the *Creative Health* report in 2017, has made me acutely aware of how widespread and interconnected this inter-disciplinary space has become. As Laura Drysdale says in her chapter entitled 'Walking with intent: Culture Therapy in ancient landscapes', heritage is only briefly touched on in the *Creative Health* report, and after this conference I would say that archaeology should have had a place in it too.

When Laura Drysdale participated in Arts & Health South West's *Culture, Health and Wellbeing International Conference* in Bristol in 2017, I was struck by the importance she placed on participant's 'voices'; the Human Hengers themselves. This was very evident in the presentations we heard at the 2018 Bournemouth conference. The personal testimony, performance, and story-telling were powerful and moving, reaffirming for all of us why we do the work we do. The values inherent in this approach are embedded in the National Lottery Heritage Fund's support for work that ensures access to heritage is inclusive, as in the Workers' Education Alliance Digability project that enabled over 300 people to experience community archaeology. In Daniel O'Donoghue's reflection on the Human Henge project, he artfully weaves in the words of participants to bring the project alive and writes:

'We all have fond memories of Flo's marvelous and unexpected singing on the final day.

If I sing
let it be like fire
in dry brush.'

Flo's singing at the conference is still the single strongest, most visceral memory I have of that day. But other powerful memories remain from two presentations that were a revelation to me: 'The Archaeological Imagination' by Rebecca Hearne, and 'Waterloo Uncovered' by Mark Evans. Archaeology in the transitional space between the imagination and embodied experiences; veterans experiencing intense moments of connection with soldiers from the past through the regimental buttons unearthed. Time is not linear, as in T S Eliot's eternal words from *Four Quartets: Burnt Norton*:

'Time present and time past are both perhaps present in time future, and time future contained in time past.' (Eliot 1944: 7)

We are at a time of great connectedness. We are finding threads of thoughts that weave us together, binding us into a shared understanding across and between disciplines. The arts and heritage and cultural experiences and narratives, provide the space in which we find this rich understanding. We connect with each other through the work and experience that thrill of creating community and shared endeavour. Laura writes that:

'Human Henge's music, photography, clay work and creative writing activities, occupy what Winnicott (1971) called 'potential space'. This is the place between subject and object that he saw as the crucible of creativity, where frustration can be tolerated and thought can thrive. Expanding into potential space from the restrictions of mental illness, enables people to be playful, curious and rebellious, private, spiritual and sensual. If we share these characteristics with the ancestors who made and used these irreducibly mysterious places, perhaps Human Henge echoes something of their existence in its physical embodiment of an interior landscape.'

Of course, research provides another misty lens through which to connect with the past and ourselves; the conference was a fine example of research, practice and personal testimony occupying a happy space together, enriching our understanding and interpretation in 360 degrees. Connection is a strong thread here too, and Vanessa Heaslip identifies that:

'Exploring data from the personal reflections, highlighted themes around 'knowing oneself' and 'connections'. In 'knowing oneself', participants expressed their improved understanding of challenges associated with their mental illness, and also their potential for recovery. They also acknowledged the inner strength they had found through engagement with the programme. This strength enabled them to reconnect both with other individuals and also with their local communities in which they lived.'

Earlier in the week, while taking part in a research group planning a randomized controlled trial on stroke and the arts, also at Bournemouth University, I was introduced to Les Todres and Kate Galvin's 'Dwelling-mobility: An existential theory of well-being' (2010). This theory draws on Heidegger's notion of *Gegnet*, or abiding expanse, which indicates both a sense of adventure and a 'being-at-home-with' as the basis of human well-being. To quote the paper:

'The western metaphysical tradition posits neutral space within which one can "put" beings and things, and time is the neutral context in which all things happen sequentially. But Heidegger was concerned that this metaphysical framework missed a "cosmos" in which Being was not just space and time (merely a neutral context), but a wholeness that was more intimately implicated in the way beings are related to one another and Being-as-a-whole.' (Todres and Galvin 2010: 2)

Or in more poetic terms, to end with another quote from the *Four Quartets: Little Gidding*:

> 'We shall not cease from exploration and the end of all our exploring will be to arrive where we started and know the place for the first time.' (Eliot 1944: 43)

Bibliography

Eliot, T.S. 1944. *Four Quartets*. London: Faber and Faber.

Todres, L. and K. Galvin 2010. "Dwelling-mobilty": An existential theory of well-being. *International Journal of Qualitative Studies on Health and Well-being* 5(3): 1–6.

Winnicott, D.W. 1971. *Playing and reality*. London: Tavistock Publications.